The Black Stork

The Black Stork:

Eugenics and the Death of "Defective" Babies in American Medicine and Motion Pictures Since 1915

MARTIN S. PERNICK

New York   *Oxford*
OXFORD UNIVERSITY PRESS
1996

Oxford University Press

Oxford   New York
Athens   Auckland   Bangkok   Bombay
Calclutta   Cape Town   Dar es Salaam   Delhi
Florence   Hong Kong   Istanbul   Karachi
Kuala Lumpur   Madras   Madrid   Milbourne
Mexico City   Nairobi   Paris   Singapore
Taipei   Tokyo   Toronto

and associated companies in
Berlin   Ibadan

Published by Oxford University Press, Inc.,
198 Madison Avenue, New York, New York 10016

Oxford is a registered trademark of Oxford University Press

Library of Congress Cataloging-in-Publication Data
Pernick, Martin S.
The black stork : eugenics and the death of "defective" babies in
American medicine and motion pictures since 1915 /
Martin S. Pernick.
p.   cm.   Includes bibliographical references and indes.
ISBN 0-19-507731-8
1. Infants (Newborn)—Diseases—Treatment—Moral and ethical aspects.
2. Eugenics in motion pictures.
3. Abnormalities, Human—Treatment—Moral and ethical aspects.
4. Euthanasia—Moral and ethical aspects.
5. Eugenics—United States—History—20th century.
6. Infanticide—Moral and ethical aspects.
7. Black stork (Motion picture)
I. Title.   RJ255.P394   1995
179'.7—edc20   94-47668

1 2 3 4 5 6 7 8 9

Printed in the United States of America
on acid-free paper

For
Marie R. Deveney
and
Benjamin William Pernick

Preface

The history of medical motion pictures cannot be researched simply by filling out call slips in well-catalogued archives. I discovered the only surviving viewable print of *The Black Stork* in a film collector's garage in New Jersey. The collector, an affable bear of a man then in his seventies, pulled a reel from a rusty metal can. The decomposing film had lined the can with highly explosive nitrate dust. He mounted the movie on a pair of hand-cranked rewinds so I could run it through a flickering monitor. Then he leaned back and leisurely flicked his cigar ash into the dust-filled can.

I've always figured that that was a test. If I hadn't gasped, I would have revealed myself as too ignorant about old film for him to bother with. If I had run out the door, I would have shown myself too timid to accomplish anything in the chaotic firetrap that housed his wonderful collection. I shuddered, and stayed, and got to see *The Black Stork*—a startling and provocative long-lost motion picture that illuminates many otherwise dark and unknown dimensions of American medicine and culture.

Early motion pictures proved critically important in communicating to the lay public the tremendous medical and public health revolution of the turn of this century. But their role is almost unknown today, because for decades almost nothing was done to study, index, or even preserve these fragile images. More than half of all films ever made have been lost, and for early titles on offbeat topics like medicine, the mortality rate was thought to be near 100 percent. Simply to learn how many and what kinds of health-related films were made requires laborious page–by–page searching of medical, film, and mass-circulation periodicals, because until recently there were no subject indexes to old films, and even now such research tools are limited to full-length features.

My research over the past decade has gradually helped change that. My research assistants and I have identified over 1300 specific films made between 1897 and 1928 on health topics for lay audiences, and we have located, restored, and preserved almost 300 surviving prints. The overall story will be told in a future volume, *Bringing Medicine to the Masses: Motion Pictures and the Revolution in Public Health, 1910–1928.*

The Black Stork book began as the eugenics "chapter" of that larger study, but soon took on a life of its own as the tremendous medical and cultural significance of early eugenics films became clear. It is meant as a work of social and cultural history, combining the history of medicine with film studies and comparing past events with medical ethics, health policy, and mass culture today. It is intended to provide a useful model for integrating contextual history, mass culture, and medicine.

The book contains two parts: one on the medical controversies and one on the movies. But the distinction is more in structure than substance. Film provides much of the evidence about the meaning of medical ideas discussed in Part I; medical and eugenic concepts are central to the analysis of films in Part II. A reader interested only in medicine might skip the end, and one focused just on film might start with the middle, but each would bypass much material of specific interest, and each might miss a central point—that medicine and the media evolved together in the context of a common culture.

This interweaving of medicine, movies, and culture provides the book's separate strands with much of their meaning and significance. When I first saw *The Black Stork,* I found it almost unintelligible because I knew little about its origin (and because I watched it on a two-inch monitor, with one anxious eye on that cigar). Without knowing the specific medical and cultural contexts, the film made little sense. But without the film to focus my curiosity, I might never have discovered the dramatic, long forgotten medical and cultural conflicts on which it provides unprecedented illumination.

Ann Arbor, Michigan   M.S.P.
February 1995

Acknowledgments

Undergraduate research assistants Aaron Han Joon Park, Christine Ahn, Robert Kashangaki; high-school volunteer intern Bryan Chen; and graduate student research assistants Matt Schaefer and Victor Hugo Lane contributed greatly to the preparation of this book and to the larger project on which it is based. I am especially grateful to Aaron for his more than two years of enthusiastic and insightful assistance. Others who helped research the early stages of the larger project on silent-era health films include Barbara Howe, Carol Pollard, and Joelle Stein.

A University of Michigan Rackham Research Partnership made it possible for Peter Laipson to contribute many helpful insights, especially on sexuality, class, and representation. The section of chapter 3 titled "Defects and Desires" particularly reflects his comments and suggestions.

Research for the project was supported by National Library

of Medicine Grant 1-R01-LM 04259-01, National Endowment for the Humanities Grant RH-20629-85, the Spencer Foundation, and the undergraduate research initiatives of the University of Michigan.

My wonderful colleagues at the University of Michigan's Program in Society and Medicine heard this project develop over the years and provided much useful advice along the way. Many other colleagues, friends, and strangers helped, and I have tried to acknowledge their specific contributions in the notes.

Without the personal effort and guidance of many archivists and librarians, the project would never have been possible. I owe special debts to the following: film archivists Pat Sheehan, Bob Summers, Sarah Richards, Rick Prelinger, John E. Allen (père et fils), Paul Spehr, Barb Humphrys, David Parker, Kathy Loughney, Pat Loughney, Audrey Kupferberg, Lawrence Karr, Ron Magliozzi, Eileen Bowser, Bill Murphy, Paul Killiam, John Kuiper, Betsy Harris, Chris Horack, Jeff Hopkinson, Elizabeth Tape, and James W. Moore; and librarians and manuscript archivists Gretchen Sachse, Bill Wallach, John Parascondola, Ed Weber, Susan Davis, Adrienne Noe, William Verick, William P. Gorman, William Wiedman, Margaret Clark, Dorothy Czarnik, Andrea Hinding, and David Klaasen.

Particularly insightful and thorough critiques of the entire manuscript were provided by those colleagues who span several worlds: filmmaker-historian Laurie Block, who knows the unique community of children with disabilities and their parents; physician-historian Joel Howell; and biologist-historian Nina Stoyen-Rosenzweig. Others whose comments on portions of earlier drafts and other suggestions were especially helpful include the following: film historians Lisa Cartwright and Kevin Brownlow; historians David Hollinger, Maris Vinovskis, Sandra Herbert, Susan Lederer, Bert Hansen, Juan Leon, Nick Steneck, Pat Spain Ward, Barry Mehler, Stefan Kühl, Saul Benison, Daniel Fox, Harvey Young, Lily Kay, and Anne Hanson; pathologist Gerry Abrams; and ethics and legal scholars Yale Kamisar and Art Caplan. To you all, thanks.

Attorney, constitutional scholar, and art historian Marie Deveney contributed valuable comments on each draft as we awaited the birth of our first child, Benjamin William Pernick. Contemplating his arrival made me more aware of the personal and emotional impact of the controversies discussed in this book, and my desire to be with him as he grows up meant I had to finally complete writing it.

Contents

PART I

Withholding Treatment

The Birth of a Controversy

The Public Death of Baby Bollinger

At 4:00 A.M., November 12, 1915, in Chicago's German-American Hospital, Anna Bollinger gave birth to a seven-pound baby boy. Dr. Climena Serviss, who delivered the infant, quickly awakened Dr. Harry J. Haiselden, the surgeon who headed the hospital staff. Haiselden diagnosed multiple physical anomalies in the infant, including absence of a neck and one ear, deformities of the shoulders and chest, very slow reaction of the pupils to light, and an imperforate anus. X rays revealed prematurely hardened skull and leg bones, and a membrane blocking the lower bowel, although the digestive tract seemed otherwise normal. The rectum extended to within half an inch of the surface (Fig. 1). Haiselden concluded that surgery could correct the intestinal defects and thus save the infant's life, but that gross physical and mental abnormalities would remain, and he urged the parents not to request an operation. The Bollingers agreed, and five days later the baby died.[1]

Subsequently, Haiselden revealed that he had secretly permitted many other infants he diagnosed as "defectives" to die during the decade before 1915. And over the next three years, he withheld treatment from, or actively speeded the deaths of, at least five more abnormal babies.

Only two weeks after the Bollinger baby's death, Mrs. Julius Werder gave birth at Haiselden's hospital to a hydrocephalic girl. The infant's head was swollen to a sixteen-inch diameter, and her legs were paralyzed. The attending doctor believed that surgery to drain fluid from the head could save the child's life, but Mr. Werder refused permission. Haiselden, contacted by telegraph during a lecture tour in New York, authorized withholding treatment, and the infant died on December 2, 1915.

In a case with a different twist, the Grimshaw family wanted Haiselden to operate on their severely deformed seven-month-old girl. He told the parents that their baby was probably too frail to live through corrective surgery, but they all agreed that unless the deformities could be corrected, "it would be better for her to die." Haiselden operated on December 11, 1915. The baby did not survive.

On July 23, 1917, William and Eva Meter brought their newborn girl to German-American Hospital. The infant had an abnormally small head (microcephalic) and an incomplete skull. The membranes of her brain were almost completely exposed. After consulting a large number of medical colleagues, Haiselden decided not to attempt a skin graft that might protect the brain from infection. Instead, he removed a ligature that had been used to stop an umbilical hemorrhage and let the baby bleed to death. At this time, he also claimed to be withholding treatment from several similar cases, but he did not announce their names.

On the second anniversary of the Bollinger baby's birth, Haiselden revealed that he was giving a narcotic drug to ease and, he implied, to speed the impending death of two-year-old Paul Hodzima, a microcephalic who was reportedly choking from a constricted windpipe. The mother stopped administering the drug a week later, after considerable public pressure, but the subsequent fate of the child apparently was never announced. On January 27, 1918, two-month-old quadriplegic Emma Stanke died of undisclosed causes after Haiselden had refused potentially lifesaving treatment.[2]

Parents of handicapped children around the country wrote moving letters of support to Haiselden and requested his help in allowing their children to die. A mother in St. Louis begged Haiselden to "perform some kind of operation that either would cure or kill" her six-year-old institutionalized mentally and physically handicapped son.

In one widely publicized incident, Joseph E. Roberts of New York, father of a newborn girl with the congenital spinal defect called spina bifida, cited the Bollinger case as precedent for allowing his daughter to die and requested a consultation with Haiselden. The physicians in the case, including noted pediatrician L. Emmett Holt, agreed not to treat the baby. Although critics charged that Holt's position was analogous to Haiselden's, Holt claimed that his refusal to operate was based solely on the belief that surgery was too risky and denied that he was influenced by the father's appeal to Haiselden. Haiselden did travel to New York, but Holt refused to consult with him or let him see the baby. The girl died without treatment.[3]

Newspapers reported a spate of similar parental requests. A father from Des Moines, whose two-month-old girl had a seriously misshapen jaw and mouth, warned that "unless somebody does kill the baby I'll have to." Told of the need for a triple limb amputation to save the life of her six-month-old boy, a Baltimore woman refused to permit the operation, reportedly because she preferred that he "should die than go through life a helpless cripple."[4]

Most of these cases riveted the attention of the nation, in large part because Haiselden vigorously publicized them. In an effort to rally public support for his campaign against the treatment of defective newborns, Haiselden displayed the dying infants to reporters and allowed the still-hospitalized mothers to be photographed and interviewed (Fig. 2). He wrote a six-week-long series of articles for Hearst's *Chicago American*, delivered public lectures, and posed for movie newsreels. Across the country, the stories made page-one headlines for days on end. At times the Bollinger case pushed even World War I to second billing (Fig. 3).[5]

In collaboration with muckraking Hearst journalist Jack Lait, Haiselden also wrote and starred in a feature motion picture, *The Black Stork*, a polished, fictionalized dramatization based loosely on the Bollinger events. The main plot of this remarkable film begins with Claude, who has an unnamed inherited disease. Despite repeated graphic warnings from Dr. Dickey (played by Haiselden himself), Claude marries his sweetheart, Anne. Their baby is born so severely disabled that it needs immediate surgery to save its life, but Dr. Dickey refuses to perform the operation. Anne is torn by uncertainty until God reveals a lengthy vision of the child's future, filled with pain, madness, and crime. Her doubts resolved, she accepts Dr. Dickey's judgment, and the baby's soul leaps into the arms of a waiting Jesus (Figs. 8–24; chapter 8).

Despite the objections of many film regulators and censors, *The Black Stork* was shown commercially in movie theaters from 1916 through the 1920s, after 1918 under the title *Are You Fit to Marry?* It was slightly revised and rereleased in 1927, and, though no sound track was added, it continued to be shown in small theaters and traveling road shows perhaps as late as 1942.[6]

Debates and Investigations

Haiselden's extraordinary propaganda evoked hundreds of reviews, letters, articles, and editorials from around the nation. As a result, his cases provoked the first and, prior to the recent "Baby Doe" cases, the most extensively documented public debate over medical refusal to save impaired newborns.

A substantial number of very prominent early-twentieth-century Americans favored letting deformed infants die. Supporters included such leading progressive reformers as settlement worker and nurse Lillian Wald, family-law pioneer Judge Ben Lindsey, civil rights lawyer Clarence Darrow, and historian Charles A. Beard.[7] Not surprisingly, men like Charles Davenport, Raymond Pearl, and Irving Fisher, leaders of the movement to "improve" human heredity known as eugenics, championed Haiselden's refusal to preserve supposedly hereditary defectives.[8] But remarkably, so did the celebrated blind and deaf advocate for the disabled, Helen Keller, and the Catholic cardinal of Baltimore, James Gibbons.[9]

Well-known medical backers included Food and Drug Administration founder Harvey Wiley and diphtheria antitoxin pioneer William H. Park. The National Medico-Legal Society voted a ringing endorsement of Haiselden's position.[10]

Other doctors revealed that they, too, let disabled infants die. Dr. Simon Baruch, a popular promoter of municipal public baths, professor at New York's College of Physicians and Surgeons, and father of financier Bernard Baruch, revealed that he once allowed a "monstrosity" to die at birth, and proclaimed that, were he to attend a case like the Bollinger baby, he "would not hesitate" to act as

Haiselden had done. A past president of the Washington State Medical Society, a professor of obstetrics at Northwestern University, and a respected Washington, D.C., obstetrician each announced that they, too, had allowed similar cases to die untreated. They claimed that physicians had been following this course routinely, but had never before discussed the practice in public. Officials of six New York City hospitals refused to confirm or deny charges that their institutions secretly permitted deformed babies to die.[11]

Haiselden won editorial endorsements from the *Chicago Herald, Tribune,* and *American; Detroit News* and *Free Press; Baltimore American; Philadelphia Ledger; New York American; Washington Herald;* and the *New Republic.*[12]

While a surprising number of prominent Americans supported Haiselden, his critics included such eminent physicians as Hugh Cabot of Massachusetts General Hospital, University of Michigan medical dean Victor C. Vaughan, industrial-health crusader Alice Hamilton, suffragist Anna Howard Shaw, medical educator and future senator Royal Copeland, obstetricians Fred Adair and Joseph De Lee, pediatrician Abraham Jacobi, and popular health advocate John Harvey Kellogg. Joining these medical leaders to urge treatment for all infants were renowned social-work pioneers Jane Addams of Hull House and Julia Lathrop of the Federal Children's Bureau.[13] Their position won editorial support from the *Boston Globe, Washington Post, New York Sun, St. Louis Post-Dispatch, Chicago Evening Post, Survey Magazine, Ann Arbor News,* and *New York Times,* though the *Times* later changed its stance to oppose only Haiselden's publicity-seeking.[14]

Haiselden's critics instigated a barrage of official investigations. Cook County Coroner Peter M. Hoffman and Chicago Health Commissioner John Dill Robertson ordered two separate autopsies on the Bollinger baby and conducted a lengthy inquest before a coroner's jury of six distinguished doctors. Although the panel found that the infant's physical defects were even worse than Haiselden had diagnosed, they emphasized that a doctor's duty is to "save or prolong life." But while they strongly criticized Haiselden's actions, they concluded that he was "fully within his rights in refusing to perform any operation which his conscience will not sanction."[15]

Despite the inquest's conclusion that no crime had been committed, Illinois Attorney General Patrick J. Lucey demanded that Haiselden be indicted. But State's Attorney Maclay Hoyne refused to file charges. Hoyne, who lived a few blocks from German-American Hospital, personally endorsed Haiselden's actions. He ruled that the Bollingers had the right to withhold their consent and that parental consent would have been required to operate.[16]

Dr. George U. Lipshulch, a state legislator from Chicago, then urged the State Board of Health to revoke Haiselden's medical license. After some deliberation, the board refused to act, on the rather curious grounds that Haiselden had been only a consultant, not the attending physician. (No action was suggested against the attending Dr. Serviss.)[17]

Each of Haiselden's later cases received similar official scrutiny, but none resulted in any legal action. Hoyne again blocked calls for Haiselden's prosecution in the Meter case. In the Hodzima case, Coroner Hoffman launched a Chicago Police Department probe. His threat to bring murder charges probably influenced Mrs. Hodzima's decision to stop giving Haiselden's narcotic to her child; however, no legal action was taken against her.[18] A recent history of euthanasia laws concluded that in 1915 strong grounds existed to prosecute both Haiselden and these parents for neglect of their respective duties to the babies. Yet in no instance were such charges ever filed against Haiselden or any of the parents.[19]

One organization did take disciplinary action, however. In March 1916, Haiselden was expelled from the Chicago Medical Society, not because he let babies die, but because he publicized the cases. The decision reaffirmed the profession's long-standing mistrust of the mass media, but it had no immediate impact on Haiselden's practice. Six months later, he claimed to be performing twenty major operations a week.[20]

The Doctor and the Parents

The man at the center of these events, Harry J. Haiselden, was born in March 1870 in Plano, Illinois, a village of well under 2000 inhabitants about 50 miles west of Chicago. His autobiography and scattered family records depict a small-town boy who sought success in the big city, a man devoted to his profession and to his mother but who had few other personal attachments. His relations with his father remain an enigma.

His father, George W. Haiselden, had been born in New Jersey to English immigrant parents. Harry's mother, Elizabeth Dickey, came from an old Pennsylvania family. Both parents were in their early thirties when Harry was born. They had one other child, a girl named Jessie, five years older than her brother. George, a painter, estimated his worth at $1100 the year of Harry's birth, a figure near the median for those in Plano who reported their assets to the census-taker. A decade later, the family lived on the town's Main Street, and George reported his occupation as "foreman in a paint shop."[21] When Harry was ten, the family moved from Plano to Chicago. George continued to work as a painter or foreman over the next fifteen years, though in 1890 he and Harry briefly owned a flour business together.

What happened next is puzzling. In 1895 George reported no occupation in the city directory, and in 1896, the year Harry completed his medical residency, George disappeared permanently from the listings, at the age of about fifty-six. Perhaps he died in 1896, though there is no Cook County or Plano death certificate for him, and Elizabeth did not report herself as his widow until 1909.[22] Harry's autobiography is uncharacteristically silent about his father. His mother, with whom he remained extremely close, died in 1915, a few months before the Bollinger case.[23]

Harry's education had begun in the Plano public school. Plano had a substantial German community, and though the Haiseldens were not German, when the family moved to Chicago Harry attended a German elementary school until he entered public high school. In high school he was more interested in playing sports than studying, and he ranked near the bottom of his class. But at a time when Chicago medical schools rarely demanded even a high-school diploma for admission, Haiselden took several college-level science courses before entering the Chicago College of Physicians and Surgeons, from which he received his M.D. in 1893. "P&S" ranked as one of only three acceptably scientific institutions among Chicago's fourteen medical schools, according to Abraham Flexner's 1910 survey of American medical education.[24]

The school had clinical privileges at Cook County Hospital, where Haiselden attracted the attention of Chicago's preeminent surgeon and medical educator, Christian Fenger. Although postgraduate hospital residencies were still quite rare in 1893, Haiselden spent 1893 to 1896 as Fenger's resident at German Hospital. In 1896, when Fenger established German-American Hospital, he took Haiselden along as his assistant. And on Fenger's death in 1902, Haiselden replaced his mentor as chief surgeon and hospital president. At the time of the Bollinger case, German-American Hospital was a forty-bed institution at 817 Diversey Parkway. By 1918 Haiselden had enlarged and moved the hospital to a seventy-five-bed facility a block closer to Lake Michigan at 741 Diversey. The old building was retained as a residence for the hospital's nurses.[25]

Haiselden traced his interest in eugenics to his childhood love of sports and to his reading of pioneer Harvard physical educator Dudley Sargent.[26] The same year he joined German-American Hospital, Haiselden also established his own Bethesda Industrial Home for Incurables. Virtually nothing is known about this institution, though eugenicists[27] of the time often advocated institutional "segregation" as a way to prevent people with hereditary disabilities from reproducing.

By 1915 however, Haiselden had become a bitter opponent of institutionalization. Haiselden's future *Black Stork* collaborator Jack Lait had written an exposé of poor conditions at the nation's second-largest institution for the retarded, the Illinois State Institution for the Feebleminded at Lincoln, in the early 1910s. In 1915 Lait cited the Lincoln facility's defects to support his claim that the Bollinger baby was better off dead. On July 24, 1916, Haiselden went to Lincoln to see for himself. He gained access under the alias Henry Jones and two days later published a dramatic muckraking account of his findings. Like Lait, Haiselden used his Lincoln experience to provide examples of the horrors of institutionalization from which he was saving impaired babies by letting them die.[28]

Haiselden claimed to be a pioneer in several different aspects of the new technological medicine. "I am essentially an X-ray man. Years ago I was instrumental in equipping our Cook County Hospital with an X-ray department," he boasted in 1915.[29] X rays were sometimes used as a non-surgical method of sterilizing those judged unfit to reproduce, a technique first developed in 1899 by Albert Ochsner, who became professor of surgery at the Chicago College of Physicians and Surgeons shortly after Haiselden's graduation. Haiselden also claimed expertise in brain surgery, a field in which his mentor Fenger had been an early specialist.[30]

A tall attractive man, Haiselden never married, though he adopted two children. The first, Dorothy Riggs, had been sent west by a New York City charity in 1905 at age five. The second, whom he named Beulah Hope Wesley, had been abandoned at birth at his hospital in 1914.

Haiselden's personal and professional lives were completely intertwined. During his "residency" he boarded not at Fenger's hospital but at home or with another physician, Benjamin Haiselden, perhaps a relative, whose name appears in the Chicago directory only in 1893 and 1894. After adopting the two girls, Haiselden lived with them and his mother at his own hospital. Haiselden's sister, Jessie, married Clarendon Rutherford, a physician who lived a block from the family's first Chicago residence, and Haiselden appointed Rutherford an officer and his successor as head of German-American Hospital.[31]

Although Haiselden's life can be reasonably well documented, only scattered details are known about the families of the babies he let die. Allen Bollinger, William Meter, and Stephen Hodzima were all Chicago mechanics; Julius Werder retired to Chicago after teaching in a school for defective children; the Grimshaw baby's father was a livestock breeder from Lake Villa, near the Illinois–Wisconsin border. Only the Hodzimas were described as being among the working poor. The Bollingers were a German-Irish couple; the Hodzimas, Austrian. No information was published about the background of the final case, but the family name of Stanke suggests a Germanic ancestry for them as well. The Bollingers had three older children, as did the Werders. The Meters were only twenty years old. Eva Meter had five more daughters before her husband died at about age forty.

At least two of the mothers reportedly experienced later regret over their decisions. Tracked down by a reporter with a very long memory in 1938, Mrs. Meter advised a family facing a decision similar to her own to "do everything they can to give their baby a chance." Anna Bollinger, who died in 1917 during the debate over the Meter case, allegedly never recovered from her grief at losing her baby.[32]

Although these events sparked more than two years of intense controversy, after 1917 Haiselden and his cause rapidly dropped from public view. His last reported nontreatment case, in January 1918, received only a single column-inch buried deep inside the *Chicago Tribune*, a paper that had supported him editorially and given front-page coverage to all his previous cases. Mass-media preoccupation with novelty and impatience with complex issues clearly played a role in this change, as did the altered political agenda of wartime and postwar America. But as Part II will show, the disappearance of public debate also reflected a growing consensus among social, medical, and media leaders that the topic itself was unfit to discuss in public.[33]

In April 1919 Haiselden left Chicago for Cuba, accompanied by two German-American Hospital nurses. The sketchy sources disagree wildly about what he was doing there. One newspaper reported that he was conducting unspecified human experiments that "could not have been made without interference in the United States." His family, however, denied that he was involved in any research other than photographing disabled slum children in Havana; they claimed he was simply on extended holiday. Other accounts say he became a recluse, living in a cave in Matanzas. About the only point of agreement is that in mid-June 1919 Harry Haiselden died suddenly in Cuba of a cerebral hemorrhage, at the age of forty-eight.[34]

Haiselden's hospital continued to prosper under his brother-in-law. During World War I, both German-American and German Hospitals found it expedient to rename themselves after their street addresses; they became Diversey Parkway and Grant Hospitals, respectively. After the war, the former German-American changed its name once again, to Chicago General. It closed in 1931, like many such proprietary hospitals a victim of the Depression. The site the hospital had occupied from 1918 to 1931 was taken over by the Pinel Sanitarium and in 1988 housed the Lakeview Nursing Home. The earlier location, where Haiselden's young patients died, was by then a vacant lot.[35]

His movie continued to be shown, and occasional references to him appeared in the papers from the 1920s to 1950. But by the 1970s, when a new generation began to discuss the issue again, almost no one recalled that an American doctor had ever publicly permitted impaired newborns to die.[36]

Haiselden and History

These events can be read as a fascinating but irrelevant oddity, rich in human interest but lacking any visible impact on the course of history. Yet these cases, isolated as they turned out to be, offer far more than just a novel and dramatic story. They constitute one of those rare moments when people attempt to examine and express what are ordinarily unarticulated assumptions and to debate in public what are usually private acts. These cases thus provide a unique window on important attitudes and practices shared by many people in early-twentieth-century America, but which they rarely discussed in public before the so-called Baby Doe cases of the past decade and which therefore left few other traces in the historical record.

Haiselden's actions, and the controversy that exploded over

them, cast a brief but piercing light on many otherwise hidden dimensions of progressive-era American culture, in areas as diverse as medicine, motion pictures, education, journalism, politics, race, gender, ethics, eugenics, and euthanasia. They illuminate the history of American attitudes toward infants, the disabled, doctors, disease, and death; the impact of the mass media in medical controversies; and the antecedents of current dilemmas in genetic therapy, health promotion, and health policy.

Further, these incidents highlight a crucial defining moment in the history of these issues. Many ideas, organizations, and technologies now taken for granted were only just taking shape in early-twentieth-century America. Although Haiselden's cases may not have directly influenced present debates, they illuminate that critical period in which many present attitudes and assumptions first took their current form.

My purpose in recovering these long-forgotten incidents is not to pass judgment on Haiselden according to present-day standards of science or ethics, but to comprehend the events in context, to envision how things looked in that world. But to accomplish that purpose, it also will be necessary to clarify whether and how his times differed from our own. And that process of comparing may increase our understanding of modern times as well.

To anticipate, my major conclusions will include the following. First, contrary to a common current assumption, modern right-to-die and Baby Doe debates are not unprecedented products of new lifesaving technologies. The general wisdom, nicely summarized by *New York Times* medical correspondent Lawrence K. Altman in May 1990, holds that "because ancient physicians could do so little for patients they did not share the modern physician's problem of differentiating between what can be done and what ought to be done."[37] However, the question of what ought to be done arose whenever past healers had techniques that *they* believed were efficacious, regardless of whether or not *we* conclude their methods really worked. Indeed, Haiselden drew on nontreatment precedents from the dawn of medical obstetrics in ancient Greece. Of course, contemporary technical advances have dramatically altered the dimensions and context of the debate. But if any of the ethical problems plaguing contemporary health care are simply the products of new technology, withholding treatment is definitely not one of them.

Second, Haiselden's actions illuminate a crucial early stage in the emergence and convergence of two deeply controversial social applications of biology—eugenics and euthanasia. I will argue that the meanings of each movement were shaped by an intense struggle among many different groups who fought to impose their concepts on mass culture.

The professionals who led the eugenics campaign frequently attacked the mass media for what they considered vulgar distortions of their scientific programs. Historians have focused on the ideas of these leaders, and many have implicitly adopted the leaders' contempt for mass culture.[38]

But this book will show that such an approach misses the vital role of mass culture in constructing both the meanings and the memory of these movements. "Mass culture," which includes any production made for a mass audience whether or not it was demonstrably "popular" in origin, constituted a crucial battleground on which professionals, popularizers, journalists, censors, and audiences struggled to shape the meanings of "eugenics" and "euthanasia" and to define the connection between them.

Mass culture did not "diffuse" scientific definitions to a passive public, nor did it simply dilute once–precise technical terms as it filtered them down to the masses. Rather, the responses to Haiselden's campaign reveal an intense, active struggle among various lay and professional groups to control the construction of these concepts. Audiences read their own meanings into official movement propaganda and in turn, the ideas of the leadership sometimes changed in response to their grudging dialogue with their audiences. As a battleground for competing concepts, mass culture itself generally did not create new definitions. However the terrain of this battlefield—the technical limits and social structure of the era's mass media—often did influence the success or failure of the different groups who fought to define eugenics and euthanasia.[39]

Because eugenics had many different meanings there is no one answer to the debate over whether and when most scientists repudiated the movement. The Haiselden controversy reveals that it was common to reject one aspect of eugenics while endorsing others. The term eugenics covered three distinct topics: goals, methods, and powers. Thus some who rejected Haiselden's methods supported his goals, while others who opposed medical decisionmaking favored empowering someone else to eliminate the unfit.

Almost no one today remembers that Americans ever died in the name of eugenics, much less that such deaths were highly publicized and broadly supported. Yet in the wake of Haiselden's campaign, death became a widely discussed and often advocated measure for dealing with the unfit. To overlook the support for eugenic euthanasia in the late 1910s is to seriously skew the dimensions of both movements.[40] Both eugenics and euthanasia provided assessments of which lives were not worth living. "Eugenics" could mean judging who was "better–not–born,"[41] and "euthanasia" could mean deciding who was "better–off–dead." The extent to which eugenics had come to include the death of the disabled can be seen most clearly in the startling number and diversity of Haiselden's supporters.

Third, a close look at how this movement judged who was unfit to live provides important new evidence about when and why a supposedly scientific movement to fight hereditary disease became associated with racial, class, ethnic, and gender hatreds that eventually would be invoked to justify genocide. There were no logically necessary links between fighting genetic disease and such specific prejudices, and each of these hatreds long predated both Haiselden and eugenics.[42] Haiselden's supporters brought their biases along with them from their individual lives and their wider culture, including many once-common prejudices now generally repudiated. And they changed some of their prejudices remarkably quickly in response to cultural changes. Furthermore, they represented a surprisingly broad spectrum of social opinion, from socialists to business leaders, feminists to misogynists, nativists to immigrants.

This ideological diversity and fluidity was possible because Haiselden successfully argued that such subjective and emotional disputes could be eliminated by science. He appealed to a faith common among turn-of-the-century Americans who considered themselves "progressive"—the belief that science constituted an objective method for resolving social and ethical questions, such as the quality-of-life decisions eugenics and euthanasia required. His backers could even simultaneously love and loathe those they labeled unfit, without acknowledging much emotional conflict, because they believed their attitudes were products of an objective method that had resolved such ethical and emotional contradictions. Haiselden and his supporters did not consider their decisions to be value free, but they insisted that their choice of values was derived from and proven by objective methods.

But faith in objectivity did not cure the value conflicts inherent in such decisions; it only camouflaged them. Both "eugenics" and "euthanasia" contain the Greek prefix meaning "good." Their etymology reflects the fact that they are deeply value-laden terms. That does not automatically make them unscientific; no science is value free. Nor does it make logical discussion and agreement impossible.

However, the common progressive belief that science provided objective means for distinguishing good lives from bad ones hid the subjectivity of the values people actually used to make such judgments. And because they believed their values to be objectively proven, they could dismiss ethical or political criticism as biased, unscientific, and therefore irrelevant.

While eugenicists used their preexisting values to judge who was unfit, Haiselden's crusade shows that the movement was not a completely indiscriminate filter-feeder, passively soaking up whatever values floated by in the surrounding culture.[43] Eugenics selectively attracted those who shared its progressive faith in objectivity. In turn, they brought with them specific preferences and values associated with modernity, in areas from aesthetics to sexuality, and these preferences directly shaped decisions about the diagnosis and treatment of "defectives." Furthermore, propagandists like Haiselden led the mass media to identify these particular preferences with eugenics, and thus helped to selectively recruit additional followers who shared these values.

Eugenicists like Haiselden not only believed their decisions to be objective; they considered objectivity itself to be an ethical imperative of almost mystical power. Science not only banished outdated traditional moral beliefs, it provided a new and better set of social and moral duties. Such assumptions made it difficult for eugenicists to reason ethically about their own judgments, while they impelled them to act on these unexamined beliefs.

Fourth, although their faith in the objectivity of science led many progressive-era Americans to expect that scientists would impartially agree on issues such as which lives were not worth saving, in practice experts drawn from different specialties with competing goals, values, and interests rarely reached a consensus. The effort to select which infants should live provides an early illustration of how a shared faith in the scientific method proved too fragile a bond to counter the increasing specialization that soon fragmented both the scientific community and the progressive political movement and that threatened to undermine their belief in objectivity itself.

Fifth, although eugenics led to control by male professionals over aspects of life previously considered women's sphere, Haiselden's crusade reveals that this outcome was in part an ironic side-effect of medicine's professionalization, one which many women and doctors opposed. Professional leaders often did not want this particular new power, while many women had hoped medical authority would increase rather than diminish their own status and autonomy.

Sixth, comparing the 1910s with the present reveals both striking similarities and significant differences. One key difference is the strong current commitment to individual choice in the use of genetic technology. But the differences are not as great as might be assumed. The economic, political, and cultural barriers that circumscribed reproductive choices in Haiselden's time have hardly been eliminated. As in the 1910s, today's medical genetics operates in a culture of resurgent racial nationalism, from Bosnia and Berlin to Brooklyn. Most important, belief that the objectivity of science is our best defense against these values remains strong and, I will argue, remains as dangerously deceptive today as it was in Haiselden's time.

Finally, then as now, the issue of withholding medical treatment became enmeshed in controversy over the role of the mass media in medical disputes. For many of his lay and medical critics, Haiselden's refusal to treat imperiled infants proved less troubling than his efforts to publicize and popularize the process of medical decision making. This dispute also played a major, previously unrecognized role in shaping the evolution of the mass media, by provoking the rise of what I term "aesthetic censorship."

The sudden prominence and equally swift erasure of Haiselden and his crusade also demonstrate the emergence of both newspapers and film as powerful new forces in early-twentieth-century medical controversies. Historians long have noted the episodic nature of the debate on euthanasia, but only in the most recent cases have scholars considered the role of the mass media in fostering such cycles. The periodic forgetting and rediscovery of eugenic euthanasia suggests that changing public awareness of many issues in medical ethics may be as closely related to changes in media coverage as to changes in actual medical practice.[44]

A Word about Words

To understand past attitudes and perceptions, people's words must be understood in context. Today, to describe someone with a disability as a "monstrosity" or "monster" could only be viciously pejorative. Yet at the start of this century, these terms had a specific technical meaning and were seen as acceptable scientific labels for newborns with severe congenital malformations. Likewise, "idiots," "imbeciles," and "morons" composed three distinct and specific levels of measured mental impairment. In both medical and popular discourse, "cripple" was the accepted term for someone with impaired mobility. "Defective" was the commonly used medical term for a person with any serious disability, primarily but not necessarily a birth defect. No irony or offense was intended when Jane Addams reportedly called Helen Keller a "great defective."[45]

These professedly neutral labels were often adopted to distance objective medical science from the pejorative value judgments associated with older words like "freak" or "sport." But the use of objective-sounding terminology also attempted to exclude from medicine the benevolent sentimental overtones of such previous euphemisms as "afflicted misfortunates."[46]

As we shall see, use of these new labels did not succeed in removing value judgments from the discussion of disabilities.[47] But it would be a mistake to impute consciously hostile motives to past individuals based solely on their use of words that in context, were intended to be objective, technical terms.

Whenever possible, I have tried to present early-twentieth-century concepts and controversies in the words of the participants, both because the changing meanings of words and images are a major topic of the book, and because no paraphrase or summary could capture the richness of the originals. I use terms like "defective" to examine, not to endorse, the values implicit in past terminology.

Contexts to the Conflict

Before Baby Bollinger:
Infanticide, Eugenics, and Euthanasia

When he refused to operate on the Bollinger baby, Harry Haiselden became the first Western physician in modern times to publicly permit the death of a potentially savable newborn. But he
was neither the first to openly advocate such a policy nor the
first to implement it in private.[1]

Infanticide had been practiced in much of the ancient world.
Greek and Roman fathers legally could kill their babies for any
reason at all. Common motives ranged from domestic economics
to religious ritual, but selective destruction of the unhealthy was
among the most widely-approved. In classical Greece, exposure
was used both to dispose of visibly impaired newborns and to
weed out those with invisible weaknesses. Both Plato and Aris-

totle recommended legally requiring the death of clearly deformed infants. Such a compulsory system existed in Sparta and under the Laws of the Twelve Tables in Rome. But exposing apparently healthy babies in order to detect hidden defects was officially discouraged as too unselective.

Although fathers or the state controlled the fates of impaired newborns, physicians also participated in infanticide as they became more involved in obstetrics. In his pioneering gynecology text, the second century A.D. Greco-Roman physician Soranus provided explicit instructions for diagnosing which infants were "not worth rearing." He condemned the "barbarian" practice of immersing newborns in cold water to test for hidden weaknesses, not because he rejected infanticide, but because he felt that the technique also killed healthy babies.[2]

Ancient Judaism condemned all forms of infanticide and attempted to suppress the practice.[3] This attitude was retained by the early church, and following the rise to political power of Christianity in the fourth century, the intentional killing of infants was rejected by religion, law, and medicine throughout much of Europe.

Despite this change, it remained acceptable for parents to leave children in public places or churches in the hope someone would take them in, even though the practice was understood to result in many unintended deaths. Likewise, placing a newborn with a wet nurse carried a recognized but legitimate risk to the infant's life. Those parents who intentionally killed a child might now be prosecuted, but those found guilty were often punished less severely than those who murdered an adult.

And the lives of deformed newborns remained particularly vulnerable. "Monsters" so misshapen they lacked human form and such "unnatural" horrors as "changelings" (imps left behind by demons who had stolen the "real" baby) might not be considered human beings. Thus killing them might not violate the ban on infanticide, a view endorsed by no less an authority than Martin Luther.

Doctors are not mentioned by modern historians as having played much of a role in these decisions, probably because the vast majority of births were attended by neighbors and midwives. But physicians might have been consulted by midwives, parents, or the authorities to diagnose whether a particular impaired infant was indeed a disposable nonhuman monster or to determine whether its particular deformity was the product of supernatural forces outside the previous experience of natural science.[4] The seventeenth-century

English vicar Robert Burton's medical classic, *The Anatomy of Melancholy,* cited with approval classical and primitive examples of selective infanticide, as well as the castration of men with inheritable diseases and the killing of heritably diseased women who became pregnant.[5]

From the seventeenth century on, physicians did become increasingly involved in efforts to repress lay infanticide. In Britain and perhaps elsewhere, the initial goal was to prevent unwed mothers from destroying the evidence of illegitimate childbearing. By the late nineteenth century, other factors also motivated the growing number of doctors who denounced lay infanticide. Their motives included the rise of organized humanitarian movements against cruelty, the start of professional efforts to control midwives and abortionists, and the growth of a life-insurance industry vulnerable to fraudulent claims.[6]

Yet the mid-nineteenth century also constitutes the first period since antiquity for which medical records document that, in at least one or two specific cases, doctors privately withheld treatment from impaired infants. In a fascinating, privately published account of 1834, Dr. Charles T. Hildreth reported the case of a "monstrosity," an infant born without a spinal cord and with evident brain damage. On his arrival after the birth, the doctor found the baby's head tightly enveloped in membranes that prevented it from breathing. Two "female friends" who had attended the delivery had done nothing to the infant, and Dr. Hildreth decided not to remove the membranes nor to attempt any form of resuscitation.[7]

Beginning about 1870, a few physicians and others first publicly advocated killing or not treating defective newborns. These proposals marked the initial convergence of two increasingly important concepts, eugenics and euthanasia.

The word "euthanasia," which previously had meant efforts to ease the sufferings of the dying without hastening their death, now also came to include both passively withholding treatment and active "mercy killing." As early as the 1870s, several British physicians and lay supporters publicly advocated active euthanasia in a variety of incurable conditions, to be administered by means such as inhaling chloroform.[8] Such discussions reflected a major reassessment of medical responses to suffering. The introduction of new painkillers such as morphine, anesthetics, and aspirin was associated with a new utilitarian view of professional duty that accepted some risk to life proportional to the amount of suffering relieved. And as medicine gained new power to cure some pains, it made the remaining incurable pains seem even less tolerable, both for the sufferers and for those who empathized with them.[9]

Most early discussion of euthanasia focused on cases of painfully and terminally ill adults who voluntarily chose to die. But ever since the earliest proposals to speed death, "euthanasia" could mean not only "mercy killing" but any "painless killing," whether voluntary and benevolent or not. The second meaning can be seen in Anthony Trollope's 1882 novel *The Fixed Period*, a satire on reform zealotry, whose narrator urges compulsory "euthanasia" for the elderly. This usage gained enormous notoriety in the United States when the eminent Dr. William Osler appeared to endorse Trollope's proposal in 1905. In the same vein, Herbert Spencer described his new device for humanely executing stray dogs and criminals as "euthanasia."[10]

From the start, euthanasia occasionally overlapped with eugenics. An applied science and a popular crusade, eugenics sought to improve human heredity and eradicate hereditary disease. The term was coined by Charles Darwin's cousin Francis Galton, and the movement claimed roots in Herbert Spencer's effort to apply Darwinian natural selection to human societies. But while Spencer's "Social Darwinism" implied that the "fittest" would survive if people simply permitted nature to weed out society's losers, eugenics favored active intervention to assist natural selection, to offset medical and charitable activities that had artificially preserved the unfit, and to streamline the slow, wasteful, and cruel aspects of natural competition.

The early twentieth century was the heyday of organized eugenics in America and throughout the Western world. The movement promoted activities ranging from statistically sophisticated analyses of family pedigrees to "better baby contests" modeled on livestock shows at rural state fairs. By the 1920s, eugenic reasoning also led many American states to legislate the compulsory sterilization of criminals, the insane, and the retarded, and prompted Congress to selectively restrict the immigration of "inferior" nationalities and races.[11]

Before Haiselden, most prominent British and American eugenicists denied that they sought the death of defectives, arguing that preventing reproduction by the unfit would suffice. But the convergence of eugenics and euthanasia had begun as early as 1868, and proposals to kill the unfit grew in frequency from 1890 on. From the first, impaired newborns were singled out as prime targets for selective elimination. German zoologist Ernst Haeckel, whose philosophy of monism attempted to apply Darwinism to society, first suggested killing impaired infants in 1868. The proposal was amplified by his disciple Adolf Jost and by pioneer race hygienist Alfred Ploetz in 1895.[12]

Writing in German, Hungarian child-welfare pioneer Sigmund Engel appealed to the "joint outlook of Socialism and Darwinism" to demand that "cripples, high-grade cretins, idiots, and children with gross deformities" "should be quickly and painlessly destroyed," a process he termed "euthanasia." "For the present we may leave the question open whether the consent of the parents should first be obtained," because "the interest of the species is more important than that of a few individuals useless to society." In a book translated in America in 1912, Engel rejected the "ultra-Darwinian" view that spontaneous infant mortality played a useful role in natural selection, noting that most causes of infant death killed fit babies too. By contrast, "infanticide" could be rigorously selective, used only when "medical science indicates, beyond the possibility of a doubt, that it is impossible for them ever to become useful members of society," or when "it is obvious that their existence is directly harmful to the species."[13]

Early British eugenicist Dr. Robert Rentoul favored selective infanticide in 1906. A prominent British health official, Dr. Charles E. Goddard, proposed killing idiots, imbeciles, and monstrosities.[14] That doctors already routinely practiced selective infanticide was assumed by Swedish inventor and chronic invalid Alfred Nobel, who reportedly described himself around 1887 as a "pitiful creature" who "ought to have been suffocated by a humane physician when he made his howling entrance into this life."[15]

In the United States, Chicago dental surgeon and medical professor Eugene Talbot quoted with approval calls for selective infanticide in his 1898 treatise *Degeneracy*. The 1899 presidential address to the American Social Science Association by Yale law professor Simeon Baldwin urged surgeons not to operate on physically defective infants if the "operation can only save the life by making it a daily and hopeless misery."[16] In 1900 Dr. William D. McKim called for killing institutionalized hereditary defectives, among whom he included the retarded, epileptics, alcoholics, and burglars. Noted psychologist G. Stanley Hall denounced medical efforts to save the "moribund sick, defectives and criminals, because by aiding them to survive it interferes with the process of wholesome natural selection."[17] Further evidence of increasing interest in the issue may be found in the growing number of scholarly medical and sociological publications about ancient and primitive selective infanticide practices.[18]

As part of a sweeping 1906 call to restructure medicine and society, Chicago surgeon G. Frank Lydston proposed both sterilizing the unfit and gassing to death "the driveling imbecile." Lydston was a colleague of Talbot and professor of venereal diseases and urinary surgery at the College of Physicians and Surgeons when Haiselden was a student there. And just prior to the Bollinger case, New York physician Edward Wallace Lee demanded the "extermination" of dependent defectives, urging that criminals, the insane, and idiots should be "eradicated."[19]

Support for legislating such proposals was particularly strong in the Midwest. A law to electrocute mentally defective infants was proposed by Michigan state representative Link Rodgers as early as 1903. Rodgers, a thirty-seven-year-old harness manufacturer from Muskegon, moved his proposal as an amendment to the budget for the state home for the feebleminded. The *Detroit News* suggested Rodgers probably got the idea from "scientists," "for the same proposition has been heard from in scientific quarters." The plan was prominently reported in the Chicago papers, where it aroused concerned discussion.

During 1906 legislative debates on euthanasia bills in Iowa and Ohio, well-known forensic psychiatrist Dr. Walter Kempster urged that any euthanasia law include "lunatics and idiots," and Dr. R. H. Gregory proposed requiring that "hideously deformed or idiotic children should be put out of existence by the administration of an anaesthetic."[20]

In discussing Kempster's proposal, a writer for body-builder Bernarr Macfadden's magazine *Physical Culture* quoted with approval a newspaper article demanding that "infants born to deformities, idiocy and suffering should be mercifully put out of the way." His list of candidates for euthanasia began with a pain-ravaged terminal burn victim, but focused thereafter on eliminating a wide assortment of those he termed "degenerates."[21]

Haiselden's refusal to treat defective newborns thus did not initiate the convergence of eugenics and euthanasia. But his campaign focused unprecedented attention on these issues at a critical moment in their relationship, and it produced endorsements of euthanasia from mainstream eugenic leaders who previously had publicly rejected such measures.

U.S.A., 1915

By 1915 the United States was in the midst of a drastic social and cultural transformation, the result of unprecedented immigration, industrialization, and urban growth. Earlier Irish and German migrations were largely replaced by a "new immigration" from eastern and southern Europe. More divided among themselves and more alien to native eyes, these newcomers pushed immigration to a record 1.2 million arrivals in 1914. A prolonged agricultural depression fueled a massive farm-to-city migration within the United States as well, and among these internal migrants were many rural southern blacks.[22]

New concepts of organizational efficiency and the switch from water- to combustion-powered machinery produced vast business "trusts" and mass-production industries. Andrew Carnegie and J. P. Morgan assembled U.S. Steel; John D. Rockefeller built Standard Oil; Henry Ford combined steel and oil with the assembly line to revolutionize both production and transportation. At the same time, low-capital piecework "sweatshops" proliferated.

Not surprisingly, such vast changes provoked raw and brutal conflicts. Strikes were generally illegal, and labor disputes sparked violent repression, with scores killed between 1912 and 1914, from the mines of Michigan and Colorado to the mills of New Jersey and Massachusetts. The election of 1912 produced nearly a million votes for Socialist Eugene Debs. A combination of economic and racial fears led Congress to ban Asian immigration. The 1915 Stone Mountain rally launched a resurgent Ku Klux Klan on a lethal crusade of terror across the South and much of the Midwest against immigrants, non-Protestants, and blacks.[23]

In response to these dramatic upheavals, a disparate group of largely middle-class native-born reformers created what they and later historians called the "progressive" movement. From Jane Addams's settlement house to Gifford Pinchot's forest conservation, from antitrust legislation to direct election of senators, women's suffrage and feminism to prohibition of alcohol, a broad range of personalities and causes claimed the label "progressive." Crossing party lines, the term was applied to Republican Theodore Roosevelt, Democrat Woodrow Wilson, and Farmer-Labor Independent Robert LaFollette. This diversity raises questions about what if anything progressivism really meant.

But one thing many progressives did share was a faith in the methods of modern science to produce efficient technical solutions for social problems. If science was objective, then scientific experts would be impartial and fair, and their social decisions would carry moral weight. The new experimental sciences also provided a model for activist government, and a conception of causality that favored specific attributions of responsibility for specific social problems. Indeed, much of the confusing diversity of progressive causes may reflect their conscious imitation of scientific specialization.[24]

Among the sciences whose progress progressives most admired were medicine and public health. In a series of stunning discoveries, microbe hunters such as Louis Pasteur, Robert Koch, and their disciples isolated the organisms responsible for dozens of dread diseases. They developed many new vaccines and other preventive techniques.

These discoveries initially produced few new cures for those already sick. Penicillin and other antibiotics were still decades in the future. But effective new treatments were developed for two widely feared infections—diphtheria and syphilis. Specific dietary changes were discovered to cure what turned out to be nutritional deficiency diseases, such as pellagra. And the gradual improvement of Joseph Lister's antiseptic methods enabled surgeons to operate successfully on the chest and abdomen, and made it safer to develop new surgical repairs for a variety of congenital deformities, from harelip to clubfoot and hunchback.[25] Recognition that many institutionalized mental patients owed their symptoms to nerve damage caused by syphilis or pellagra even made it possible to hope that many of the insane might soon be cured, though this optimism did not extend to those with other mental impairments.[26]

These therapeutic results were relatively few, but they were virtually unprecedented. And they seemed based on generalizable scientific methods that promised unlimited future applications. Koch popularized the concept that his discoveries were based on simple methodological "postulates" that emphasized the laboratory isolation of unique microscopic causes for each specific disease. When Pasteur produced his very first vaccine, for the cattle disease anthrax, he predicted the impending eradication of all infections, not because anthrax was particularly important, but because he had discovered the method for making vaccines.[27]

Even before these scientific advances bore practical fruits, American physicians had begun to redefine medical professionalism, to emphasize technical expertise over previous social and personal qualifications. In the late nineteenth century, most states passed new medical licensing laws. And with the financial support of major foundations, medical schools reorganized themselves around the new science. These changes began to reduce the number of practitioners and raise the power and prestige of the profession. They also gradually repressed the competing medical sects of the nineteenth century and standardized the previously disparate methods and contents of medical training.[28]

These medical discoveries also helped inspire the formation of new national associations to fight tuberculosis, cancer, mental illness, occupational injuries, and other particular diseases. Such groups united patients, professionals, and publicists in a number of targeted disease-specific crusades.[29]

One such group, the American Social Hygiene Association, founded in 1913, took aim at venereal diseases. A disparate coalition, the social hygienists disagreed over whether science had proven or supplanted traditional sexual morality, and over which expert specialties should control sex diseases, but they were united by their faith that scientific methods would produce an objective solution to "social" diseases.[30]

The organized campaign for artificial contraceptives began in this period as well. Effective spermicides, condoms, and diaphragms had been invented decades earlier, but it took a prolonged political movement to overcome obscenity laws that banned their discussion and to convince doctors to promote them. Early promoters of "birth control" such as Dr. William J. Robinson, Emma Goldman, and Margaret Sanger linked the crusade for contraception to broader issues of feminism, sexuality, socialism, and eugenics, but like many other progressive health reforms, Sanger's "planned parenthood" movement soon adopted a single-issue focus and a greater reliance on medical experts.[31]

Among the most popular progressive movements were those affecting the health and welfare of children: child-labor regulation, compulsory schooling, juvenile courts, home economics, milk inspection, school nursing, school health education, and more. Progressive reformers contributed both to the professionalization of obstetrics and pediatrics and to the growth of research into child development and pedagogy. The efforts of a largely female group of reformers trained in the settlement movement led to creation of a Children's Bureau within the federal Labor Department in 1912.[32]

Progressive health-reform campaigns contributed to dramatic reductions in childhood mortality and a large improvement in life expectancy, but they also fostered the growing intervention of technical experts and the state in the lives of individual families. Many progressives, such as John Dewey, hoped the methods of science would give ordinary people the tools for greater self-determination, to let them better achieve their own goals. But others used the authority of the state to compel compliance with measures the experts determined to be in the public interest.[33]

Examples of both trends can be seen in progressive-era medical law. In 1905 the United States Supreme Court first upheld compulsory smallpox vaccination, a decision that rapidly became the precedent for many other involuntary medical procedures, including eugenic sterilization. Yet in 1914, future Supreme Court Justice Benjamin Cardozo upheld a New York patient's right to refuse even potentially lifesaving treatment, an important precedent in the evolution of concepts of patient autonomy.[34]

Like medicine, mass communications experienced a radical transformation caused by technological and organizational innovations in the turn-of-the-century decades. Photoengraving, the high-speed press, telephone, phonograph, movie projector, and radio were introduced. William Randolph Hearst, Joseph Pulitzer, and their rivals built nationwide networks of low-priced, mass-market newspapers. And a variety of new professions, from psychology to public relations, specialized in the study and control of mass motivation.

One result was the development of modern propaganda. As defined by many progressive reformers, "propaganda" did not imply deception or distortion; it was simply the use of information to influence public opinion and behavior. What distinguished propaganda from information was not the content but the intent—the desire to control the audience's response. Progressives embraced propaganda as an attractive middle ground between technocracy and "dumb-ocracy," a modern technological method to produce popular compliance with expert advice, without the need for direct coercion.

The growth of medical knowledge magnified both the importance and the difficulty of communication between doctors and the public. In response, progressive public health reformers were among the most enthusiastic pioneers of mass-media propaganda, including motion pictures. In 1910, only about five years after the introduction of commercial movie theaters, Thomas Edison made the first health propaganda film for the tuberculosis association. Within four years, almost every aspect of health reform reached the screen, including venereal disease, infant mortality, and eugenics. By 1928 over 1300 silent films on medical topics had been produced for lay audiences.[35]

At the hub of American transport and the border between industry and agriculture, Haiselden's Chicago experienced the full force of almost all the era's changes. Chicago was the White City of the 1893 fair, the lyrical brawn of Carl Sandburg's poems, the oppression and filth of Upton Sinclair's *Jungle*, the hard-boiled cynicism of Ben Hecht's *Front Page*. It was home to Jane Addams's Hull House, national headquarters for the American Medical Association and the Socialist Party. The election of 1915 ousted a civic-reform coalition and began the long reign of Mayor William Hale "Big Bill" Thompson's Republican machine, though the town was not yet the gangland capital it soon became during Prohibition. A major destination for the great migration of southern blacks before and during World War I, Chicago was a volatile mix of rural native whites, Germans, Slavs, Italians, Jews, and African-Americans that exploded in the murderous antiblack riot of July 1919. Haiselden's Chicago was at the center of modern America.

Taking Sides: Some Rough Images of the Debate

Haiselden publicized his cases partly to get others to take a public stand on treating impaired infants. He hoped to demonstrate that his ideas enjoyed widespread support among those who had no previous chance to express their opinions in public, and to compel those who previously had no opinions to choose sides.[36]

An extraordinary number of Americans took this opportunity to record their positions on a topic never before this widely debated. Their responses provide a completely unique glimpse at how public impressions of eugenics and euthanasia were constructed in this formative era.

From newspapers, magazines, and professional journals, I compiled a list of 333 people who took a public stand on Haiselden's refusal to treat impaired newborns, and a partly overlapping list of 47 individuals who commented publicly on Haiselden's propaganda activities. Many wrote long articles, while others responded briefly to a journalist's questions. Another 53 people recorded their opinions in response to an unpublished private survey and will be discussed separately from the published comments.

While these responses provide unique and important insights, they must be interpreted with extreme caution. None of these groups constituted a random sample, and no claim that they accurately represented any larger body of opinion would be justified. Modern concepts of polling were unknown in 1915. Some publications deliberately sought "balance" by publishing equal numbers of advocates for each side, while others seem to have featured primarily those who agreed with the editor.

Nor was the list of publications I examined random or representative. It drew heavily on English-language northeastern and midwestern big-city and college-town newspapers and on national lay and professional periodicals. These sources were supplemented by local Catholic, radical, and African-American publications. Many of the responses were carried by nationwide news services and were reprinted across the country, but there may have been considerable local variation in what portion of these opinions were seen in any one locality.[37]

Furthermore, published comments are not even definitive evidence about the opinions of the individuals quoted. Journalists unfamiliar with the issues often hurriedly extracted a few punchy phrases from haphazardly transcribed recollections of hastily arranged interviews. They reported what they considered important about what they remembered hearing, not necessarily what the person may have said. Thus even the editors of the *New York Times* mistakenly attributed to one source their own view that Haiselden should not have publicized his actions, when what that source actually wrote was that Haiselden's published arguments were unconvincing.[38]

Others may have deliberately misrepresented their private opinions to the press. Newspapers across the country quoted eminent Boston physicians Richard and Hugh Cabot as attacking Haiselden. Richard Cabot reportedly declared, "I don't think any physician or surgeon should take into his own hands the question as to whether any human being deserves to live. Our business as doctors is to further life, never to diminish it." Yet both men privately supported euthanasia within their own family. In November 1893 Richard Cabot helped to chloroform his incurably diabetic brother, Ted; in July 1918 Hugh argued against prolonging the life of his twin brother, Phillip. Richard Cabot was an advocate for unflinching medical honesty toward patients. If newspaper accounts about the Cabots' opinions could differ so sharply from their private actions, then such accounts cannot be relied upon as accurate depictions of any individual's personal beliefs unless corroborated by other evidence.[39]

Although such "straw polls" cannot provide an accurate picture of public opinion, the published results did shape the image that was presented to the contemporary public about who held what positions, and these surveys were often seen at the time as gauges of public opinion.[40] Thus a collective analysis of these individual responses can still be historically useful as a summary description of what significant portions of the contemporary public were being told about the reaction to Dr. Haiselden's acts. Although they are not measures of public opinion, they are valuable rough summary outlines of the images presented to the public about who took what side.

One issue on which these images cast new light concerns the strength of support for radical eugenic measures in 1910s America. Although recent studies have noted that America led the world in compulsory sterilizations for the first third of this century,[41] none have suggested the extensive support for eugenic euthanasia portrayed by the published reactions to Haiselden's cases.

Of the 333 people identified who publicly took a stand on the issue, more than half endorsed letting at least some impaired infants die, including 14 who called for actively killing defective babies. Only a bit over one-third favored attempting to save every newborn. Most of the remainder granted doctors the discretion to make such decisions without explicitly stating what course they personally supported (Table 1).

Another crucial topic illuminated by these responses is the political image of early eugenics. Since the 1930s, eugenics has been identified almost exclusively with far-right politics, but the political

Table 1.[a] Publicly Stated Position on Treating Impaired Newborns

	Number	*Percentage*
Treat all	116	35
Don't treat some	153	47
Actively kill	14	4
Up to doctor[b]	32	10
Other[c]	15	4
Total	333	100

[a] For each of the tables, please note the many limitations discussed in chapter 2.

In each table, the percentages are read vertically, showing what proportion of the group named at the top of each column reportedly took each position.

[b] Includes those who say that they can't condemn Haiselden, or that he was within his discretion, but don't indicate whether they personally agree or disagree with his decisions.

[c] Includes those quoted as opposed to active killing without commenting on withholding treatment, and those whose quoted views cannot be summarized easily.

complexion of the early movement is a subject of intense controversy. The first American eugenics advocates were radical utopian socialist-communitarians like John Humphrey Noyes. In Europe and the United States, prominent socialists continued to support eugenics at least until the 1920s, including many who saw the movement as linking feminism, birth control, and political radicalism. Yet from Galton onward, eugenics drew on "Social Darwinist" and neo-Malthusian explanations of poverty that socialists considered anathema.

Eugenics also appealed to many political progressives. It drew upon the same faith in scientific expertise, modernism, and state activism that characterized many progressive reformers. But eugenicists often opposed the health and welfare measures promoted by progressives, considering that such efforts would only increase the numbers of the unfit.[42]

The public debate over Haiselden's actions thus provides important new evidence on this puzzling and controversial topic. (Table 2). Those who called themselves "progressives" or "independents" generally were quoted as opposed to Haiselden's cause. Two-thirds of them called for treating all impaired newborns. Among Haiselden's most outspoken critics was the best-known woman progressive, Jane Addams, who had denounced proposals for killing defective children as early as 1903.[43]

But people who adopted the Progressive Party label comprised only one portion of those who identified with progressivism as a social philosophy or a reform ideology. Thus pioneer public health nurse and settlement leader Lillian Wald, whose career exemplified progressive reform, appears in Table 2 as a Democrat, the party whose candidates she supported from 1912 on.[44] Wald backed Haiselden.

Table 2. Publicly Stated Position on Treatment, by Known Political Party, Distinguishing Known Catholics from Other or Unknown Religious Affiliations

	Democrat		Independent or Progressive	Republican	Socialist
	Catholic	Others			
Treat all	4 (80%)	5 (29%)	10 (67%)	15 (43%)	0
Don't treat some	0	10 (59%)	4 (27%)	13 (37%)	9 (82%)
Actively kill	0	0	1 (7%)	1 (3%)	2 (18%)
Up to doctor	1 (20%)	2 (12%)	0	3 (9%)	0
Other	0	0	0	3 (9%)	0
Total (N = 83)	5	17	15	35	11

The socialists quoted on the issue strongly supported not treating impaired infants. The *Call*, New York's leading socialist newspaper, commissioned front-page articles by Haiselden and Mrs. Bollinger and printed them more prominently than news of the execution of radical I.W.W. union organizer Joe Hill. Socialist physician William J. Robinson and his son Frederic, founding secretary of the Voluntary Parenthood League, portrayed Haiselden's actions as supporting their efforts to legalize birth control, while Anita Block, editor of the *Call*'s women's page, backed Haiselden in stridently eugenic terms. In a series of essays, poems, and cartoons, other socialist writers linked his actions to pacifism and class conflict. They ridiculed as hypocrites those who got worked up about the lives of defective infants while ignoring the lives crushed out or crippled by poverty and war.[45]

All eleven identified socialists who spoke out on the issue supported allowing impaired newborns to die, and two favored actively killing them. But while socialists figured disproportionately in this portrait of Haiselden's supporters, the vast majority of those quoted in his cause were not politically radical. And many noted radicals, even among those deeply involved with feminism and birth control, kept silent on Haiselden's crusade. Anarchist Emma Goldman and her Chicago-based manager Dr. Ben Reitman were touring the Midwest lecturing on birth control and were speaking in Chicago at the height of the Bollinger case publicity. Yet neither the published accounts of her appearances nor her private correspondence mentions Haiselden or the treatment of impaired babies. Likewise, Margaret Sanger, mourning the death of her own daughter, kept silent about the issue of letting other children die, even after Helen Keller publicly equated Sanger's crusade with Haiselden's.[46]

The Chicago-based *American Socialist* confined its coverage of the controversy to short summaries without commentary in its news-of-the-week section. Chicago's anarchist monthly, *The Alarm*, reversing the priorities of the *Call*, covered Haiselden only as a footnote to the Joe Hill execution, denouncing the Utah governor who refused to commute Hill's sentence as a "monster" who should have been allowed to die at birth.[47] Such political metaphors had been used by the left even before the Bollinger case. Ironically, Joe Hill himself wrote one example, a song that suggested strikebreaking company thugs should have been abandoned by their mothers.[48]

Even the editors of the *Call* expressed misgivings about the uses to which Haiselden's eugenics might be put. So long as capitalists controlled society, there was a real danger that allowing defectives to die could lead to "murder" of the poor for "economic considerations."[49]

The Democratic Party in early-twentieth-century America drew considerable support from immigrant and Catholic communities, especially on such cultural–moral issues as alcohol prohibition. By 1915 the church had already denounced abortion, birth control, eugenic sterilization, and active euthanasia, while eugenicists had already begun to campaign against immigration.

Public statements on saving impaired newborns portray the Democrats as sharply split along religious lines. Four-fifths of Catholic Democrats quoted demanded treatment for all babies. Just over one-quarter of the non-Catholic Democrats who spoke out favored that position.

These comments also depicted Catholics of all political stripes as committed to defend any impaired infant's "right to life." Over three-fourths of Catholics quoted urged that doctors should try to save every baby, a position attributed to less than half the Protestants, less than one-third of the Jews, and just over one-quarter of those with no known religious affiliation (Table 3).

Catholic opposition to Haiselden was expressed in particularly vehement terms. One Chicago Catholic newspaper headlined its front-page coverage of the Bollinger case, "Human Life is Being Dragged Down to . . . the Stud Farm and Cattle Pen." The New Orleans diocesan paper labeled Haiselden's actions "monstrous, unchristian, damnable." In a nationally reported incident, a Catholic lay church worker admitted attempting to kidnap the Bollinger baby from the hospital to obtain treatment for it. She also reportedly led a group of women who broke into the Hodzima home and turned over to the police a bottle of the allegedly lethal painkiller Haiselden had prescribed. In turn, Haiselden's supporters sometimes attacked the Catholics in equally vehement terms. Socialist

Table 3. Publicly Stated Position on Treatment, by Religion

	Catholic	Jewish[a]	Protestant/Other	Atheist/Unknown
Treat all	14 (78%)	6 (33%)	36 (44%)	60 (28%)
Don't treat some	0	10 (56%)	31 (38%)	115 (53%)
Actively kill	0	0	3 (4%)	11 (5%)
Up to doctor	4 (22%)	2 (11%)	6 (7%)	20 (9%)
Other	0	0	5 (6%)	10 (5%)
Total (N = 333)	18	18	81	216

[a]Includes those with confirmed affiliation and those with surnames that in Europe had been legally designated for Jews.

Anita Block proclaimed the church "eager to have millions of idiots and imbeciles born, so long as it can only get them baptized."[50]

Whether Catholic or Protestant, Christian clergy were the occupational group most often quoted as opposed to letting impaired infants die. (No comments from rabbis or other non-Christian clergy were found. The Jews quoted were disproportionately doctors.) Sixty percent of the clergy but only one-quarter of the lawyers favored treating all newborns. Social workers and doctors were about halfway between these two extremes (Table 4).

Among the doctors there were striking differences in the reported opinions of different specialties. Almost two-thirds of the obstetrician-gynecologists and both of the orthopedic surgeons were quoted as favoring treatment. Only a bit over one-third of general surgeons or public health physicians felt that way. And though eugenics appealed to progressives' faith in specialized expertise, these public responses did not portray Haiselden's medical supporters as primarily specialists. While specialists constituted more than two-thirds of all doctors quoted, they comprised barely half of those reported as opposed to treating defectives. By contrast, of the nonspecialists whose views were published, only 14 percent reportedly favored treating all impaired newborns (Tables 5 and 6).[51]

Eugenics also overlapped with many issues of gender politics. The campaign for "better babies" allied eugenics with an important "women's issue," while its support of birth control for the poor and opposition to religiously based morality furthered the appeal of eugenics to many feminist sexual reformers. Yet like other progressive reforms, eugenics increased the authority of male experts over female reproductive decisions. And eugenics often seemed to ratify the claim that women's biology determined their role in society.[52]

Published comments on the deaths of Haiselden's patients conveyed this complexity. The press identified the question as a gender-based issue. Newspapers featured discussions of whether mothers or

Table 4. Publicly Stated Position on Treatment, by Selected Profession

	Clergy	*Social Workers*	*Doctors*	*Lawyers*
Treat all	15 (60%)	7 (47%)	74 (40%)	5 (25%)
Don't treat some	4 (16%)	6 (40%)	78 (42%)	8 (40%)
Actively kill	1 (4%)	2 (13%)	5 (3%)	2 (10%)
Up to doctor	4 (17%)	0	23 (12%)	3 (15%)
Other	1 (4%)	0	6 (3%)	2 (10%)
Total (N = 246)	25	15	186	20

Table 5. Publicly Stated Position on Treatment, by Selected
Medical Specialty

	OB-GYN	Pediatrics	General Surgery	Public Health[a]
Treat all	34 (62%)	6 (50%)	7 (39%)	6 (38%)
Don't treat some	12 (22%)	5 (42%)	5 (28%)	8 (50%)
Actively kill	2 (4%)	0	0	0
Up to doctor	5 (9%)	1 (8%)	5 (28%)	2 (13%)
Other	2 (4%)	0	1 (6%)	0
Total (N = 101)	55	12	18	16

[a]Includes venereology, at that time considered a branch of dermatology, but very closely involved in public health campaigns.

doctors should decide which babies to treat, and of how Haiselden's actions would affect other campaigns for women's causes.

But among those quoted, men and women favored treating impaired newborns in virtually the same proportions (Table 7). Those identified with women's rights issues were similarly divided. While some argued that a mother should not have to sacrifice her own life in caring for a severely defective baby, others like Julia Lathrop regarded any action that diminished the sanctity of motherhood as a serious threat to the position of women.[53] Among nonphysicians, women who opposed treatment were portrayed as slightly more likely than men to support simply withholding therapy, while more men than women supported active killing and trusting the doctor's decision. But among doctors, even these gender differences appeared muted.

Promoters portrayed both eugenics and euthanasia as progressive modern measures that questioned the authority of tradition. Not surprisingly, among those quoted on the issue, people 35 years old or younger in 1915 were most supportive of Haiselden, with only

Table 6. Publicly Stated Position on Treatment, Specialists
and Nonspecialists

	All Known Specialties	Generalists or Unknown[a]
Treat all	66 (51%)	8 (14%)
Don't treat some	41 (32%)	37 (66%)
Actively kill	2 (2%)	3 (5%)
Up to doctor	18 (14%)	5 (9%)
Other	3 (2%)	3 (5%)
Total (N = 186)	130	56

[a]Since virtually all the doctors identified were listed in a medical register or directory that included specialty information, it is fairly safe to assume that those who did not give a specialty thought of themselves as generalists.

Table 7. Publicly Stated Position on Treatment, by Gender Where Known, Physicians and Others

	Physicians		Others	
	Women	*Men*	*Women*	*Men*
Treat all	5 (50%)	65 (41%)	17 (29%)	20 (28%)
Don't treat some	4 (40%)	66 (42%)	34 (59%)	35 (49%)
Actively kill	0	3 (2%)	2 (3%)	6 (8%)
Up to doctor	1 (10%)	20 (13%)	1 (2%)	7 (10%)
Other	0	4 (3%)	4 (7%)	4 (6%)
Total	10	158	58	72

one-sixth urging treatment for impaired newborns. For the elderly, the implications of the issue appeared more ambiguous: A precedent allowing mercy killing of infants might be extended to free the elderly from fear of a prolonged and painful final illness, but the old also could become special targets if Haiselden's actions served to legitimate killing of the weak and burdensome. Among those quoted, people 56 and over were not as supportive of Haiselden as those under 35, although only one-third favored treating all sick newborns. The age group seen as most hostile to his crusade were those 36 to 55 (Table 8).

To guide their decisions about *The Black Stork,* the National Board of Review of Motion Pictures (NBRMP), a private body drawn from the film industry and various social agencies, solicited the opinions of 90 community leaders from around the nation, generating a total of 53 replies. This "national advisory committee" was intended to represent the views of "the best people"—a reformist moral and cultural elite—not a cross-section of public opinion at large. But unlike those quoted in print, these respondents recorded their views privately and in their own words, unfiltered by reporters or editors. And while their comments were not representative of any other group, they comprise an apparently complete record of the

Table 8. Publicly Stated Position, by Age in 1915, Where Known

	Age 56 and Over	Age 36–55	Age 35 and Under
Treat all	15 (33%)	41 (44%)	4 (17%)
Don't treat some	18 (40%)	39 (41%)	14 (61%)
Actively kill	2 (4%)	1 (1%)	3 (13%)
Up to doctor	7 (16%)	11 (12%)	3 (13%)
Other	3 (7%)	2 (2%)	1 (4%)
Total ($N = 162$)	45	94	23

ideas expressed within this particular group, whose opinions played a crucial role in deciding what the nation would get to see about this issue.[54]

Many of the NBRMP advisers stuck to the specific question of judging Haiselden's film (these replies will be discussed in Part II), but just over half also took a stand on treating impaired infants. These 27 individuals were a socially homogenous group, more than one-quarter of whom were Protestant clergy. They included no Catholics, one Jew, two physicians, and only three women.

Two-thirds of this group of self-defined moral leaders favored treating all impaired babies. Yet even among them, almost one quarter opposed saving defective infants, including 2 who urged actively killing them. The clergy did not disproportionately support treatment, nor did those who professed a religious affiliation, and the 3 women favored treatment in roughly the same proportion as the men (Tables 9, 10, 11).

Tabulating these cumulative responses provides an intriguing new snapshot of how the support for eugenic euthanasia was portrayed to the public in the 1910s, a subject on which we have virtu-

Table 9. Privately Surveyed Position on Treatment, by Occupation

	Clergy	Other Known Occupation	Unknown	Total
Treat all	4 (57%)	12 (71%)	1 (33%)	17 (63%)
Don't treat some	0	2 (12%)	2 (67%)	4 (15%)
Actively kill	0	2 (12%)	0	2 (7%)
Up to doctor	2 (29%)	0	0	2 (7%)
Other	1 (14%)	1 (6%)	0	2 (7%)
Total	7	17	3	27

Table 10. Privately Surveyed Position on Treatment, by Known Religious Affiliation

	Religion known[a]	Religion unknown
Treat all	8 (62%)	9 (64%)
Don't treat some	1 (8%)	3 (21%)
Actively kill	1 (8%)	1 (7%)
Up to doctor	2 (15%)	0
Other	1 (8%)	1 (7%)
Total	13	14

[a] 26 Protestant, 2 Jewish

Table 11. Privately Surveyed Position on
Treatment, by Sex Where Known[a]

	Women	Men
Treat all	2 (67%)	11 (61%)
Don't treat some	1 (33%)	1 (6%)
Actively kill	0	2 (11%)
Up to doctor	0	2 (11%)
Other	0	2 (11%)
Total	3	18

[a] Six people whose names included only their first initials could not be identified from other sources.

ally no other records. But even aside from their severe statistical limitations, such data alone cannot capture the process by which people struggled to make sense of a series of unprecedented events. It is not enough therefore to count up who favored treating defectives without also asking questions such as how the category "defective" was created and how its meanings changed when "treating them" or not became the question to resolve.

In the following chapters, close readings of the words and images used in this debate will probe how early-twentieth-century Americans came to decide not only whether they favored Haiselden's actions, but what Haiselden's activities meant, at a crucial point in the history of eugenics and euthanasia when these meanings were still novel, fluid, and contested.

3

Identifying the Unfit: Biology and Culture in the Construction of Hereditary Disease

"The chief significance" of the Bollinger case, "is the eugenic question," asserted Yale economist Irving Fisher. "Eugenics? Of course it's eugenics," Haiselden patiently explained to a reporter. New York's Commissioner of Charities John Kingsbury agreed, "This is eugenics in the concrete." Drawing on what had become the classic eugenic example of a defective family pedigree, Haiselden asked rhetorically, "Which do you prefer—six days of Baby Bollinger or seventy years of Jukes?" His film *The Black Stork* was even advertised as a "eugenic love story."[1]

To accomplish its goal of improving human heredity, eugenics claimed to answer a number of related but conceptually distinct questions. Among the most important were the following: First, what human differences are influenced by heredity? Second, what counts as an improvement—which human traits are good and which are not? Third, what techniques are best to produce the desired improvements? And fourth, who should have the power to answer the other questions? Much historical confusion over who supported and who opposed eugenics results from conflating these separable questions and from overlooking the struggles that took place over which answers to these questions would count as "eugenics."

Haiselden's crusade confronted Americans with each of these four questions at a critical point in the effort to define eugenics. This chapter uses the resulting controversy to examine the construction of what counted as an hereditary defect. Chapters 4 and 5 focus on methods and on power respectively.

Eugenicists perceived an astonishing array of human variations as inherited defects. The list included conditions still seen as genetic diseases today, but it also included many differences no longer considered hereditary illnesses. Some of these differences, such as syphilis and poverty are still usually seen as bad things to have, but are no longer generally attributed to heredity. Others, such as dark skin color, are still generally attributed to heredity but are no longer labeled inferior. Still others, such as the trait eugenicists called "nomadism," are no longer seen as either inherited or undesirable and may not even be perceived as a meaningful category any more.

In other words, changes in what counts as an hereditary disease since 1915 have been the result of changes in both science and cultural values. To understand who early eugenicists considered "hereditary defectives" thus requires examining both what they meant by "hereditary" and what they considered to be "bad." The controversy over saving defective infants provides an opportunity to observe how science, social conditions, and cultural values intersected to shape professional and lay conceptions of what constituted hereditary defects.

Heredity, Environment, and the Scope of Eugenics: Scientific Conceptions to 1915

During the first years of the twentieth century, German biologist August Weismann's view that individual heredity was permanent, and the rediscovery of Austrian monk Gregor Mendel's work on the transmission of specific traits, produced a vast transformation in scientific concepts of human heredity. Though these scientific changes are not sufficient to explain early-twentieth-century eugenic concepts of heredity, they were a key component of such meanings.

To understand this scientific transformation, it is essential to recognize that before this century, calling a trait "hereditary" did not necessarily imply that it was permanent. Many nineteenth-century biologists believed that inherited traits could be altered by a person's life experiences and that these alterations would be passed on to the next generation. To inherit health, for example, was similar to inheriting money; both constituted a legacy from your parents that determined your starting point in life. If you built up your body or your bank account, not only would you become stronger and richer, but you would leave your children a better inheritance than you had received. But if you lost your biological assets to bad habits or unhealthy conditions, your children's inheritance would be as devastated as if you had squandered or been robbed of your financial assets. "Heredity" meant anything children got from their parents; it was no guarantee that they would retain it.[2]

Belief in the malleability of individual heredity is today associated with the eighteenth-century French biologist Jean-Baptiste Lamarck, who appealed to the "inheritance of acquired characteristics" as the causal mechanism for his pre-Darwinian theory of evolution. But while such beliefs are widely labeled "Lamarckian," Lamarck and his supporters neither originated nor monopolized the belief that life experiences reshaped a person's heredity.[3]

According to the oldest recorded version of that belief, specific shocks during conception or pregnancy could leave recognizably similar "marks" or "impressions" on the offspring. The Bible tells how Jacob cheated Laban by placing colored sticks in front of Laban's pregnant cattle to change the identifying markings of their offspring.[4] In the nineteenth century, such maternal impressions provided a purely natural explanation for birth defects, an alternative to seeing such events as manifestations of divine punishment or of witchcraft. Mothers were still held responsible for defects, for not having been more careful to avoid harmful impressions, but their fault was negligence not sin.[5]

Twentieth-century science sharply distinguishes between the influence of "heredity" and "environment." But it is both meaningless and deeply anachronistic to try to force nineteenth-century concepts of heredity into that dichotomy.[6] It is true that belief in hereditary malleability did emphasize the extreme importance of heredity. This view depicted an infant not as a blank slate, but as a blackboard covered with directions on which the infant's ancestors had been writing for centuries. But it simultaneously insisted on the ex-

treme importance of environment. It saw inheritance as a pre-
written blackboard, not a pre-engraved tablet. The individual's actions and surroundings continuously erased and rewrote the slate
before bequeathing it to the next generation.

Similarly, the nineteenth-century debate over the relative influence of "nature" versus "nurture" cannot be directly translated
into modern distinctions of "heredity" versus "environment." "Nature" usually included only those inborn traits that were believed to
reflect the ideal type designed by the Creator, and which had not
been altered by subsequent human activity. A hothouse hybrid or
an alcohol-induced birth defect were products of nurture, not nature, even if the resulting traits could be transmitted by heredity.[7]

Even nineteenth-century references to "breeding" cannot be
equated with modern meanings of heredity. A "well-bred" child was
polite through the combination of inborn gentility and careful training. "Good breeding" combined good ancestry with good upbring-
ing; even a good twig had to be properly bent. The phrase "born and
bred" was not a redundancy.[8]

Belief that an individual's heredity could be changed made biological contributions to social improvement seem both practical and
urgent. Even the victims of hereditary diseases could be helped by
better surroundings, but if they were not assisted now, they would
pass on worse problems to their children.

These concepts of heredity fostered a version of eugenics that
emphasized improving the environment, not simply selectively controlling reproduction. Undesirable hereditary traits could be eliminated from future generations by improving the lives of their parents now, not just by stopping people with bad traits from becoming
parents. Faith in the malleability of heredity thus appealed to a diverse assortment of biologists who wanted to remold humanity,
from Benjamin Rush in Enlightenment America to T. D. Lysenko in
the Stalinist Soviet Union.[9]

Although many nineteenth-century scientists believed a person's heredity could be changed, they disagreed over how much
change could be produced in how short a time. The pace of change
might depend on how long the trait was believed to have existed,
how strong the environmental pressure, or how far the change devi-
ated from an image of God's originally created natural type. Over
the course of the nineteenth century, scientific opinion became more
pessimistic on these points. In the 1790s Benjamin Rush had insisted that a temperate climate, freedom from slavery, and skin-
blanching bloodletting could "cure" even black skin color within a

single lifetime. A century later most believers in hereditary malleability concluded racial differences might take millennia to erase.[10]

Even more pessimistically, the pace of change was not directionally symmetrical. The most recently acquired, least ingrained "higher" characteristics were the easiest to lose. Therefore while evolutionary progress through hereditary malleability might be excruciatingly slow, deterioration could be devastatingly swift. Any relaxation of the environmental supports for the hereditary transmission of advanced civilized characteristics would permit the rapid reemergence of vastly older primitive traits, a process variously called "atavism," "degeneration," or "reversion to type."[11] Thus by the 1890s, some "Lamarckian" eugenicists were as vigorous as their "Weismannian" rivals in promoting rigidly selective control of reproduction, because they concluded that any environmentally induced changes in heredity would be either glacially slow or severely deleterious.[12]

The suspicion that changing an individual's heredity was impractical gradually shaded into the conviction that it was impossible. From the 1880s to the 1910s, August Weismann slowly convinced a majority of biologists that individual heredity was permanent. Weismann sharply distinguished the "germ plasm"—the substance of heredity—from the rest of the body, and held that the germ plasm was unaffected by environmentally acquired traits.

On Weismann's view, treating individuals with inherited diseases would confer no benefit on their offspring. Selective control of reproduction, not environmental improvement, was the only means of improving heredity.

But since individual heredity was permanent, any improvements produced by eugenic selection would be permanent as well. On the older concept of hereditary malleability, without constant environmental support, undesirable traits could reappear even after they had been eliminated. Benjamin Rush believed he could "cure" hereditary blackness, but nineteenth-century doctors also feared the hot sun and uncivilized conditions of the tropics would turn colonists' children into Negroes. For Weismann, once a trait had been eradicated it would stay eradicated. With the acceptance of Weismann's view of heredity, it first became possible for eugenics to promise "final solutions."

Weismann's rejection of "Lamarckian" heredity thus paralleled Pasteur's refutation of spontaneous generation for microscopic organisms. Both seemed to show that the causes of disease could not originate from nothing. Thus both made it possible to envision the permanent complete eradication of disease through a one-time sterilizing effort to eradicate all pathogenic germs or genes.[13]

Unlike Pasteur, however, Weismann could never fully prove his claim—no experiment in a human timescale ever could. Weismann's most famous demonstration, in which he showed that rats whose tails had been cut off did not produce short-tailed offspring, did not disprove the malleability of individual heredity. It provided less proof than the far more extensive history of human ear-piercing or circumcision, especially since rats use their tails more than humans use their earlobes and foreskins. But Weismann's experiments were extremely effective propaganda, because laboratory rats and precise measurements conveyed the aura of scientific rigor, and because the results could easily be repeated in elementary biology courses.

Supporters of Weismann singled out the ancient belief that birth defects were caused by "maternal impressions" as a particular target of their attacks on the malleability of heredity. By the 1890s physiologists attributed most birth defects to disruptions in normal embryonic development. The notion that a specific defect might bear the recognizable imprint of its specific environmental cause thus seemed akin to the outdated faith in correspondences among other natural phenomena, from the homeopathic belief that "like cures like" to the astrologers' correlation of celestial and earthly events. Weismann's supporters used the discrediting of "maternal impressions" to cast scorn on the whole idea that environment could influence heredity, while his opponents generally tried to distance themselves from this now-embarrassing belief.

Yet well into the 1920s, maternal impressions continued to be invoked by physicians and patients, who still found the idea a satisfying, if exceptional, explanation of striking individual birth defects.[14] And while most American scientists appear to have accepted the permanence of heredity by the early 1900s, belief in hereditary malleability remained evident well into the 1930s. Though one speaker told the 1914 National Conference on Race Betterment that Weismann's view had won "almost complete acceptance by biologists," prominent University of Michigan pathologist Aldred Scott Warthin testified at the 1928 Conference, "I believe absolutely in the transmission of acquired qualities."[15]

In addition to the transforming effect of Weismann's views, early-twentieth-century concepts of heredity were also profoundly reshaped following the 1900 revival of ideas first published in 1866 by Gregor Mendel. The distinctive ratios of specific traits he observed in cross-breeding different varieties of pea plants led Mendel

to conclude that heredity was governed by discrete, separately inherited units, and that every individual inherited two sets of these
units, one from each parent. To manifest some traits, called recessive, an organism had to inherit unit factors for that trait from both
parents, but to manifest other traits, called dominant, it was sufficient to inherit at least one unit factor for that trait.

In 1909 Danish scientist W. L. Johannsen proposed calling Mendel's units of heredity "genes." He also coined the terms "genotype"
and "phenotype" to distinguish an organism's genetic makeup from
its manifest traits. Early British Mendelian William Bateson used
the term "genetics" to describe this approach to the study of heredity.[16]

Many early-twentieth-century followers of Darwin resisted the
Mendelian concept of discrete genes. They saw variation as a contin-
uum, best described mathematically by continuous bell-shaped
curves, not fixed ratios among sharply discrete categories. This dispute between "biometricians" and Mendelians was not synthesized
until the 1930s. Especially in Britain, eugenicists tended to favor the
biometric over the Mendelian view.

One of the most pressing practical problems facing Mendelian
eugenics was how to diagnose healthy "carriers" of undesirable recessive genes. Strict Mendelian genetics implied that a person with
one gene for a recessive disease and one dominant healthy gene (a
heterozygote) could only be distinguished from someone with two
copies of the healthy gene by the results of their reproduction—too
late for preventive eugenic measures. And between 1915 and 1917,
British geneticist R. C. Punnett calculated that, for any reasonably
uncommon recessive disease, eugenic measures to prevent reproduction by those manifesting the symptoms would miss so many undi-
agnosable healthy carriers that selective breeding would be useless
in reducing the incidence of that disease.[17]

Eugenicists who accepted the Mendelian view of heredity therefore might have to dramatically expand the scope of their preventive measures. To wipe out recessive diseases, a ban on reproduction
would have to include not only those who currently have these diseases, but all healthy people with any family history of such mala-
dies. In practice, the absence of genetic disease for three generations
back was felt to be sufficiently stringent, though longer scrutiny
might be needed for those from small families.

Most early eugenicists sought to avoid such a drastic dragnet
by finding some way to identify healthy carriers. Biometric eugenics
was attractive because it implied hybrids would manifest an inter-

mediate blending of healthy and unhealthy traits. On this view, the slightly subnormal population constituted an especially dangerous problem—not deficient enough to be considered sick themselves, but bearers of a vast reservoir of defective germ plasm in the population. The effort to diagnose defective hereditary tendencies carried by healthy people also helps explain the continuing interest by eugenicists in nineteenth-century anthropologist Cesare Lombroso's efforts to identify specific stigmata of degenerate heredity.[18]

Heredity, Environment, and the Scope of Eugenics: Haiselden and Mass Cultural Meanings

These transformations and conflicts in the science of heredity deeply influenced eugenics, but science alone never fully controlled the definition of "heredity" or the scope of "eugenics." Haiselden's cases reveal that, in early-twentieth-century mass culture and medical practice, "heredity" was a much more inclusive term than would be suspected from the era's science alone, expansive enough for eugenics to claim as its domain the entire range of human imperfections. The controversy over Haiselden's crusade demonstrates how scientific concepts of heredity evolved in a complex dialogue with alternative cultural meanings.

Biologists and eugenics leaders saw themselves as struggling to impose their definitions of heredity and eugenics on an uncomprehending public. From the early 1900s, geneticists like Johannsen and Thomas Hunt Morgan attacked lay concepts of heredity as a key obstacle in establishing their profession. By 1938 one frustrated British observer proposed requiring that only "experts should ever use the word 'heredity.' That word had better be left to the geneticists."[19]

"Eugenics is one of the few cases in which a scientific term has come into popular use," but "it is subject to a great deal of misconception," Irving Fisher complained in 1915. Echoing other eugenic leaders, Fisher and Eugene Lyman Fisk railed against "erroneous" uses of the term, promoted by "uninformed publicists." The Illinois State Charities Commission in 1914 quoted Karl Pearson:

> Eugenics, in Sir Francis Galton's mind was to be a science . . . , with its academic center in every university. . . . It has become a subject for buffoonery on the stage and in the cheap press. We are treated to "eugenic" babies, and to "eugenic" plays, which have nothing to do with the problem of race welfare.

Fisher urged a campaign of "eugenic work and propaganda . . . to remove these misunderstandings."[20]

But media accounts of Haiselden's views reveal that the struggle to define heredity and eugenics was more complex than the top-down effort depicted by Fisher. Mass culture included alternative concepts that were not simply erroneous distortions of science, and which sometimes even modified scientific views.

Although scientists by 1915 generally shared Weismann's dichotomization of environment and heredity, in mass culture the terms "heredity" and "eugenics" continued to be used in connection with traits that were attributed to environmental causes. Haiselden blamed every one of his published cases on environmental causes. For example, he found the Bollingers to have "unusual vigor and natural health." The *Chicago American* declared that the Hodzima baby was "not the victim of a hereditary disease," and that the parents were "fit to pass any eugenic test." And in three of his cases, the parents had prior offspring, all healthy.[21]

Although the parents' heredity was not to blame, Haiselden warned that each baby "would reproduce its kind, and these initial deformities in time would become multiplied," if he had not let them die in infancy.[22] He invoked a variety of mechanisms to explain how these defects could be inherited. Some could be explained as instances of "atavism"—the sudden loss of recently acquired higher traits and the reemergence of primitive heredity that had remained dormant for many generations without being expressed. Thus Haiselden considered it possible that these defective offspring of healthy parents might be "a throw-back to the darkest jungle days."

But rather than blaming the babies' ancestors for their defects, Haiselden usually pointed to a range of environmental factors that affected the mothers during pregnancy, including invoking the ancient belief in "maternal impressions." Julius Werder, a former teacher of disabled children and father of the second child allowed to die at Haiselden's hospital, attributed his baby's hydrocephalus and paralysis to "the sight of a hopeless paralytic in a wheelchair which gave my wife a nervous shock." Haiselden pronounced the explanation plausible. Similarly, in 1917 Haiselden gave qualified public support to the Meter family's opinion that their baby's microcephaly and exposed brain might have resulted from the mother's having witnessed a man who "fell from a third-story window and dashed out his brains at her feet." The case should "interest those physicians who hold this sort of thing impossible," Haiselden asserted.[23]

It is not clear whether Haiselden's cautiously ambiguous statements on the issue were framed to camouflage his own belief in a
theory his colleagues might have scorned, or whether they were intended simply to avoid depriving his patients of a comforting source
of meaning for their pain.[24]

In addition to "maternal impressions," Haiselden explained that
many other acquired conditions could cause inheritable birth defects, especially parental infections and hormonal disorders. Thus
he attributed the defects of one of his patients to typhoid fever and
another to thyroid problems. Like his newspaper articles, the original version of *The Black Stork* blames the birth of one "pitifully deformed" baby on "an overworked mother," while another girl who
elopes with her consumptive boyfriend gives birth to a deformed
baby as a result of his tuberculosis. Drawing a graphic if not very
attractive link between heredity and contagion, the film complains,
"A man may be fined for spitting on the floor but if he is suffering
from a transmissible disease he may spit on (kiss) the lips of a
healthy girl or marry, and nothing is done about it."[25] Though the
disease that mars Claude's ancestry is never named, the film shows
his baby with the shrivelled, wasted look that in other films signi-
fied congenital syphilis (Fig. 16).[26] The film urges passage of a "eugenic law" prohibiting the marriage of "people with transmissible
hereditary diseases."

Historians from Mark Haller to Daniel Kevles have dismissed
these concerns with environmentally-caused conditions as not really
eugenic, but the result of mass culture's misunderstanding of heredity, or of the colonization of eugenics by unscientific moral concerns.[27] But such distinctions both overly dichotomize science and
mass culture and draw anachronistically sharp lines among glands,
germs, and genes. They overlook an important alternative meaning
of "heredity," and miss the complex interplay between scientific and
lay concepts. In 1915 the scope of eugenics included infectious, hormonal, and other acquired diseases for two important reasons.

First, many scientists felt Weismann's views still left room for
environmental contributions to hereditary disease. In 1915, such beliefs were neither unscientific nor limited to mass culture. Thus,
while a 1914 magazine detective story by science popularizer Arthur
B. Reeve explained about the thyroid: "[T]he gland seems to tell on
the germ-plasm of the body," the leading eugenic scientist Charles
Davenport likewise attributed hereditary criminality to glandular
defects.[28] *Wood B. Wedd and the Microbes,* an anti-eugenic farce
filmed by Thomas Edison in 1914, equated eugenics with germ-

fighting. But so did eminent psychologist G. Stanley Hall. His plan for a Children's Institute featured a "Department of Eugenics" whose concerns specifically included infectious diseases and milk inspection.[29]

Among infections, venereal diseases, especially syphilis, aroused particular eugenic concern. Eugenics played an important role in the construction of "social hygiene," as the campaign against sexually linked diseases was euphemistically called.[30] The association pervaded mass culture, including many of the over a dozen social hygiene motion pictures produced in the period. One example, *S.O.S.: A Message to Humanity* (Sunshine 1917), was billed as a film about "eugenic marriage" although it apparently dealt exclusively with congenital syphilis.[31] State legislatures in this period also promoted the link, often including venereal diseases (VD), tuberculosis (TB), and other "transmissible" diseases in the list of disorders whose carriers could not legally marry under laws usually labeled "eugenic."[32]

In their 1917 attack on popular misconceptions, Fisher and Fisk insisted, "Eugenics is not simply sex hygiene, as many have come to consider it." Yet the association was not confined to the ignorant public. In 1919 Johns Hopkins University public health professor Reynold Spaeth wrote that syphilis was caused by Mendelian "defective unit characters." Likewise, the anti-VD leaders defined their task to include eugenics. In 1916 the Chicago Society for Social Hygiene divided its work into two divisions: one to combat VD and the other to restrict reproduction by "irresponsibles," including the feebleminded and criminals.[33]

Such views were not confined to the remaining Lamarckians. Many of Weismann's followers accepted that certain environmental "germ poisons" could directly damage the germ plasm and that the damage done could be inherited. By 1917 considerable evidence indicated that infections and chemicals, especially fevers, syphilis, and alcohol, could induce birth defects, and that these conditions appeared to run in families. The term "racial poisons" was coined in 1906 by London physician C. W. Saleeby. A 1921 survey of 1000 scientists and science educators found that 58 percent believed alcohol and syphilis were racial poisons, and 50 percent believed hormones had a similar effect.[34] The modern concept of "mutations" was only just emerging in the 1910s, and its eventual evolutionary significance was not resolved until the 1930s. Thus some specific acquired diseases were still scientifically accepted as causing inheritable damage.

Conversely, the work of British physician Sir Archibald Garrod strongly suggested that many hormonal disorders were inherited, and that inborn errors in the production of metabolic enzymes such as hormones might be the mechanism underlying most inherited diseases.[35]

In addition, although dramatic late-nineteenth-century discoveries in microbiology did discredit the view that diseases such as TB and VD could be directly inherited, as opposed to being caught from, one's parents, bacteriology did not rule out the possibility that inherited factors still influenced who was most susceptible to infection. Microbe hunters generally saw killing bacteria as a more efficient and practical solution than the eugenic effort to build up hereditary resistance. But eugenicists were not rejecting Pasteur's science when they insisted that eliminating hereditary susceptibility to microbes provided the best long-term strategy for eliminating infectious diseases.[36]

Second, broad linguistic and cultural associations shared by scientists and non-scientists alike also linked heredity and contagion. Infection was caused by "germs"; inheritance was governed by "germ plasm." In both cases, a "germ" meant a microscopic seed. Such seeds enabled both infectious and hereditary diseases to propagate, spreading lethal contamination from guilty to innocent bodies. And the transmission of each kind of "germ" could be halted by "sterilization."[37]

Venereal diseases in particular were linked to hereditary defects in this broader cultural and linguistic sense. Both were transmitted through sexual reproduction, hence both were considered "sex diseases." Thus the *New York Times* film reviewer explained to readers that one early eugenic movie was about "sex questions." Conversely, "eugenic" could sometimes be used as a code word to signal that a movie was about sex or VD. Likewise, gland diseases were linked to sex because the best-known glands were the ovaries, testes, and mammaries. The U.S. Public Health Service high-school biology film *The Science of Life* (Bray 1922) began its reel on social hygiene and eugenics by explaining the endocrine system.

The linguistic association between heredity and VD was further promoted by the 1905 introduction of blood tests to diagnose syphilis. Blood, long a metaphor for heredity, was now seen as a vehicle of infection too. Thus "bad blood" came to mean tainted ancestry, whether contaminated by syphilis germs or by defective genes.[38]

Most important, in ordinary usage calling something "hereditary" meant that you "got it from your parents," regardless of whether "it" was transmitted by genes, germs, precepts or probate.[39] Although scientists' technical terminology distinguished between "hereditary" and "congenital" conditions, and although Weismann had drawn a sharp scientific line between "heredity" and "environment," scientists and lay people still shared a much broader language in which "heredity" encompassed everything obtained from one's forbearers, no matter how they conveyed it. Thus, *The Science of Life* defined a man's heredity as "what he receives from his ancestors." In this inclusive usage, eugenics, the science of improving heredity, meant scientifically protecting children against getting anything bad from their parents, and assuring that parents gave their children nothing but the best.

Concepts of scientific causality are intimately linked to attributions of moral responsibility.[40] To cause something is to be responsible for it and to take the blame if it turns out poorly. Thus, in ordinary language, what defined "heredity" was the parent's moral responsibility for producing the trait, not simply the biological mechanism through which the parental influence operated. On this definition of "heredity," "eugenics" meant the science of being a good parent.

When the Chicago Eugenics Society introduced a bill in 1917 in the Illinois legislature to require premarital syphilis testing, Kellogg's *Good Health* magazine revealingly struggled to reconcile the purely technical with the broader general meanings of heredity. "Laws of this kind do not, strictly speaking, come under the heading of eugenics, but . . . since they protect the unborn child, they have in this sense real eugenic significance."[41]

Many films explicitly defined "eugenic" as "fit to marry," that is, capable of being a good parent. From the film's earliest showings, ads for *The Black Stork* featured the question "Are You Fit to Marry?" and by 1918 that question had become the film's new title. Some films, such as Haiselden's, made ancestry part of such assessments, but others judged parental fitness by purely personal traits, regardless of their origin. True, a muscular physique was easier to show on screen than a vigorous ancestry, but whether the reasons were cinematic or more general, the implication was that eugenic fitness to procreate could be judged by viewing the individual without examining the pedigree.[42]

The 1923 U.S. Children's Bureau film titled *Well Born* focused entirely on teaching good prenatal care. Likewise, the only movie made by the Eugenic Film Company, the remarkable 1917 production *Birth*, concentrated solely on providing women with information on childbirth and neonatal care. It included scenes demonstrating natural and Caesarian birth, premature babies in incubators, and even concluded with a baby "dead when born" being "brought to life" by the "heroic measures" of a surgeon. What made all these films "eugenic" was their goal of having all children get good care from informed parents.[43]

Although seen most frequently in the mass media, this expansive view of eugenics as good parenting was not simply a popular error. It was part of a broader nontechnical language that experts spoke too. In discussing a 1921 paper that linked venereal disease with eugenics, R. A. Fisher explained, "There may be something very much like inheritance, in the practical sense. Whether there is inheritance in the biological sense is not the only matter. We are anxious to make a more perfect mankind and we are interested in the practical side of it." New Jersey physician Theodore Robie declared at the Third International Eugenics Congress in 1932 that "it would . . . be conducive to racial improvement to sterilize even those feeble minded who do not necessarily fall in the hereditary group," since *mental defectives tend to maintain inferior homes in inferior environments, and they quite generally rear their children in an inferior manner.*[44]

If eugenics could apply to any trait acquired from a parent or capable of transmission to a child, it could be used to improve almost any human characteristic. In this nontechnical discourse, "eugenics" could mean opposition to all forms of human weakness, not just to defects with any visible link to ancestry.

Reviewers of the 1914 movie *The Eugenic Boy* took "eugenic" to mean strong and pure; they made no connection whatever to ancestors. Drawing on this broad meaning, one 1915 contender for Chicago alderman billed himself as the "eugenic candidate." The label referred neither to his views on heredity nor to his pedigree, paternal skills, or physique. Rather, he apparently meant to convey that he was pure, uncorrupted, fit for office. (He lost.)[45]

In this language, eugenics represented not just "good heredity" but goodness itself.

Constructing the Socially Defective: Crime, Race, and Class

Since almost any human difference could be seen as "hereditary" and within the scope of "eugenics," what counted as improving heredity depended on which traits were judged good or bad. To many progressive-era eugenicists, social disorder, racial differences, and class conflict ranked among the worst pathologies of the age.

A eugenically inspired panic over hereditary criminality and the "menace of the feebleminded" gripped the nation in 1915, just as Haiselden's refusal to treat defective babies hit the headlines. "Half Wits Peril Many," warned a front-page headline in the *Chicago American* within a fortnight of the Bollinger case. The accompanying article reported police plans for the "roundup of all defectives in Chicago" following the arrest of an allegedly subnormal Persian immigrant for murder. Shortly afterward, a judge blocked the marriage of an allegedly defective Chicago couple on the grounds that three-quarters of all crimes were caused by hereditary defects.

Haiselden explicitly cited these and many similar cases of crimes committed by defectives to demonstrate why such babies should not live.[46] "The average physician today saves imbeciles at birth. This adds to the crime waves of the city's future," he explained.[47] Helen Keller endorsed the decision not to save the Bollinger baby, noting that a mental defective "is almost sure to be a potential criminal." According to Mrs. Bollinger, Haiselden persuaded her to let her baby die by warning her the child would "be an imbecile and possibly criminal"; a vision of the fulfillment of this prophecy constitutes the dramatic high point of *The Black Stork*.[48]

That the Chicago murderer was a "Persian" was not an irrelevant detail. Many early-twentieth-century eugenicists regarded non-Anglo-Saxon ancestry as another important form of hereditary defect, involving class, race, and ethnicity.

Race played a key role in many early eugenic constructions of the unfit. An article on "The Race Problem" by Chicago doctor Charles S. Bacon in a mainstream northern medical journal of 1903 noted that "the tendency to negro degeneracy and eventual elimination is I believe apparent." The author predicted that "the 'Black Belt' will be defined by the government as a negro reservation similar to Indian reservations," this being "the plan . . . that has worked so well in its treatment of the Indian question until it has practically eliminated the question with the race."[49] As early as 1888, one Boston physician reportedly advocated extending the same "solution" to "the problem of the feeble-minded" that had been applied "practically to the Indian question." "I would stamp out and kill the whole brood."[50] Motion pictures invoked Darwinian competition to explain the impending extinction of the Native Americans, both in fictional features like *The Vanishing American* (Paramount 1925) and in educational films like *A Vanishing Race* (Edison 1917) or *The Vanishing Indian* (Sioux ca. 1920).[51]

Eugenics also transformed the category of race, both by linking it to Weismann's concept of heredity as immutable, and by expanding it to label dark-skinned European ethnic groups as separate and permanently inferior "races." Dr. J. G. Wilson, a U.S. Public Health Service doctor in charge of examining immigrants on Ellis Island in New York, wrote in *Popular Science Monthly*, "If the science of eugenics deserves any practical application at all, it should insist upon a careful study of the . . . Jews," because "the Jews are a highly inbred and psychopathically inclined race," whose defects are "almost entirely due to heredity." That Jews tended to disagree with such objective "scientific" observations only confirmed their validity: "The general paranoid attitude of the race is shown in an almost universal tendency to fail to appreciate the point of view of the one who opposes them."[52]

Several of Haiselden's supporters were among the leading popularizers of racial eugenics. Nine days after its ringing endorsement of the Bollinger baby's death, the *Detroit Free Press* editorial page carried an article by a physician titled "The Race Peril at Our Doors," which warned that "the original, sturdy Anglo-Saxon and Germanic stocks are dying out or being replaced by . . . a vast influx of degenerates . . . wholly undesirable for parenthood, to mate with our clean children." Another Haiselden backer, federal Food and Drug Administration founder Harvey Wiley, told the readers of *Good Housekeeping* magazine in 1922 that "it is universally acknowledged that descendants of the Scotch and Irish Presbyterians . . . have always shown themselves to be a superior people." And the classic text of eugenic race theory, Madison Grant's *The Passing of the Great Race*, published a few months after the Bollinger case, endorsed "the elimination of defective infants" as the first step in "the obliteration of the unfit," a process Grant advocated extending "ultimately to worthless race types."[53]

The Black Stork links class, ethnicity, and race to hereditary defects, both overtly and more subtly. In its original version, the film traces Claude's baby's impairments to his grandfather's liaison with "a slave—a vile filthy creature who was suffering from a loathsome disease." The film industry, still reeling from the massive protests triggered by D. W. Griffith's offensive portrayal of blacks in *Birth of a Nation*, demanded that this depiction be deleted. Movie trade spokesmen feared that any mention of race could be inflammatory to someone and that any depiction of miscegenation would outrage southern whites. Reviewing the February 1917 version of the film, the movie trade journal *Moving Picture World* warned, "The story shows the source of the taint to have been in a slave woman, which, of course, means the contamination is of a double character. The inclusion of the color question will give Southern exhibitors pause." *Motion Picture News* agreed, "A scene showing a Southern 'gentleman' just out of the embrace of a diseased slave . . . should be eliminated before the reformers get a chance to condemn the whole business for it." Thus sometime between 1918 and 1923, the scene was reshot to substitute a white servant girl for the slave.[54]

Despite this deletion, the film retained other closeups of a severely handicapped black child (Fig. 15), the only other black person depicted. And in addition to these explicit references, subtler racial images pervade *The Black Stork*. The title itself evokes associations between blackness and genetic deficiency. And the metaphor was graphically interwoven throughout the film; each intertitle was framed by a drawing of two black storks. In his writing as well as his film, Haiselden repeatedly associated the word "Blackness" with words like "Weakness—Pain—Disease—Degeneracy—Vice—Crime—Filth—Loathsomeness— . . . Ugliness."[55]

The studio that produced *The Black Stork* was no stranger to racial fear-mongering; in fact, it was simultaneously shooting the notorious Hearst serial *Patria*, utilizing some of the same cast for both pictures. *Patria*'s graphic depiction of a brutal Japanese-Mexican invasion of the United States dramatized the danger of the "yellow peril." A formal protest from Japan and the prospect that the film would incite anti-Japanese riots prompted President Woodrow Wilson to successfully demand that the film be made less inflammatory.[56]

Replacing the slave in *The Black Stork* with a white servant changed the source of the contaminating defect from race to class. In its vision of the deformed baby's future, the revised film graphically depicts his socioeconomic atavism, his fall from the family wealth into which he is born to the poverty from which his flawed heredity originated. "Pauperism breeds paupers," the 1916 film declared. One early scene struck a populist note by depicting poor but normal children who could have been helped by some of the "millions" wasted caring for the hereditarily ill. But all the other characters portrayed as poor were labeled as defectives.

Although bad heredity caused "poverty and misery," wealth was not a reliable indicator of good heredity, especially among the dissipated rich, as portrayed in the film by Claude. The film's model of fit parents was neither rich nor poor, but the solidly middle-class private secretary Tom and his wife Miriam, a nurse. White-collar and professional workers were portrayed as the best guardians of the nation's germ plasm, not such other possible groups as captains of industry, sturdy yeomen farmers, or productive industrial workers.[57]

While race and class were key interlinked components of what Haiselden meant by defectiveness, he did not actually target racial minorities or the poor in withholding treatment from infants, at least not in his publicly reported cases. The parents were either middle-class eugenics enthusiasts or industrial workers, of British or Germanic extraction. At least in these cases, the goal was to keep the Northern European stock pure, rather than to limit the reproduction of other groups.

Gender preferences have also played an important role in the histories of infanticide and eugenics. British and American scientists often used Darwinian concepts to argue that men were more highly evolved than women. American eugenicists generally thought it more efficient to sterilize women defectives rather than men, especially after the mid-1920s.[58] And in Asian and other cultures in which girls have been considered less valuable than boys, selective infanticide has been used to dispose of the unwanted sex.[59] But though Haiselden claimed to admire Japanese infanticide, he never mentioned its use for sex selection. Neither Haiselden nor his supporters ever seem to have discussed using eugenic selection to favor male babies. Two of Haiselden's six reported cases involved males.[60]

For Haiselden and many other eugenicists, race, class, and social order were key factors in distinguishing the fit from the defective. These views need to be understood in a broader social context, not to dismiss eugenic racism as simply the normal values of another time, nor to condemn the entire era as hopelessly benighted, but to help understand how these social values came to play such a crucial role in shaping eugenics.

For example, belief in white superiority was not unique to supporters of eugenics. Scientific justifications for racial slavery predated Darwin and Galton. And some of the most violent white supremacists of Haiselden's time rejected eugenics as unscriptural. Even in its early-twentieth-century heyday, eugenics had no monopoly on scientific justifications for race distinctions. Infectious diseases and public health also provided extensive metaphorical support and scientific evidence for policies such as immigration exclusion and racial segregation. Treating other races as "germs" was at least as common as labeling them genetic defectives.[61]

Nor were Haiselden's judgments of racial eugenic worth particularly extreme in the context of 1915 America. In an era when southern lynchings averaged one a week, Haiselden's mentor Christian Fenger had been an early patron of pioneer black surgeon Daniel Hale Williams, and Haiselden emulated Fenger's example. At a time when Williams's Provident Hospital was the only hospital in Chicago with a racially integrated staff, Haiselden hired Carl Roberts, a young black surgeon, as an extern at German-American Hospital. Haiselden also strongly identified himself with the lonely righteousness of the abolitionists' crusade against slavery. If Chicago's leading African-American newspaper, the militant *Defender,* found anything threatening to blacks in Haiselden's crusade, they remained unusually silent. The *Defender* was the only Chicago paper examined that did not cover the Bollinger baby story at all.

Haiselden's attitudes toward Asians were similarly not especially hostile at a time when Asian immigration had been banned for a decade, and Hearst was demanding race war with Japan. In terms simultaneously patronizing, competitive, and admiring, Haiselden cited alleged Japanese precedent for his own practice: "The surgeons of Nippon often fail to tie the umbilical cord" of defectives, he asserted. "As a result, the Japanese are a wonderfully vigorous race deservedly coming into world prominence."

Throughout the first half of this century, immigrant doctors, especially Jews, routinely faced discrimination in obtaining hospital staff positions. Yet Haiselden headed a hospital founded by and for immigrants, most of whose doctors were foreign-born, including Slavs and Jews in addition to Germans. The black extern Roberts and almost all the immigrant doctors publicly endorsed their boss's crusade.[62]

And Haiselden's critics also portrayed nonwhites as inferior, particularly when they equated his refusal to treat impaired newborns with the infanticidal practices of barbarous and primitive savages. To the editors of the *Christian Science Monitor,* the fact that infanticide and other "pleasantries of that nature" were practiced by "Chinese," "Red Indians," and "along the banks of the Ganges" was a major reason for condemning Haiselden's actions. Theology professor B. L. McElroy explained that "the Australians [aborigines] stand at the bottom of the human ladder." To support Haiselden, he concluded, would be "to Australianize our ethics."[63]

By emphasizing heredity as the engine of human progress, eugenics emphasized the importance of ancestry and transformed the concept of race. But the specific racial hierarchies adopted by Haiselden and his backers were not intrinsic to eugenics. Instead, they reflected broader cultural biases about what counts as "good" breeding. Eugenics was one of several competing scientific, religious, and political sources that were drawn upon by race theorists to legitimate their classifications and hierarchies. Its ability to justify these preexisting prejudices helped to legitimate eugenics even as eugenics helped to reinforce these specific racial distinctions. It was because class, ethnic, and race-based value distinctions were already so powerful that they were so readily adopted and amplified by progressive-era eugenics.[64]

Successive versions of *The Black Stork* graphically illustrate how easily eugenics absorbed and adapted to the changing prejudices of the surrounding society. For Haiselden in 1916, Germans and Britons comprised the hereditary elite among immigrants. Thus in his original film, the innocent girl who marries the tainted Claude had the phonetically spelled German name Annye [Anja] Schultz. But in February 1917, as war with Germany became a clear possibility, her name was changed to the more Americanized Anne Schultz. And following the virulent anti-German hysteria unleashed by the war, the character became fully naturalized as Anne Smith.[65]

These changes do more than simply illustrate the linguistic war in which sauerkraut was renamed "liberty cabbage." Like the switch from black slave to white servant, the Americanization of Annye Schultz illustrates how responsive eugenic assessments of good and bad heredity could be to even rapid fluctuations in the tide of social prejudices.

But Haiselden and his supporters did not simply and passively reflect whatever judgments of human worth they found in their culture. The next two sections of this chapter illustrate how eugenics selectively appealed to specific groups in society, who brought with them very particular value judgments.

Defects and Desires: Eugenics, Aesthetics, and Sex

Beauty

Eugenics promised to make humanity not just strong and smart but beautiful as well. Being hereditarily fit included being visually attractive. Ugliness was an hereditary disease. "An attractive appearance goes hand in hand with health," explained the U.S. government film series *The Science of Life* in a segment linking good grooming with good breeding.[66]

Scientists' efforts to explain the evolutionary role of beauty began in 1871 with Darwin's extensive analysis of sex selection in *The Descent of Man*. Eugenics founder Francis Galton began his scientific career by compiling a "beauty map" of Britain based on the ratio of attractive to plain and ugly women he encountered at various locations. Although these leading scientists studied the aesthetic component of eugenic "fitness," such concerns appeared more frequently in the mass media. Albert Wiggam, a major eugenic popularizer, even dedicated one of his books "To the health, intelligence and beauty of the unborn."[67]

While historians of Germany such as Sander Gilman and George Mosse have explored eugenic aesthetics, studies of the American movement generally overlook this aesthetic dimension, in part because such concerns appeared more clearly in the mass media than in professional texts, and in pictorial rather than written sources. Eugenicists' insistence on the objectivity of their science also made the movement seem hostile to emotions and art. Thus James Joyce's Steven Daedalus contrasted "eugenics" and "esthetic," and accused eugenics of trying to reduce beauty to its biological functions.[68]

But eugenics had a powerful aesthetic dimension, best seen in mass culture. Wiggam even claimed that beauty was the *best* indicator of overall hereditary fitness. He regarded health, intellect, morality, and attractiveness as "different phases of the same inner . . . forces." Thus he concluded, "If men and women should select mates solely for beauty, it would increase all the other good qualities of the race."[69] Eugenic publicists, including Haiselden, sometimes treated aesthetic preferences as nature's instinctive guide to selecting the fittest mate. Such views were especially suited to the technical limits of silent film, which placed a premium on inferring a character's inner worth from externally visible signs.[70]

But eugenic leaders and popularizers generally were skeptical that truly healthy beauty could be recognized by the untrained eye. Scientists since Darwin found beauty problematic precisely because aesthetic preferences in choosing a mate often seemed to favor clearly maladaptive traits.[71] That beauty did not always correlate with health was also a matter of common experience and cultural commentary, from Edgar Allan Poe's romanticization of consumptive women, to the social hygiene movement's campaign against alluring but infected prostitutes.

Thus eugenicists did not simply endorse existing cultural preferences, but actively attempted to "improve" current standards. Irving Fisher and Lyman Fisk explained that careful propaganda was needed, to "unconsciously favorably modif[y] the individual taste . . . in mate-choosing." Wiggam emphatically agreed. "If their ideals of human beauty are properly trained" by "artists and educators," young people will "unconsciously reject the ugly," and will "fill their homes with beautiful wives and handsome husbands."[72]

The content of this aesthetic propaganda can be clearly seen in the only two surviving pro–eugenic full–length American motion pictures of the era, Haiselden's *The Black Stork* and the government health education series *The Science of Life*.[73] Both films equated beauty with fitness, and both attempted to influence audience conceptions of beauty. But each presented internally–conflicting aesthetic standards, an ambivalent mix of modernism and romanticism.

The Science of Life primarily emphasized stark mechanical images of beauty. An attractive body was a sleek streamlined engine, whose beauty became manifest in powerful motion and efficient function. Such artistic values enhanced the image of eugenics itself as dynamic, modern, and powerful. The film equated the attractive fit body with a gleaming locomotive. Photographed in a low-angle tilt shot that swept upward from wheel level, the engine's sharp clean lines and powerful mass appeared starkly silhouetted against the sky. Similarly, athletes of both sexes displayed their exemplary bodies in shots that emphasized sharp-edged unadorned outlines, looming mass, and efficient motion. The film urged "THE WOMAN OF TOMORROW" to develop strength and beauty through vigorous exercises, demonstrated by a short-haired woman whose hard flat body was accentuated by stark black tights and knee-level photography.

Earlier eugenic texts had identified beauty with athleticism, but the availability of motion pictures first made it possible to display the beauty of bodily action directly. The desire to depict the poetry and science of motion contributed to the development of cinema, while the use of film helped reshape modern beauty in terms of physiology not anatomy, as active function not just static form.[74]

Although *The Science of Life* emphasized industrial modernism, it also drew on other older standards of beauty, from the poise and proportionality of classical sculpture to visions of primitive vitality and bucolic nature inspired by nineteenth-century romanticism. For example, the starkly modern woman's exercises were set against a backdrop of classical columns and potted plants. And these scenes were intercut with shots of a round-cheeked outdoorsy girl, smiling freckle-faced in soft focus while brushing her full wavy hair. Similar efforts to link modernism to older concepts of beauty characterized the "physical culture" movement. Physical culture's founder, eugenics enthusiast Bernarr MacFadden promoted modern exercise equipment while dressed in a savage leopard skin and classical sandals. This distinctive aesthetic mix reached its peak in *Way to Strength and Beauty*, a 1925 German film shown in the United States, which combined dramatically modern steep-angle cinematography with scenes of both classical and primitive Teutonic athletes.[75]

The Black Stork's images of beauty drew heavily on the naturalistic modernism of Thomas Eakins. And with its focus on negative eugenics, *The Black Stork* emphasized depictions of horrific ugliness as well as beauty.

The whole first reel of the film contrasts attractive healthy bodies with ugly defective ones. Most often, beauty is illustrated by athletic adolescents in outdoor settings. Five naked boys dive into a swimming hole, three bare-chested boys wrestle, gauzy-gowned young women dance around a flowerbed, a woman in a swimsuit does handstands on the beach. Haiselden used these scenes to introduce what the film considered to be the prime exemplar of physical attractiveness—himself. "I am regarded as a big man—a strong man. I am more than six feet and one inch tall. I am muscular. Years of hard training in all forms of sport and play have made my muscles like iron," he wrote.[76]

Unlike the 1922 *Science of Life*, the original 1916 version of *The Black Stork* explicitly attacked any equation of beauty with efficient machinery. The film uses a speeding motorcar to represent the not mechanical beauty but the false allure and superficial attractions of the "fast" life.

Yet when the film was rereleased in 1927, industrial modernism dominated. The subplot linking fast cars to loose living was completely cut, and a long new prologue was added, in which beauty was represented by a massive new automobile owned by a "professor of heredity".

This ambivalent aesthetic vision exemplified what Thomas Mann called "a highly technological romanticism." Eugenics promised to create a romantic utopia by means of modern science, and its aesthetic propaganda reflected this uneasy mix of goals.[77]

Haiselden presented images of beauty not simply as inspiring role models, but to heighten the emotional impact of his depictions of ugliness. His portrait of the Bollinger baby was, he admitted, "not a pretty one. It mars the pages of this book—as I intended it should mar them. It is better that the deformities of this tiny castaway should sear themselves into the minds of thinking men."

The ugliness of defectives was as much a disease as any of their other impairments. "It was terribly ugly," Haiselden wrote. Such ugliness was not "light or superficial"; it was a true "handicap." "To be hideous, utterly hideous is a dreadful curse." Such a defective "is not a beautiful thing. It is a monstrosity. It is not to be saved." Ugliness deprived the defective of "it[s]" humanity and justified depriving "it" of life.[78]

Both films selectively highlighted the repulsive ugliness of defectives, in dimly lit shots of dingy beggars, stark clinical scenes of retarded and physically handicapped patients, and closeups of babies severely disfigured by congenital syphilis.

The Black Stork sometimes photographed defectives from above, exhibiting them as scientific specimens, beneath the viewer. But *The Science of Life* used an opposite approach. In one remarkable low-angle shot of a bum sitting in a doorway, the camera slowly tilted upward from his worn shoes to his grizzled face. The same camera technique used in the very next scene to highlight the power and beauty of a locomotive is first used to dramatize the looming enormity, the ugliness, and the danger of the unfit.[79]

Eugenic popularizers promoted definitions of ugliness that reinforced their judgments on other human differences, including gender, class, race, and nationality. Albert Wiggam lamented,

> We want ugly women in America and we are getting them in millions. . . . [T]hree or four shiploads have been landing at Ellis Island every week. . . .
>
> Examine these women as they are unloaded at Ellis Island. I have studied thousands of them. . . . They are broad-hipped, short, stout-legged with big feet; broad-backed, flat-chested with necks like a prize fighter and with faces expressionless and devoid of beauty.

These "draft horses" were rapidly replacing "the beautiful women of the old American stocks, the Daughters of the Revolution."[80] Haiselden too linked race and aesthetics, repeatedly equating "blackness" with "ugliness."[81] Portraying "others" as ugly supported diagnosing them as defective. Conversely, labeling "others" as diseased heightened the perception of them as repulsive.

Like race, economic class distinctions also were presented in aesthetic terms. *The Science of Life* promised that both "health and success" awaited the visually attractive. A consumptive chauffeur in the 1916 version of *The Black Stork* labels himself "poor" because he lacks both "money and good looks." In both films, the couples selected to illustrate "wise mating" exhibit their economic status and their aesthetic values by wearing tastefully conservative but up–to–date business suits and dresses on their prosperously stout bodies.

Both films bitterly attacked any aesthetic values that conflicted with their concepts of health. Any art that made disease seem interesting or attractive was denounced as decadent. Thus *The Science of Life* scorned the view that physical strength made a girl unattractive. The film used both scientific X rays and satirical cartoons to ridicule harmful fashions and to promote "sensible" tastes in dress for both sexes. *The Black Stork* warned that the pathological allure of the fast life was no substitute for true beauty. And Haiselden raged against cosmetics and plastic surgery that enabled ugliness to masquerade as beauty.[82]

These films reveal how eugenicists sought not only to enhance human beauty but to selectively define it, to promote what they considered healthier aesthetic tastes. They promised to make people more attractive while they selectively promoted the attractiveness of what they considered beautiful. They offered to eliminate ugliness while depicting as ugly everything they wished to eliminate. Their mass media propaganda reveals the internal tensions and circular logic that characterized their aesthetic distinctions between the "fit" and the "defective."

These contradictions were heightened by the ease with which viewers found alternative meanings in such propaganda. Unauthorized interpretations were common among reviewers of *The Black Stork*. Many reported that the film's exhibition of deformed bodies evoked pity, or even fascination, rather than disgust, a topic examined in Chapter 8. Others found that scenes intended to make defectives look repulsive made the film itself "repellant" and "revolting." These unintended aesthetic responses played a key role in provoking the censorship of the film. The origin and importance of such "aesthetic censorship" in response to *The Black Stork* and other eugenic films is explored in chapter 6. Although eugenic popularizers attempted to use mass culture to promote their own aesthetic values, mass media images of eugenics were shaped by the clash of many competing visions.

Sexuality

Bodily exhibitions also could be seen as sexual. Displays intended
to contrast beauty with ugliness and thus to promote aesthetic se-
lectivity might instead be seen as stimulating indiscriminate sexual
desires. For example, two remarkable photos, published in the 1921
Scientific Papers of the Second International Congress of Eugenics,
contrasted the attractive features of a young girl of the "Nordic
race" who became a prostitute because of poverty, with the swarthy,
long-nosed, low-browed face of a girl who became a prostitute "on
account of disharmonic race mixture." But since both girls were
photographed bare-breasted, scientifically unsophisticated male
readers may have missed the point that only the first was supposed
to be attractive.[83]

Haiselden's newspaper articles and film utilized nudity to convey an association among physical exercise, emotional self-mastery,
scientific detachment, and moral purity. His autobiography opens
with a paean to "The Old Dam swimming hole" of his youth. "To
wear a bathing suit was a disgrace in those days. The graduates of
that old swimming hole are strong men today—and still loyal. We
all paved the way to health and strength that would last us through
our prime." His movie exhibits a variety of naked and nearly naked
children and adolescents engaged in vigorous sports. Like the autobiography, the original version of the film opens with a group of
naked young men diving into a pond. The lengthy scene, introduced
with a passage from James Whitcomb Riley's poem "The Old
Swimmin'-hole," evokes images of Thomas Eakins's controversial
1883 painting *The Swimming Hole. The Science of Life* also included
a long scene of a naked preadolescent girl undergoing a medical
exam, in a reel shown to both sexes.[84]

Haiselden may have meant his depictions of nudity to represent
innocent beauty, but others could have found them sexual, even ho-
moerotic or pedophilic. Thus I was surprised to find that not one of
the film's critics objected to such nudity, and it played virtually no
recorded role in the decisions of the major film censors. The film
industry's National Board of Review of Motion Pictures in the 1910s
and the influential New York State Motion Picture Division in the
1920s listed pages of specific scenes they found objectionable on aesthetic, medical, and religious grounds, but they mentioned nudity
only once. In May 1918 the NBRMP requested deletion of a "view of
nude babies showing sex."[85] The only other scene they cut for being
too sexually explicit depicted a fully clothed streetwalker soliciting

men.[86] But while these regulators may not have demanded it, by the time the film was reissued in 1927, all but a fleeting glimpse of nudity had been cut.

The Black Stork's distributors and supporters clearly anticipated that some audiences would find the film sexually provocative and ostensibly sought to preempt such readings. A favorable notice in the *Exhibitor's Trade Review* reassured theater owners,

> Like Hawthorne's "The Scarlet Letter," this . . . film deals with the consequences of vice, not with vice itself. There is no glamor cast over the sowing of the unclean taint. . . . Concerning a question which is a primitive one of sex, there is no recourse to sensual presentation. The exhibitor who books this film need have no fear [it will] inflame the minds of the impressionable.[87]

The *Motion Picture News* headlined one article, " 'The Black Stork' Is Not a Sex Picture."[88]

Such pious denials could themselves be used to build audience expectations of sexual content. The ads for the film at Baltimore's Blue Mouse Theater in 1919 claimed "There is nothing . . . to offend anyone of either sex," but went on to suggest that "owing to the delicate subject" "it will be shown to separate audiences only"—women-only before 6:00 P.M., men-only after 6:00 P.M.[89] Some exhibitors apparently hoped sensation-seekers would conclude that where there is so much smoke, there might be some fire.

And even though sexual content played almost no role in the recorded decisions to censor *The Black Stork*, once the film was censored it was lumped together with films that had been banned on sexual grounds. After it was excluded from mainstream theaters, the picture was relegated to houses like the suggestively named Blue Mouse, and to distributors such as Piccadilly Film Corporation and Famous Italian Pictures, which specialized in "foreign" (i.e., "exotic") movies.[90] As film theorist Annette Kuhn has shown for the anti-VD films of the era, a film's being banned can lead audiences to see even professedly antisexual pictures as being in the same category with films intended to be erotic.[91]

But the primary reason *The Black Stork* was seen as being about sexuality was not its nudity, its advertising, or its censorship, but its subject—eugenics. Despite its appeals to objective reason, eugenics contained strong doses of fantasy, longing, and desire. As already noted, eugenics and sexuality were closely linked in mass culture. In turn, eugenicists themselves were deeply preoccupied with sex.

The eugenics movement cared about sexuality for two reasons.

First, controlling sexuality was a tool for achieving other goals, and second, eliminating specific sexual activities could be a goal in itself. For example, many eugenicists attacked sexual promiscuity both because it spread other hereditary diseases from feeblemindedness to syphilis, and because promiscuity itself could be considered an hereditary disease. Homosexuality, masturbation, birth control, sodomy, prostitution, rape, and even too frequent sex within marriage were topics of debate among eugenicists, both as to whether they increased or decreased the propagation of other diseases, and as to whether they were inherited diseases themselves.[92]

Surprisingly, many historians of eugenics either overlook this focus on sexuality or try to fit it into a simple dichotomy between repression and freedom. Mark Haller's pathbreaking book spends only four paragraphs on sexuality, mostly in an attempt to distinguish serious eugenics from "crackpot fads for sex reform."[93]

The first historians to recognize the sexual dimension of American eugenics were feminist scholars such as Linda Gordon. Their accounts emphasize that by the 1920s eugenics was repressive both sexually and politically, part of a male professional program to take control of pleasure and reproduction away from women, as it sought to limit the power and numbers of the working class.[94]

Other recent interpreters, such as Daniel Kevles, conclude that eugenics remained split between a politically and sexually repressive mainstream and a politically and sexually radical minority. The latter group included Havelock Ellis, Emma Goldman, George Bernard Shaw, Magnus Hirschfeld, and William J. Robinson.[95]

From different perspectives, Christopher Lasch and Michel Foucault see all forms of eugenics as aimed in part at controlling sexuality, in an effort to discipline previously private behavior by subjecting it to professional scrutiny. Unlike the censors who banned *The Black Stork*, eugenicists did make sex public. But whether they favored or opposed sexual pleasure, their attempt to make private lives the subject of professional surveillance could serve to undermine individual autonomy.[96]

These accounts all run the risk of imposing current categories on the past. Early-twentieth-century eugenicists were rarely for or against sexual pleasure or sexual autonomy in general; rather, they focused on determining which particular sexual pleasures to encourage and which to repress, and for whom. They did feel that professional experts should determine what counted as healthy sex, but they saw professional power as protecting rational individual autonomy, against both the irrational repression of traditional sexual morality and the slavery of addiction to sexual pleasure.[97] Most important, while eugenicists held widely differing views about sex they tended to overlook their differences, because they were focused on a shared goal of making sexuality rational and modern.

Haiselden's example reveals the anachronism in trying to separate early eugenics into distinct sexually repressive and radical camps. The response to his cases shows that a shared faith in modern science and a shared hostility toward unscientific tradition united eugenicists and other progressive-era sex reformers, despite their differences over issues of present-day concern.

On some aspects of sexuality, Haiselden took positions now usually seen as radical for the 1910s. He supported birth control without regard to marital status. His earliest and strongest backers included birth control pioneers Dr. William J. Robinson and his son Frederic, New York socialists instrumental in promoting the ideas of Havelock Ellis and Sigmund Freud among America's political and cultural avant-garde.[98] Others usually seen as radical opponents of sexual repression supported Haiselden as well, including Clarence Darrow, Judge Ben Lindsey, and Anita Block.

Haiselden's film supported similar sexual views. In contrast to movies like *The Science of Life* that urged sexual control and never mentioned pleasure, *The Black Stork* extolled sexual pleasures for the healthy as the incentive and reward for keeping fit. Between a shot of nude male swimmers and a scene of female dancers in see-through gowns, Haiselden's intertitle proclaimed that "the pleasures of the earth are only for those who are physically and mentally fit."

Yet other aspects of Haiselden's life and crusade now seem extremely repressive of sexual pleasure and hostile to heterosexuality. He never married, choosing instead to live with his mother, a fervently religious prohibition crusader. His autobiography, written shortly after her death, explained his bachelorhood as resulting from his dedication to her. (He barely mentioned his father.) "My mother lived until she was 86 years old, and during her life she ruled. I never could bear to muss up the arrangements of the home and bring some one between us," he explained. "Then, I never wished to disappoint a girl by marrying her," he added ambiguously.[99]

In *The Black Stork*, Haiselden's character is named "Dr. Dickey"; Dickey was his mother's maiden name. Dr. Dickey is the only major character without any personal attachments. The film never mentions his marital status, but he is depicted as too committed to his profession for a personal life, working alone late into the night on eugenics treatises. The autobiography's devotion to his mother becomes the film character's dedication to science and humanity. And while he may have adored his mother, his film demonized less godly women. "[D]efective women who make their living on the streets are of more danger to mankind than a plague."

Haiselden was not simply an isolated exception who managed to live on both sides of an otherwise clear borderline between radical and repressive eugenics. Rather, the response to his crusade illustrates a key point about early eugenics and a range of other progressive-era sex reformers, from Freudians to social hygienists. While sex was a significant concern, present categories of sexual politics were neither very important nor very clearly defined in the 1910s.[100]

Haiselden's backers included both Mary Ware Dennett, who was arrested for writing that sex was "a vivifying joy," and Charles Davenport, who diagnosed "eroticism" as a dangerous genetic disease. Their differences did not prevent both Dennett and Davenport from seeing Haiselden's views as consistent with their own, because in the context of the 1910s, what they shared outweighed and obscured their differences. Each was convinced that modernism would produce a new source of authority to replace traditional religion as the method for distinguishing good sexuality from bad.

For Dennett, science was less important than art and emotion as the source of modern sexual values, but she saw them all as working in the same direction, to make sex "a vital art . . . to be studied and developed."[101] As George Bernard Shaw explained in his lengthy preface to *Damaged Goods,* the controversial French stage play about syphilis, any art that destroyed sexual taboos was aiding "the scientific spirit" in its struggle to supplant "vulgar Bible worship" as the arbiter of morality.[102] Frederic Robinson, who sponsored the first American production of *Damaged Goods,* was Dennett's colleague in the Voluntary Parenthood League and published her 1918 essay on "The Sex Side of Life." He introduced it with an editorial by his brother, pioneer medical historian Dr. Victor Robinson, in which Victor explicitly framed Dennett's work as "a rational sex primer." He proclaimed her art the ally of "the new spirit . . . in medicine" in its struggle against the "Theologic School of Sexology."[103]

In some cases, such alliances were partly expedient coalitions. The male editors of the *New York Call* recognized Haiselden's goals as distinct from their own sexual and political agenda, but they supported him as a useful ally against a common enemy, moral censorship. "The Bollinger case has no direct bearing on birth control," they admitted. "But the publicity which the case has received has at last swept away these barriers of silence." [104]

But the alliance against sexual tradition was more than just a temporary convenience. Once freed from outmoded sources of authority, progressive sex reformers expected to evolve a new objectively valid sexual consensus based on the scientific method and a rational approach to modern reality. [105]

In hindsight, this faith in a new modernist consensus seems doomed. Rational methods and opposition to tradition did not suffice to reconcile these reformers' many conflicts over what constituted good sex. But in the context of the 1910s, they were engaged in a common revolt against Victorian values in the name of rational modernity. To share these views was sufficient to be seen as part of a united sexual avant-garde. Haiselden together with sex reformers of many other persuasions were all categorized as advocates of "advanced views." [106]

Elite Priorities and Mass Culture: Physical and Mental Defects

Eugenicists drew on their cultural values not only to differentiate good traits from bad, but also to prioritize which were the worst among the massive list of conditions they considered defective. Not surprisingly for people who thought of themselves as scientists and intellectuals, many eugenic leaders ranked mental impairments as far more serious than physical disabilities. Eugenicists led the development and mass employment of I.Q. testing in these years to combat the "menace of the feebleminded." That threat seemed so terrifying in part because the eugenic leaders' professional cultures particularly valued what they regarded as intelligence. [107]

This hierarchy of handicaps emerges clearly in the response of eugenic intellectuals to Haiselden's cases. Sociologist Franklin H. Giddings explained, "The idiotic child should mercifully be allowed to die. The child with a good brain, however crippled otherwise, should be saved." Helen Keller agreed that death was warranted "only in cases of true idiocy." In evaluating the utility of saving handicapped infants, "the mind is more important than the body" concluded a pioneer of special education. [108]

In contrast, Haiselden's campaign to expand the mass appeal of eugenics consistently rejected this hierarchy of mind over body.

Initially, he insisted that the question was largely theoretical, since he diagnosed his first cases as having equally serious mental and physical defects. He insisted on his "absolute certainty" that the Bollinger baby would never achieve the intelligence of an "ordinary animal."[109] Among the prognostic signs of neurological damage he cited were facial paralysis, a droopy eye, delayed pupillary responses, difficulty in swallowing, and a peculiar high thin cry. He also relied heavily on X ray photos, which supposedly showed that the infant's "forehead [was] short and slanting," and that "the femur, or thigh bones, were abnormally large." These X rays, he concluded, showed "the skeleton of a monkey. It told me plainer than anything . . . that this child was in reality a defective—an animal lower than man."[110] Cook County coroner's physician Henry G. W. Reinhardt, who conducted the first autopsy on the infant, agreed with Haiselden that "the probabilities are strongly that the child would have been a mental defective."[111]

But with the exception of a few specific syndromes, turn-of-the-century physicians disagreed over whether and how mental retardation could be diagnosed in a newborn. Following an official inquest and a second autopsy, a specially convened coroner's jury of prominent physicians concluded, "We find no evidence from the physical defects that the child would have become mentally or morally defective."[112]

In response to that judgment, Haiselden continued to insist the baby showed signs of severe brain damage in addition to bodily deformities. But he also now rejected the mind-body distinctions and priorities that many of his professional supporters had found so significant. Like fellow eugenic popularizer Albert Wiggam, for whom physical beauty indicated mental and moral fitness, Haiselden insisted that virtually all physical defects were associated with eventual mental and moral defects, due either to common underlying hereditary causes or to the psychological effects of social ostracism. "Even if the baby had the highest mental faculties, I would still be inclined to let it go," Haiselden declared. "The greater its mentality the greater would be its own humiliation over its deformity." The 1916 version of *The Black Stork* proclaims, "Unhealthy bodies often cause unhealthy minds." The film depicts Claude and Anne's baby as a mentally normal hunchbacked boy who grows up to become an insane criminal; according to the 1927 version, the transformation is the result of "the constant humiliation and embarrassment caused by his deformity." The *Washington Star* editorialized, "Physical deformity at birth . . . points almost unmistakably to mental and moral deficiency in later life."[113]

In the 1915 Grimshaw and 1918 Stanke cases, Haiselden permitted or accelerated the deaths of babies whose announced handicaps were entirely physical. He likewise hailed the death of the Roberts baby in New York, whose spinal defects were generally believed not severe enough to cause brain damage.

Thus while eugenics drew its value judgments from broader cultural currents, different strata of the movement had different values. The professional leadership placed higher value on the mind than on the body. But popularizers like Haiselden equated mental and physical defects and appealed to a mass-media audience that they expected to value physical strength and beauty as much as intellect. Haiselden's values were not always reflected in mass culture. Some films, such as D. W. Griffith's *Man's Genesis* (Biograph 1912) adopted the eugenic leaders' view that intelligence was more important than physical strength. But Haiselden's crusade demonstrates that elite values did not always dominate the discussion of eugenic fitness in mass culture.[114]

Degrees of Difference: Normality or Perfection?

Eugenics offered "better babies." But how good was good enough? Were the unfit only those who were grossly more defective than the average, or did they include those with any flaws? Did fitness mean normality, or did it require perfection?

Haiselden's crusade reveals a version of eugenics based on extreme intolerance of all imperfection. This attitude was deeply rooted in the nineteenth-century origins of American eugenics, but it was shaped by the hopes and fears of the early twentieth century. Nineteenth-century utopian followers of Robert Dale Owen, such as John Humphrey Noyes of Oneida, had conducted America's first experiments in controlled human breeding. Their eugenics combined millennial religious perfectionism with faith in unlimited scientific progress. Such anticipation of perfection remained important to Haiselden's intolerance of human defects. But Haiselden's perfectionism also reflected darker fears of regression and decline. The quest for eugenic perfection reflected both a faith in scientific utopias and a terror that, without them, mankind would sink in a sea of subhumans.

Eugenic perfectionism drew directly on turn-of-the-century genetics. Weismann's doctrine that heredity was permanent heightened both the danger of decline and the hope of improvement. If
defectives would keep breeding defectives, despite all efforts at therapy or reform, their menace was incalculable. But if unfit ancestors
were necessary to produce defective offspring, if new hereditary defects could not be created by a bad environment, then a few generations of thoroughgoing eugenic measures should suffice to purify humanity forever. The new belief in the permanence of heredity made
it both urgent and, for the first time, theoretically possible for eugenics to aim for perfect and permanent "final solutions."[115]

Mass culture highlighted the emphasis on perfection. In a 1914
detective story by Arthur B. Reeve, the head of a eugenics institute
opposes a sweeping ban on the reproduction of all defectives, explaining that "almost no one is . . . eugenically perfect." But his
zealous female assistant rejects that view, arguing, "Strength should
always marry strength, and weakness should never marry. . . .
Nothing short of that will satisfy the true eugenist."[116]

This was the context in which *The Black Stork*'s national distributor announced as the film's "basic principle" "that malformations
both physical, moral and mental should not form a part of human
existence." In a revealing phrase, one writer referred to Haiselden's
supporters as "those of us who resent *any* manifestation of human
degeneracy as unworthy of man's high mission."[117]

Haiselden's perfectionism focused on eliminating all deficiencies. Not operating on the Bollinger baby was an example of "the
Greater Surgery—the surgery that cuts away the vileness and decay
and leaves only the sweet and clean and wholesome in this life of
ours."[118]

"Sterilize defectives for three generations and," Haiselden
promised, "we shall have no Bollinger baby cases to worry us. When
parents come to realize fully that a child is deficient—I do not mean
insane to the point of idiocy alone, but whenever the child is subnormal—they should permit sterilization."[119] In his eugenic utopia, as
in raconteur Garrison Keillor's Lake Wobegon, all the children
would be above average. *The Black Stork*'s publicists aimed even
higher; they pitched Haiselden's "eugenic photoplay" as part of "his
endeavor to make the United States a nation of physically perfect
human beings."[120]

For tactical reasons, however, some of Haiselden's backers
urged that such sweeping goals be kept under wraps and only im-
plemented incrementally. Harvey Wiley called for "gradual" expan-

sion of the eugenic target population only after extensive propaganda had prepared the public for each widening of the net. As early as 1900, William McKim had developed this strategy, urging the elimination of only the most unpopular 10 percent of defectives at any one time. Madison Grant adopted the same approach. His classic of eugenic race theory, published just months after the Bollinger case, urged that "the elimination of defective infants" be seen as the start of a step-by-step process that should gradually be "applied to an ever widening circle of social discards."[121]

Opposing Expansive Concepts of Hereditary Defect: Equal Worth or Entering Wedge?

Opponents bitterly attacked Haiselden's definition of hereditary defects, in terms that illustrate some crucial tensions in their own concepts of hereditary worth and the evaluation of human differences. While some rejected his approach because it was too broad and inclusive, others rejected even the most limited and specific efforts to label any human lives as worth less than others.

The claim that all human beings were equally valuable, or at least that differences in their true worth could not be judged by earthly means, was usually expressed in explicitly religious terms. Such critics distinguished between having a defect and being a defective, and insisted that the worth of a person could not be based on external characteristics. Their point was not simply that killing defectives violated their "right to life," but that defining some people as defective denied the equal value of their lives.

New York lawyer Jean Norris explained, "Whether an imbecile or a genius, every human being has a soul" that "comes from God." Therefore, "What person dares to say that the idiot's life is not as precious as that of a normal human being?" The Catholic bishop of Helena, Montana, invoked both church doctrine and the Declaration of Independence to argue that, with respect to the value of their lives, "all men are equal."[122]

Many of these critics did not blame Haiselden or eugenics alone. Labeling defectives as worthless was instead a symptom of the most fundamental mistake of modernity—the banishing of spiritual concerns from the sciences and the desacralization of the world. For Catholic critics of modernism, the Bollinger case was the logical if horrific consequence of a secularized view of life and of a medical science that treated bodies while ignoring souls.

To deny the equal worth of people with defects was thus a form of "materialism"—the belief that life can be fully explained by the same scientific laws that govern nonliving matter, without reliance on a special vital principle such as the soul. The Chicago Catholic *New World* headlined one story on the Bollinger case, "Materialism of Grossest Sort Killed Infant." Another front-page editorial, headlined "That Baby's Right to Life," explained, "The question at stake . . . is even greater than . . . the sacredness of human life. It is the value of a soul." Belief in the equal value of all human souls constituted the central issue in the "struggle between the grossest materialism and all religion." [123] These views were voiced most prominently by conservative Catholics. But similar attacks came from sectarian medical defenders of nineteenth-century scientific vitalism and natural theology, for whom materialism was both bad religion and bad science. [124]

While insisting that possession of a soul gave each human being equal inherent value, many of these critics also argued that defectives had social utility too. Here they invoked not God but Ralph Waldo Emerson.

> If, according to Emerson's law of compensation, for everything we have missed we have gained something else, who knows but what this babe— deformed and malformed as it is said to have been—might have possessed some gift that would have added a little mite to the world's spiritual or intellectual heritage?

An editorial in the *Medical Record* of New York cited Emerson to argue that science "cannot know . . . that an infant of a few days who is physically defective may not grow up to be a useful member of society." [125]

Perhaps the most widely reprinted condemnation of Haiselden in 1915 was Jane Addams's assertion that many supposed defectives had made great contributions to the world. Her honor roll of the "world's great defectives" included Helen Keller, Charles Steinmetz, John Milton, and Talleyrand. [126] Even those who specifically attacked Haiselden for employing "utilitarian" criteria to judge the worth of human lives could not resist simultaneously pointing to the social utility of Helen Keller. [127]

Such arguments were not logically inconsistent. To point out that many defectives made useful contributions to society did not necessarily contradict anti-utilitarian claims for the equal value of all human souls. Valuing some people over others could be attacked both because it was inherently wrong and because it had bad consequences.

But in terms of rhetorical power, discussing the usefulness of defectives diminished the force of appeals to their equal spiritual value. The claim that "all people have inherent worth and many supposed defectives are also socially useful" too easily could be conflated with the view that "defectives' lives are worthless but the costs of making such distinctions outweigh the advantages."

As early as 1788, Jeremy Bentham had cited infanticide as his primary example of an act that was not itself an offense against society, but which "certainly ought to be punished as a step leading in the direction of such an offence." Even though newborns allegedly felt no fear and little pain, the act of killing them diminishes social utility because it "conduces to habits of cruelty" toward others.[128]

Those who followed Bentham's lead in their attacks on Haiselden usually employed the "entering-wedge" argument, which held that even if killing defective infants was right, it should be condemned because it would lead to bad consequences. (Since the 1930s the more common metaphor has been a "slippery slope,"[129] but that expression conveys a sense of inevitability not inherent in the act of driving in a "wedge.") Different versions of the entering-wedge argument were directed at each phase of eugenic decision making: defining the unfit, deciding what to do with them, and choosing who should control such power. The first use will be examined here; the others in chapters 4 and 5.

The entering-wedge argument against Haiselden's definition of defectiveness attacked his categories as too vague and subjective to be safe. Defining some people as defective would be the first step in an ever-widening circle. This dangerously unbounded concept of the "unfit" meant that there was no way to stop Haiselden's precedent from going "too far," from becoming "the thin edge of a wedge that would be driven too deep."[130]

"[W]ho in the future will be safe . . . , where will the line be drawn between the 'fit' and the 'unfit,' between the so-called 'defective' and the 'non-defective'?" asked the Catholic *New Orleans Morning Star*.[131] "Who can tell whose babe may next be termed 'unfit?' " warned the Reverend Mabel Irwin. "Where will we stop?" John Harvey Kellogg asked. "Who will define exactly the kind or degree of undesirability which makes . . . the individual . . . sufficiently unfit?"[132] "It sometimes seems that there are normal people whose lives are not worth preserving," noted the Superintendent of Public Welfare for Kansas City, Missouri. If defective children were allowed to die, he worried, "the same philosophy would furnish sufficient justification for getting rid of a great many people . . . who are regarded to be quite worthless by a good many of us." An

Omaha minister was concerned that "such a photoplay as *[The Black Stork]* might easily be followed by one suggesting that old people might be killed as unfit to live, or that because the mother of a family has become helpless it would be well to chloroform her."[133]

The line between physical and economic deficiency seemed especially fragile. When eugenicists like Haiselden labeled poverty an hereditary disease, they made one of the few arguments that both the Catholic *New World* and the Socialist *New York Call* could unite in condemning. The Bollinger case "will bring gradually a toleration of the murder of any who are deficient . . . in any degrees, and will eventually win even a sanction of the slaughter of those poor in worldly possessions," warned the *New World*. The *Call* supported Haiselden and declared that the poor would benefit from eugenics once the social order was controlled by the masses. But "under our present economic system," "there is no way of keeping economic considerations from creeping into" the definition of the unfit. "The fact that no line can be distinctly drawn between defectiveness that should be eliminated for the welfare of the community at large, and defectiveness of a lesser degree, that should be permitted to exist, would infallibly bring in other extraneous considerations, most of them economic."[134]

Those who used the entering-wedge argument attacked diagnosing people as "defectives," not because they felt doctors had not yet discovered how to make such diagnoses accurately, but because "defective" was an inherently subjective and relative term that could never be bounded by purely objective scientific criteria. How can we "define the degree of 'deficiency' that thus dooms beyond appeal?" queried the *New York Sun*, since the question was "not medical" but varied "according to individual opinion." One eugenicist's views on the worth of defectives were "a matter of taste," according to an article in the *Boston Herald*. "Who are the unfit?," asked the *Washington Post;* too often they were "anyone not belonging to the particular clan in which the topic was under discussion."[135]

Fitness and Objectivity

Many eugenicists admitted that their distinctions between the fit and the defective incorporated cultural, ethical, political, and aesthetic values. Yet most rejected the charge that such classifications were therefore subjective or unscientific.

Eugenicists claimed both that their values could be proven to be correct by the objective methods of science, and that their values

were products of the objective laws of nature. For example, while
Galton conducted statistical anthropometric surveys to quantify the
elements of beauty and derive its scientific laws, Wiggam insisted
that aesthetic instincts were determined by objective biological
forces.[136] From the start of the movement, such eugenicists acknowledged that their feelings and values influenced their diagnoses. They
did not generally claim to be value free, but they denied that their
feelings and values were subjective. Using the objective methods of
science, they believed, enabled them to discover objectively true
standards of beauty and goodness.

Like Galton, Haiselden and his supporters insisted that their
distinctions between the fit and the defective were derived by purely
objective scientific methods. "When a doctor examines . . . and
makes tests, he KNOWS," explained New York eugenicist Dr. Edward Wallace Lee. "How did you know?" asks Claude in *The Black
Stork*, when Haiselden diagnoses his hereditary taint. "I am a Doctor. It is written on you. I can read," Haiselden replies. His examination of the Bollinger baby led Haiselden to declare it "An inferior
animal! A lower form! An imbecile! These were my pronouncements
upon the newborn child. My science told me these things."[137] These
claims promised both that science could ferret out the stigmata of
hidden recessive defects, and that science provided purely objective
methods for defining what heredity was "bad."

William J. Robinson derided as unscientific bigots those
"pseudo-eugenicists" who diagnosed as "an abnormal . . . any body
who . . . differs in any way from the dull, smug, respectable, plati-
tudinous mediocrities," and he ridiculed those who sought to "cas-
trate or sterilize every man or woman who is not strictly moral according to *their* standard of morality." But for the truly objective
scientist, defining the unfit "is not difficult" so long as value judgments were based on nonsubjective methods. "To avoid any possible
injustice or error the eugenicists would deal only with cases about
which no doubt could be possible. All borderline or questionable
cases would be left alone and there is not the slightest danger that
anybody would be unjustly segregated or sterilized," he explained
reassuringly.[138]

Eugenicists such as Haiselden believed that scientific methods
could determine where natural selection was heading and that eugenics could help it get there more efficiently. Thus they convinced
themselves that nature, not subjective preferences, determined what
traits were valuable. T. H. Huxley had attacked such moral reifica-
tions of fitness as early as the 1890s. Huxley recognized that what's
fit for a given environment is whatever reproduces most successfully

in that specified environment, not what's good for all times. Protozoa are neither complex nor intelligent, but they are fitter to live in pond water than people are. To predict the future course of evolution without knowing the future of environmental change is simply to project one's own values onto nature.[139]

By 1917 a few other eugenicists abandoned the claim that eugenic diagnoses could be objectively derived. University of Michigan zoologist O. C. Glaser portrayed eugenics as simply a set of techniques for reaching socially set goals, not a means for deciding what the goals should be. "Society stamps this or that as good," he declared. "The eugenist can . . . tell how to proceed" to get there, but not where we ought to go.[140]

In a different response to Huxley's critique, C. W. Saleeby rejected the idea that diagnoses of fitness should be determined by the objective needs of survival. The important distinction was spiritual, not scientific, a contrast between "characters of which the human spirit approves" and "those of which we disapprove." "The business of Eugenics or race culture" is thus not simply to produce people who are fit to survive in the existing environment, but "to create an environment" in which spiritually satisfying traits can survive.[141]

Glaser's view preserved eugenicists' objectivity by leaving all value choices to others, while Saleeby's eugenics was openly subjective. But unlike most other eugenicists, both Glaser and Saleeby agreed that objective methods could never suffice to distinguish the fit from the defective.

"Good" and "bad" are inherently value assessments, reflections of a culture's social structure and ethics, not just its technology.[142] Thus eugenic distinctions between good and bad heredity inevitably reflected eugenicists' cultural values. Admitting that the diagnosis of bad heredity is based on values does not mean such judgments are illegitimate. No science is value free; every field of medicine depends on value judgments in distinguishing good health from disease.[143]

But Haiselden's claim that his judgments were derived from purely objective methods served to obscure the actual cultural sources of values he and his supporters employed, to the point of hiding from themselves their own circularity and contradictions. The claim of objectivity also selectively recruited to eugenics many middle-class reformers who shared his faith in objective methods, while marginalizing as biased those who criticized him on overtly ethical or political grounds.

4

Eliminating the Unfit:
Euthanasia and Eugenics

From Prevention to Death

Although some prominent eugenicists advocated death for the unfit as early as 1868, before the Bollinger case such ideas rarely won endorsement in public from the leaders of the movement. The most prominent eugenic researchers and spokesmen called for preventing the reproduction of the unfit and for stimulating the fertility of the fittest, rather than seeking to eliminate those already born with defects. Preventive measures included providing sex education and birth control information to the poor, confining defectives in sex-segregated institutions, or legislating compulsory sterilization.

Charles Davenport, perhaps the foremost American eugenic researcher of the period, insisted in 1911 that eugenics did "not imply the destruction of the unfit either before or after birth."

Yale economist Irving Fisher and eugenic publicist Harry Laughlin echoed Davenport's disclaimer.

At the 1914 and 1915 National Conferences on Race Betterment, America's first professedly eugenic national conventions, several noted speakers did bring up the question of eliminating those born with impairments. But all endorsed the view attributed to eminent statistician Karl Pearson, who denied "the charge that we wish the weakling killed off," and proposed instead the "fundamental doctrine . . . that everyone, being born, has the right to live," but not the right "to reproduce his kind." John Harvey Kellogg and Paul Popenoe sounded a bit wistful in their rejection of selective elimination; they noted that "to kill off the weaklings born" constituted "Nature's way, the old method of natural selection," and the only method that had been available before modern times. But since eugenic science provided preventive techniques that were more humane and efficient, these old methods "we are all agreed must be supplanted."[1] In a metaphor equal to Haiselden's least-felicitous phrases, one speaker did endorse the view that "death is the normal process of elimination in the social organism, and . . . in prolonging the lives of defectives we are tampering with the functioning of the social kidneys." But even he accepted Pearson's view that preventive eugenics was the only proper way to counteract the problem.[2]

Haiselden also believed that eugenic euthanasia would be unnecessary if other preventive measures were pursued more vigorously. He claimed to have performed eugenic sterilizations himself as early as 1900. And he collaborated with William J. Robinson to portray the Bollinger case as an unfortunate result of society's refusal to legalize contraception.[3]

He took a similar position on selective abortion, viewing it as necessary only because contraceptives were denied to those unfit for parenthood. He generally mentioned abortion only to attack the hypocrisy of those medical leaders who condemned his refusal to save impaired infants, while secretly tolerating the "dreadful practice" of aborting healthy fetuses. But in February 1916, he declared publicly that he planned to perform one voluntary eugenic abortion and would consider doing others.[4] Robinson's *Medical Review of Reviews* agreed that both selective infanticide and abortion were stopgaps made necessary by the ban on contraceptives. It used the same word, "feticide," to refer to both procedures.[5]

Haiselden even continued to search for ways to cure defectives, perhaps out of a lingering Lamarckian hope that cured patients would produce normal children. Thus he experimented with brain surgery as a treatment for both inherited and acquired behavioral disorders. In a front-page obituary, the *Chicago Herald and Examiner* reported, "He was a believer in the theory criminal tendencies could be eliminated by brain operations, and performed a number of successful operations to substantiate this theory. He believed also that insanity could be similarly cured, and backed that up by frequent operations."[6]

Psychosurgery was novel but not unprecedented at this time. Although the idea remained controversial, many physiologists believed that specific behavioral abnormalities could be localized to specific defects in the brain. In 1914 two Pennsylvania doctors even used motion pictures to demonstrate the supposed abnormalities of an insane brain.[7] Several German and British surgeons had experimented with brain operations to cure schizophrenia and syphilitic insanity as early as 1890. Others sought to control behavior through castration and through trephining, the ancient operation to remove a portion of the skull. Belief that hidden abscesses could produce deviant behavior also led surgeons to remove organs that might harbor such "focal infections," especially in regions close to the brain, such as the tonsils, adenoids, and teeth.

For example, the *New York Times* reported in 1903 that two London criminals had been restored to law-abiding citizenship by skull trephining. In 1908 a Dr. Cronin reportedly cured delinquent New York public school students by removing their adenoids. In 1914 a Philadelphia court ordered a juvenile offender to be trephined to cure his criminal behavior. The following year, a Brooklyn judge, overriding parental opposition, ordered a nine-year-old's tonsils removed as a cure for truancy. Other criminals were reported to have been successfully trephined in Philadelphia in 1916 and Michigan in 1917.[8]

The idea of curing crime surgically strongly appealed to filmmakers. In D. W. Griffith's professedly "eugenic" 1914 melodrama *The Escape*, a psychopathic sadist from a family of defectives is restored to sanity by skull trephining.[9] In a Lubin film released the previous year, *Doctor Maxwell's Experiment*, an operation to cure criminal tendencies succeeds so well that the research subject saves the doctor from committing a crime and marries the doctor's daughter. Trephining likewise cured crime in *The Surgeon's Experiment* (Majestic 1914).[10]

Despite such related precedents, Haiselden may have been the first to claim success in operating directly on the brain to cure criminality; however, exactly what Haiselden did remains unclear. Although one newspaper credited him with having performed "hundreds" of "brain" operations, the only specific case described in the article clearly involved skull trephining, not actual brain surgery. In that 1916 case, a Chicago policeman who began arresting people at random was supposedly restored to sanity after Haiselden removed a piece of bone "pressing against the brain."[11]

Haiselden's interest in such surgery did not necessarily conflict with his belief in the inheritance of criminality and the need for other eugenic measures. Nor was he unique in combining the two. A 1908 study of juvenile delinquents by Thomas Travis gushed that operations to correct the physical defects characteristic of criminality could cure even the worst young thugs, but that "adult offenders" often proved "not amenable" to such treatment. For them "there is only one realm left, and that is extirpation," through sterilization, imprisonment, or the death penalty, "as a method of prevention" against "delinquency-breeding."[12]

Haiselden considered birth control, sterilization, abortion, even brain surgery as preferable to killing. But unlike most earlier eugenic publicists, Haiselden promoted the death of defectives as a necessary backup measure at least until better methods were more widely adopted. So long as the preferred methods remained outlawed, unused, or imperfect, death would be necessary to "sterilize" the unfit, as eugenics would help sanitize death: "Death is the Great and Lasting Disinfectant."[13]

Until 1915 most prominent eugenicists carefully distinguished preventive eugenics from euthanasia. Yet when Haiselden's actions moved the issue from theory to practice, that distinction virtually collapsed. Many of the same leaders who only a few years earlier had vigorously denied seeking the deaths of defectives now trumpeted the Bollinger case as a major breakthrough in eugenics.

Irving Fisher now wrote to "emphatically approve" Haiselden's action: "I hope the time may come when it will be a commonplace" that "defective babies be allowed to die." Likewise Charles Davenport abandoned his previous position. If surgery were used for "the artificial preservation of those whom the operation of natural agencies tends to eliminate," he warned, "it may conceivably destroy the race." Echoing Haiselden's praise for the Grim Reaper, Davenport now denounced as "anti-social" those doctors who "unduly restrict the operation of what is one of Nature's greatest racial blessings—death."[14]

Several eugenicists, such as Chicago health publicist Arthur

Corwin, did reiterate Pearson's earlier distinction. "Killing weakly infants at birth is not eugenics. The principles of eugenics . . . seek to prevent the birth of the unfit altogether," the *Chicago Medical Recorder* reminded readers.[15] Almost all such critics were, like Corwin, physicians.[16] But the vast majority of eugenics advocates who publicly commented on Haiselden's actions following the Bollinger case now depicted death as just one more method to prevent the reproduction of defectives, a necessary form of birth control when other less drastic preventives had failed.[17]

Haiselden realized that by taking direct action he could prod the leaders and theorists to a more radical position, a strategy anarchists of the time popularized as "propaganda of the deed." "Eugenics had a million theories, each theory with ardent backers. . . . But it lacked drive," he explained. "I came to the conclusion that the times were crying for some one central deed—some decisive action that would draw together all these theories and beginnings of things into one definite crusade." "The answer was to be Baby Bollinger."[18]

One individual acting outside the official movement could shift the spectrum of debate to make the movement leaders seem mainstream by comparison with him, while pushing the movement to support his previously radical views. Haiselden was only one doctor, but by gaining extensive media coverage of his dramatic acts, he was able to reshape the leadership's definition of what methods were "eugenic." Conversely, no history of how the official eugenics leaders came to be accepted as a mainstream social movement can be complete without understanding how this now-forgotten provocateur altered the environment in which the movement evolved.

Killing or Letting Die

In the Bollinger case, Haiselden emphasized that he simply allowed the baby to die by withholding lifesaving treatment, without actively hastening its death. He appealed to the infant's right to die a natural death without medical interference.[19] When a supporter advocated creating a government commission to painlessly execute retarded babies, Haiselden objected, "I do not believe in taking life directly."[20]

The *Detroit News* editorial writers regarded that distinction as vital to their support of Haiselden. It was also a crucial difference in the eyes of James Cardinal Gibbons, who held that surgery on a newborn constituted the kind of "extraordinary" intervention that Catholic law considered permissible to withhold.[21]

"Haiselden Says Nature, And Not He, Killed Baby," declared a headline in the socialist *New York Call*. When he was not speaking to socialists, Haiselden sometimes attributed the death to God. "It was the will of God that the child be born defective. It is his will that the child die. Shall I set myself up as wiser than the Almighty? God does not want that child to live," Haiselden explains to Anne in *The Black Stork*. His position thus echoed a nineteenth-century faith in the divine beneficence of nature, as well as that century's skepticism about the value of artificial medical intervention. The distinction was also an effective way of shifting the responsibility for the death from his own shoulders to God's: If God wants these babies to live, let God save them.[22]

The effort to differentiate passive from active killing did not impress his critics. As they did in challenging Haiselden's diagnostic categories, they invoked both moral duties and social utility to condemn his treatment decisions.

Those critics who felt Haiselden had violated a moral obligation repeatedly charged that "allowing a child to die from voluntary neglect is murder."[23] Many simply equated the two actions without further explanation, as if the point were self-evident.[24] Others explained that both active and passive euthanasia deprived a human being of the "right to life."[25]

Such right-to-life arguments implicitly postulated a right to be saved from dying, not just a right not to be killed, but that point was also treated as self-evident. Haiselden's critics rarely explained what a "right to life" meant or what specific obligations it entailed.[26] By 1915 the phrase was already being invoked more as a familiar slogan than as part of an explicitly articulated argument.

A few of those who equated withholding treatment with active killing did explain that the two actions shared a common evil intent. Because desiring someone's death was wrong, effectuating such intentions was murder, whether the goal was reached through action or inaction. Thus a *New York Times* editorial declared the distinction between omission and commission "a quibbling difference if any," because "the known consequences of any act, including acts of abstention, can justly be held to have been intended."[27] But for the most part, those who labeled Haiselden a murderer simply stated the charge as if it required no further elaboration.

While right-to-life critics declared passive euthanasia equivalent to murder, other opponents distinguished the two measures but opposed withholding treatment because it might eventually lead to murder. The first spoke in terms of moral imperatives; the latter emphasized the likelihood of bad consequences.

"The refusal to save the life . . . is liable to be taken as tantamount to the taking of a life." "Only one more step remains—either in childhood or maturity to kill off the unfit altogether," the Reverend Mabel Irwin cautioned.[28]

In fact, Haiselden and his supporters did a great deal to make these entering-wedge concerns credible. From the start, Haiselden himself anticipated that passive euthanasia would soon lead to active killing, and left the impression that he regarded the distinction as a question of tactics rather than of ethics. "I did not kill Baby Bollinger. That day is not yet."[29]

Even in the Bollinger case, Haiselden raised the possibility he might administer opiates for pain relief in doses large enough to likely prove fatal. His subsequent cases further blurred the line. Only a few weeks later, he performed a fatal operation on the Grimshaw baby after agreeing with the parents that the child should be either cured or killed.[30] While Haiselden at first advocated that physicians simply not tie the umbilical cords of defective newborns, in 1917 he actively removed the Meter baby's umbilical ligature and the infant reportedly bled to death.[31] And in the Hodzima case of 1917, he prescribed potentially lethal doses of opiates for a microcephalic infant who was taking longer than expected to die.[32]

In defending these increasingly active measures, Haiselden discarded his previous distinction between active and passive euthanasia, and like some critics of his earlier view, now focused on the question of his intentions. If an act caused both good and harmful consequences, he argued, it should be judged by which effect was intended. This "doctrine of two effects" long provided a theological rationale for taking the inevitable risks involved in any medical treatment. Thus Haiselden now explained, the opiates he gave the Hodzima baby were intended to fight pain, not to kill, and this good intention justified the drug's likely but unwanted risk to the infant's life.[33]

Such arguments are most persuasive in the court of divine judgment, with an omniscient judge who knows people's true inner motives. In the mundane setting, however, this doctrine could become a rationalization for almost any action. A road paved over with allegedly good intentions could lead anywhere you wanted to go. When opponents attempted to block his opiate prescriptions for the

Hodzima baby, he responded by threatening to kill the baby surgically, "I may then perform an operation that will relieve the child's suffering—and remove from the world a child doomed to idiocy."[34]

In *The Black Stork*, the head of the local medical society admits to Anne that he had considered actively killing a defective infant by administering an overdose of a surgical anesthetic labeled "twilight treatment." "Twilight sleep," a highly controversial, potentially lethal technique for eliminating the memory of pain, was advocated by many feminists and physicians for use in childbirth, not in surgery. A 1914 article on the subject, in a journal for which Haiselden later wrote an article, warned explicitly that twilight sleep should not be considered as a surgical anesthetic. "It is, of course, necessary to distinguish between surgical anesthesia and twilight sleep. The distinction is clear in principle and practice." Yet Haiselden himself used twilight sleep as the surgical anesthetic in his operations to sterilize defectives. His selection of this method might indicate simply a lack of accurate information about the new procedure, but it could also have meant that he intended to actively administer overdoses, as depicted in *The Black Stork*.[35] One 1917 advertisement for *The Black Stork* quoted him as saying, "Kill defectives, save the nations, and see 'The Black Stork.'" The 1927 version included a reference to a mother who actively poisoned her mentally deficient son.[36]

Even in 1915 some of his supporters opposed making a distinction between passive and active euthanasia. The *Chicago Tribune* found no significant difference between the two and endorsed both. By 1917 the *New York Sun* claimed a significant number of New York doctors shared that view.[37]

A few eugenicists even favored active killing over simply withholding aid. John Harvey Kellogg thought Haiselden should have tried to save the Bollinger baby, but once treatment had been ruled out, he wrote, it would have been more humane to kill the infant outright than to let him die slowly. New York physician Edward Wallace Lee approved the death of the Bollinger baby but preferred active killing.[38] In endorsing *The Black Stork*, Edward D. Page added, "A number of years experience on the New Jersey Commission for the care of the mentally defective has led me to believe that it would be desirable to put a great number of these adults out of the way in a humane and sensible manner."[39]

As Page's comments indicate, Haiselden and his supporters never restricted euthanasia to immediately imperilled infants. They saw the unfit of all ages as candidates. But expanding the target population beyond infants virtually required expanding the methods to include active killing, since adult defectives were not often in immediate need of lifesaving medical treatments. Haiselden predicted "a great awakening some day" that would result in "the painless death of the hopelessly insane." In 1917, he revealed, he had also actively administered potentially lethal doses of narcotics to a seventy-two-year-old woman amputee with a broken hip and breast cancer. "Cancer of the face should always have the lethal dose" of painkiller, Haiselden added.[40]

Although Haiselden initially emphasized the difference between killing and allowing to die, his subsequent statements and actions dramatically pushed the boundaries of the distinction. I did not find even one example of someone who had supported his initial position who explicitly repudiated his increasingly active methods. But following the Hodzima case, many of his former backers stopped talking about him at all. And without mentioning their previous support for Haiselden, several important eugenicists, from Irving Fisher to William J. Robinson, suddenly restated Pearson's formulation that eugenics sought to prevent the reproduction of defectives without seeking their death. Many different factors contributed to this erosion of support and erasure of memory (to be discussed in chapter 9), but the timing suggests that key eugenicists concluded Haiselden had damaged the cause by moving from passive measures to active killing too quickly.

For Whose Benefit?

Whose interests would be served by eliminating defectives? Haiselden and his supporters portrayed his refusal to treat impaired newborns in two very different ways—both as a humanitarian effort to relieve the intense suffering of afflicted individuals and as a utilitarian attempt to protect society against costly and menacing defectives. At times, euthanasia was defined by its motive—"mercy killing"; at other times, it was simply a method—"painless killing," which could be used for a wide variety of purposes.

Historian Charles Beard, who supported mercy killing for terminally ill adults, based his opposition to treating the Bollinger baby on humanitarian grounds—to end what he called the baby's "unrelievable suffering."[41] Simon Baruch agreed that the central issue was relieving individual agony. He equated Haiselden with a doctor who refused to stop a hemorrhage in a case of advanced cancer, and concluded, "The fact is . . . the public does not understand the true physician, whom I believe to be the most perfect altruist in every community."[42]

But did defective newborns really suffer? Many nineteenth-century doctors doubted any infants experienced suffering, and partly because of such beliefs, they often concluded anesthesia was unnecessary in surgery on neonates. The ability to suffer was thought to depend upon not just the perception of pain, but the ability to remember and anticipate pain. Suffering thus required a level of memory and intelligence not available to any newborn, especially not to one whose mental processes were judged deficient.[43]

Haiselden himself held two seemingly contradictory views on whether mentally impaired newborns felt any suffering that needed relief. He insisted he was motivated by the "kindest mercy" when he allowed the Bollinger baby to be "put out of its misery."[44] Yet he also wrote of this and other defective infants, "There is no brain development to register suffering."[45]

Not only did defectives lack the ability to suffer, they lacked the capacity for life at all. Haiselden repeatedly declared that the Bollinger baby's "tiny brain . . . was not a live thing—but a dead and fearsome ounce or two of jelly." "[T]hose who have no brains—their blank and awful existence cannot be called Life." "We live through our brains."[46]

Just as Haiselden's cases reveal an unsuspected history to modern infant euthanasia controversies, they also demonstrate that the current debate over "brain death" is not an unprecedented product of new medical technology. In fact, for much of history, these two issues have been closely linked. If the inability of a person's brain to function constitutes death, then continued medical treatment is no longer appropriate.

But there is an internal inconsistency in linking the relief of suffering to the redefinition of death. Considering a mentally defective infant as already dead and desiring to put it out of its misery are two contradictory positions; the dead are beyond all earthly suffering.[47]

This ambivalence about whether or not defective infants suffer reflected a deeper uncertainty over whether their deaths were primarily designed to relieve the individual infants or to end the misery of others, including the family and society at large. As pediatrician Abraham Jacobi noted in 1912, those who advocate killing the comatose to relieve suffering must be speaking of someone else's suffering, not the patient's.[48] And determining the interests of a newborn baby was impossible anyway, the *Washington Post* declared. All claims to the contrary were simply the impermissible attribution of someone else's desires to a being who had not yet had a chance to form desires of its own.[49]

The birth of an impaired child caused real suffering to many others, especially to the family members whose expectations were shattered and whose lives had to be completely restructured. Haiselden received scores of letters and public expressions of support from parents in despair who saw him as the only person who understood or could end their sufferings. Working mothers bore a special burden. Mrs. Lewis Ohl of New York described her completely paralyzed fifteen-year-old boy as needing "constant care" and "in pain most of the time." Although he "cries when I leave," she explained to a socialist reporter, "I cannot take care of him, as I must do my own work, and he has grown . . . so I cannot lift him." "I love him . . . and because of this, I wish him dead every minute of the day."

Mothers described their greatest pain as that caused by sympathy with their children's sufferings. "It is hard, yes. But not for me. It is the child who suffers," explained one woman. Conversely, disabled children described the pain of being a burden to their mothers. "We are in every one's way but mother's, and her poor heart aches with ours," a teenaged "little crippled girl" told Haiselden.

That girl concluded her letter with a common terror for both mothers and disabled children: "What will become of me when mother dies?" "Life is hard on the poor," the mother of a handicapped child from New York's Lower East Side reminded an interviewer. "When the mother dies there is no one to care for deformed babies."[50]

In Haiselden's view, the same principle that justified aborting a fetus to save the mother would justify his refusal to save infants whose defects threatened the lives or emotional health of the parents, or adversely affected the health of normal siblings. "It is our duty to prevent idiotic malformed babies from killing their mothers by overwork, worry, shame."[51]

In addition to the suffering their conditions caused themselves and their families, defectives allegedly posed enormous costs to society, now and in the future. Politically conservative eugenicists like Charles Davenport expressed their support of Haiselden in terms of the collective welfare of the "race." "The functions of the individual must be subordinated to the best interests of the race."[52] Haiselden's socialist supporters usually made the same point in the interests of "society," or "humanity," though they too sometimes spoke in terms of the "race." As Helen Keller put it, "Our puny sentimentalism has caused us to forget that a human life is sacred only when it may be of some use to itself and to the world."[53] Writing in the avant-garde *Medical Review of Reviews*, socialist Anita C. Block proclaimed, "The time is here when Society will refuse any longer to pay out millions of dollars . . . in the care of this racial menace." She lauded Haiselden for "the ultimate socializing of the individual for the greater glory of the race."[54]

Many doctors and clergy considered this willingness to sacrifice impaired individuals for the collective good to be among the most objectionable aspects of Haiselden's campaign. Though physicians had benefitted greatly from government activities such as licensing and public health, in 1915 the American Medical Association was just beginning to formulate an anticollectivist ideology on issues from health insurance to reporting of contagious diseases. By 1920 it would become a central dogma of American medical professionalism to equate government involvement in medical decisions with sacrificing the care of individual patients for the collective good of society.[55]

Haiselden's campaign coincided with this critical period of transformation in professional attitudes toward government and the public welfare. Medical reaction to his collectivist goals both illustrated and helped precipitate the emerging professional crusade against "socialized medicine."

Industrial hygiene reformer Dr. Alice Hamilton warned that Haiselden's collectivism raised "a question of enormous importance, involving . . . the whole relation of the physician to society." She denounced the "growing number of radicals" outside the medical profession who held it to be the doctor's "duty . . . to bring about death in the interest of society." Dr. Kellogg declared "the first principle" of civilized ethics to be "The state is for the man, not the man for the state."[56]

Religious opponents, too, contrasted their concern for the individual soul with what the Catholic *New World* called Haiselden's deification of the state. The *New World* devoted a full article to publicizing the fact that some socialists had endorsed Haiselden's actions. The meaning of the Bollinger case according to the Reverend Mabel Irwin was that "individualism and socialism have grappled in a life and death struggle, and socialism appears to be the victor."[57]

Such allegations linking Haiselden's eugenics to "socialism" are very revealing but cannot be taken out of context. The debate over Haiselden's actions was part of a struggle to control the meanings of both "eugenics" and "socialism." A number of Haiselden's prominent supporters did identify themselves with the Socialist Party. But in this debate, neither Haiselden's backers nor his critics confined the word "socialism" to the doctrines of a specific political movement. The term included any actions that subordinated the interests of individuals to the good of society as a whole. This kind of "socialism" was not limited to the collective ownership of the means of production, but included any collectivist utilitarianism, especially if the greatest good for the greatest number was defined by the state. Used in this sense, the label "socialism" lumped together many varied opponents of libertarian individualism without distinguishing between the left and the right.[58]

Ironically, even some vocal critics of Haiselden's collectivism relied on implicitly collectivist utilitarian assumptions themselves. In the same article that proclaimed the struggle against Haiselden to be a last-ditch defense of individualism, the Reverend Irwin also rejected passive euthanasia because it would lead to active murder. Such entering-wedge arguments implicitly deny relief to individuals who might be helped by passive euthanasia, in order to protect society at large against abuses.[59] The Catholic *New Orleans Morning Star* blasted Haiselden for even considering that defectives posed a "burden upon society," while at the same time warning that his actions posed great dangers "to society at large."[60] But in 1915 no one commented on any inconsistency in attacking both the collectivism and the collective consequences of Haiselden's campaign.

Haiselden's backers never denied that their desire to eliminate defectives derived in part from their concern for the interests of society. But several of his physician supporters, including some professed socialists, tried to minimize the relative importance of such collectivist motives. Although in another context socialist Dr. William J. Robinson had written that defectives had no individual rights, when supporting Haiselden he labeled the "racial" argument for nontreatment "timid," and found it far less compelling than the relief of "individual" suffering. Hearst health columnist Dr. Woods Hutchinson asserted, "The main question was, 'What's best for the child?' " "The question of his becoming a burden on the community," was "entitled to consideration," but it merited "only secondary and minor emphasis." Hutchinson claimed "at least two-thirds" of Haiselden's supporters would put their concern for the individual ahead of collective concerns.[61]

While some debated the relative importance of society and the individual, most of Haiselden's backers simply asserted their desire to terminate what Lillian Wald called both the "misery" and the "menace" of defectives, without making any effort at all to distinguish or prioritize between the two motives. "By the weeding out of our undesirables," Haiselden explained, "we decrease their burden and ours."[62]

Historians and philosophers who have studied the developing early-twentieth-century link between eugenics and euthanasia have pointed to this blurring of social and individual goals, benevolent and utilitarian values, as a critical logical error in ethical reasoning. Historian Robert Proctor criticizes German race hygienists of the 1920s and 1930s for their tendency "to confuse these two very different senses of euthanasia: . . . the one based on relieving suffering, the other based on minimizing medical costs." "The logic in each case is different: in the first, the goal is to provide individual happiness in the final moments of life; in the second, the goal is . . . to relieve society of the financial burden of caring for lives considered useless to the community."[63]

Efforts to end suffering can also conflict with the exercise of individual freedom. As Aldous Huxley argued in *Brave New World*, to eradicate individual pain would require extensive social control.[64]

But the interests of society and the individual, while logically distinct and potentially in conflict, are not necessarily incompatible. Often they do coincide.[65] Many of Haiselden's backers focused on those cases in which euthanasia might end individual suffering, enhance personal freedom, and cut social costs at the same time, rather than trying to choose among these goals in cases where they conflicted.

Loving and Loathing

Haiselden's crusade did not combine logically incompatible goals, but it did appeal to fundamentally irreconcilable emotions: His supporters were motivated by a jarring combination of compassion and hatred.

Haiselden himself lurched sharply from affirmations of love to expressions of loathing. *The Black Stork* appealed to the audience's empathy with the deformed child's future life of suffering and ostracism, and even drew upon religious imagery to portray euthanasia as merciful and humane. Haiselden insisted he allowed defectives to die "because he loves them."[66]

But while empathizing with the individual defective, Haiselden emphasized the need to protect society from what he termed "lives of no value."[67] "We have been invaded," Haiselden warned. "Our streets are infested with an Army of the Unfit—a dangerous, vicious army of death and dread," composed of "horrid things that drag themselves through our streets by day and night." The Bollinger baby was "dangerous as dynamite," the Hodzima baby a "menace to society." Looking at them Haiselden saw all the "foulness of the world." He ended his autobiography with a challenge: "Horrid semi-humans drag themselves along all of our streets. . . . What are you going to do about it?"[68]

The menace of defectives derived in part from the fear of contamination; thus, hereditary diseases were as threatening as contagious epidemics. He likened eugenic sterilization to "shoot[ing] down a slobbering cur in the streets to prevent it from spreading its rabies."[69] The unfit themselves were denounced as infectious parasites. Referring to both defectives and capitalists, one self-professed Christian Socialist predicted that "the day of the parasite, who eats his bread without earning it, will soon pass." The unfit did not simply *have* a disease; they *were* the disease.[70]

Haiselden's propaganda routinely combined sympathy with hostility, even when the mix seems logically contradictory. To prove he acted benevolently and spared defective babies untold misery, Haiselden and *Black Stork* coauthor Jack Lait graphically described the miserable conditions they had seen in institutions such as the one at Lincoln, Illinois. "The great state of Illinois in order to save money allowed hundreds of windows to go without screens," permitting flies to swarm over the patients, Haiselden charged. "Worse still, I found that the inmates were fed with the milk from a herd of cattle reeking with tuberculosis." Yet when they discussed institutionalization in *The Black Stork*, they completely reversed their previous picture. "Our defectives are housed in palaces costing fortunes while our unfortunate normal children live like maggots in filthy hovels," the film now insisted, as the camera cut from sweeping panoramas of a spacious tree-lined hospital campus to closeups of poor slum children.[71] Their newspaper exposé portrayed the institutionalized retarded as suffering victims of state neglect, while their film depicted the same patients as state-coddled parasites living at the expense of working families.

The important point is that Haiselden and his supporters did not seem to see these attitudes as contradictory. They repeatedly combined expressions of love and sympathy for the suffering of individual babies with attacks on defectives as loathsome evil creatures engaged in a war against society. Haiselden fantasized that his hospital

"was some mediaeval torture chamber, and that Baby Bollinger, lying naked there on the great table, was the victim of some unspeakable cruelty. And yet as this thought flashed over me I saw another vision. This was no chamber of horrors. Here at last men and women were gathered together for the purpose of performing a deed full of the kindest mercy."[72]

Some of Haiselden's backers emphasized love more than hate; others quite the opposite. But his position easily accommodated both. Some of the protestations of love ring hollow to modern ears, and may well have been intentionally deceptive. But most of his supporters slid easily and unselfconsciously from one emotion to the other. Without a word of transition, Helen Keller described the Bollinger baby as "the hopeless being spared from a life of misery. No one cares about that pitiful, useless lump of flesh." Clarence Darrow's comments revealingly captured the full ambiguity of this appeal. "Chloroform unfit children. Show them the same mercy that is shown beasts that are no longer fit to live."[73]

Haiselden's supporters could combine such contradictory feelings without experiencing much conflict, because they believed they were being entirely rational, that all their emotional responses were derived from objective science. "This is clearly a matter where scientific fact should take precedence over maudlin sentimentalism," declared Detroit health officer Dr. William Price. Hearst columnist Dr. Woods Hutchinson cited Haiselden's example as demonstrating, "The world really is becoming rational at last, thanks to science." A *New York American* editorial contrasted Jane Addams's "wholly emotional" opposition to Haiselden with his supporters' reasoning from "the facts to the logical conclusion." "This is no time to grow sentimental over the misfits of the world," Haiselden warned. "[C]old hard logic . . . cannot be overturned by false and sickly sentiment."[74]

For Haiselden, the urge to eliminate defectives was itself a primal instinct, an objective force of nature. In a particularly striking passage in his autobiography, he recalled that he first became aware of the retarded when, at the age of eight, he joined the gang of boys who regularly assaulted "Crazy Mary," the village idiot. In words that evoke images of a witch, he described how she would "fly through the streets, her gray hair flying in the wind, brandishing her arms, and screaming at the crowd of young brutes that pursued her with sticks and stones." But significantly, while he now felt "sorry" for such attacks, he did not feel responsible for them, because he saw such actions as being beyond his control, dictated by the laws of nature. He did not deny having strong emotions, but attributed them to an innate and universal biological imperative. Even a child "instinctively sees the menace in these wretched beings and adopts this means of fighting against it." As a result, beatings were "only part of the price that the inferior forms of human life must pay if they wish to live among their more fortunate brothers."[75]

Literary critic Leslie Fiedler has argued that physical deformities evoke both love and hate, because they force us to confront our internal conflicts between self and otherness.[76] Haiselden and his supporters clearly exhibited this dichotomy, but their insistence that their emotions derived from objective science left them particularly incapable of recognizing the conflict.

Objective Science and Moral Obligation

Critics equated Dr. Haiselden with Dr. Frankenstein, someone whose "coldly scientific" views excluded any concern for morality or feelings. "Science has long sneered at these qualities in men and women as weaknesses, arguing that for race betterment pity and sympathy must be suppressed," explained a Washington clergyman.[77] Even one of Haiselden's patient's parents saw the issue as part of the warfare between science and religion. "My religion tells me that I am committing a crime," admitted Mrs. Hodzima. But "medicine and religion must be kept separate."[78]

But such comments overlooked what others saw as a crucial element in Haiselden's appeal. Haiselden never claimed to be value free. He insisted his cause was ethically as well as medically correct. He did not try to banish values from science; he offered science as a superior source of value. He did not reject emotion or religion as unscientific; he substituted objective science for traditional religion as the true basis for benevolent feelings and moral obligations. "I was acting according to the passionate dictates of my conscience," he insisted, but he believed his moral judgments were determined according to the objective methods of science.[79]

Scientific methods provided an objectively true basis for both emotions and ethics, far superior to those false sentiments whose only basis was irrational social conventions. Allowing baby Bollinger to die was not a victory of cold logic over love, Haiselden insisted, but a victory of objective love over sentimental love. "[K]indness took the highest form," triumphing over "false sentiment, false manhood, false humanity," he proclaimed. The *Philadelphia Ledger* called his decision "the highest benefaction."[80]

Thus Haiselden was not antagonistic to all religion, but only to those faiths he saw as based on outdated tradition and illogical mysticism. He viewed the scientific method as the foundation of a new objectively true religion, in which the laws of nature were truly morally binding "laws"; not neutral facts but ethical imperatives. "It is an unfortunate thing that Science and Religion do not often go together. In my life the two always have harmonized," Haiselden insisted. A lifelong "devout" Methodist, he even named one of his adopted daughters Beulah Hope Wesley. But the God he worshipped was a scientist, "the Chief Surgeon of us all."[81]

Those critics who accused Haiselden of playing God were much more on target than those who accused him of opposing all religion. Haiselden compared the Bollinger baby to the Christ child, explaining that the infant's sacrifice revealed a new rationally based testament to supercede the old religion. More often, Haiselden cast himself as the martyred messiah; he even called his vigil over the Bollinger baby his "Gethsemane."[82] A Detroit physician termed Haiselden God's co-worker in the task of creating a new humanity.[83]

Haiselden's assertion of moral and spiritual authority for eugenics illuminates several crucial developments in the evolving relationship between science and religion. In part, his rhetoric reflected the survival of nineteenth-century natural theology, the belief that the laws discovered in nature and the laws revealed in religion each manifested the goodness and authority of their common Creator. And in part, his higher benevolence sounds like an anticipation of George Orwell's "newspeak," in which the actions people had called evil were simply relabeled the higher good.[84]

But Haiselden's religious claims also embodied important early-twentieth-century concepts that were neither mere echoes of the past nor anticipations of the future. For many of Haiselden's contemporaries, the objectivity of science made it the best source of moral and spiritual values.

"Objective" meant "impartial." To be impartial also meant to be fair, to be just. Fairness and justice were moral virtues and ethical imperatives. Objective methods also produced the truth, and thus were the foundation of honesty. And honesty was the most basic duty if ethics was to avoid comfortable self-delusions and be applicable to the world as it really was. Objectivity was thus both a virtue and a duty. Promoted by writers from Sinclair Lewis to Walter Lippmann, this "intellectual gospel" preached the scientific method as a spiritual and moral replacement for traditional religions.

From the start, Galton himself called for making eugenics a new religion, to imbue the movement with the sense of moral imperative that religion provided. By 1928 the Third Conference on Race Betterment featured the sermon "A Biologic Philosophy or Religion," in which Dr. Aldred Scott Warthin preached on the text, "Our Duty to the Immortal Germ Plasm." "[S]imple biology, the simple facts of life, can become an adequate philosophy, an adequate religion."[85]

This was the context in which Haiselden proclaimed the moral duty to implement the judgments of eugenics. In intellect and influence, Haiselden was no Lippmann, but his depiction of eugenics as a religion both reflects and illuminates one way the "intellectual gospel" preached by progressive intellectuals like Lippmann could be received.[86] If eugenic euthanasia was based on objective science, then its implementation could be considered morally binding. Because he invested the methods of science with the moral force of a religion, Haiselden considered it his moral duty to eliminate those whom science had proven unfit to live.

5

Who Decides? The Ironies of Professional Power

Doctors, Families, and the State

Eliminating the unfit required that someone have the power to make life-and-death decisions. Who could be entrusted with such authority? Supporters of withholding treatment suggested several possible decision makers, such as individual doctors, committees of experts, individual parents, or the state, but the vast majority of them urged giving this power to the medical profession.

Haiselden's crusade coincided with a dramatic expansion of medical authority over many aspects of American cultural life, including such previously private domains as reproduction and the family. In the early decades of this century, obstetricians supplanted midwives, pediatricians professionalized childrearing, and allied professions from psychology to home economics "medicalized" the home from the kitchen to the toilet and the bedroom.[1]

In 1915 child care was largely a female responsibility, whereas the medical profession was overwhelmingly male. Thus any growth of medical power over reproduction and childrearing meant an increase in men's authority over what had been women's work.

Some of these changes resulted directly from concerted efforts by the profession to market its own new expertise. But the debate over treatment of impaired newborns demonstrates that the medicalization of private life could be a much more complex process. At least in this case, medical control over family life resulted from choices made by mothers and fathers, social reformers, and the state, as well as physicians. And lay supporters of nontreatment were more vocal than the physicians in their desire to give doctors this power.

Those who opposed allowing doctors to make nontreatment decisions predictably included lay opponents of professional power in general, but the primary resistance to giving doctors this particular power came from medical leaders themselves. They included some doctors who opposed anyone having the power to withhold treatment and a significant group who did not care if someone else made such decisions, so long as it wasn't them. These professional leaders portrayed their opposition to assuming this particular power as necessary for the defense of professional authority in general.

Alice Hamilton perceptively observed the ironies of her profession's reluctance to assume this new social role: "Curiously enough it is not the medical profession which is seeking an extension of its rights; it is the laity which is trying to force upon physicians a power over life and death which they themselves shrink from."[2]

But while lay people played a central role in trying to medicalize this decision, their stand was based on a broad progressive faith in the objective methods of medical science, a faith that was actively promoted by professional leaders. Ironically, lay support for giving doctors powers they did not especially want derived in part from the profession's own propaganda on behalf of professional authority in general.

Support for Medical Power

The great majority of those quoted in favor of letting defectives die felt the decision should be left entirely to the medical profession.

The *New York Times* strongly urged that nontreatment decisions should be "kept strictly within professional circles," "without the horrified exclamations of unenlightened sentimentality."[3] One common suggestion was to create special medical committees, what Helen Keller called "physicians' juries for defective babies." The idea won extensive support within days of the Bollinger case. One early proposal by the Chicago coroner called for "a commission of medical experts . . . to decide, with the physician in charge, whether 'hopeless' children shall live or be allowed to die," a process he termed "passing sentence on the patient." The plan was endorsed by Haiselden, and adopted in the official inquest verdict. Another proposal would have empowered the U.S. Public Health Service to set a national standard. A Chicago realtor called for "legislation creating a commission authorized to put to death painlessly hopelessly imbecile children," though he thought it "desirable to obtain the consent of parents."[4]

Of 71 people quoted publicly about who should make nontreatment decisions, more than one-third felt it should be up to the individual doctor, and another third endorsed having an expert committee make the decisions. Less than one-quarter felt the parents should have any say. Those quoted included 38 physicians and 33 others. The quotes attributed to lay people were much more likely to trust individual physicians and less likely to trust parents than were the views attributed to doctors (Table 12). The literal handful (5) of respondents who spoke about this question in their private responses to the NBRMP split in the same proportions as those quoted in public, with 2 each favoring individual doctors and medical committees, and only 1 supporting a parental role, subject to the individual doctor's concurrence.

Table 12. Publicly Stated Position on Who Should Decide, Physicians and Others

	Physicians	*Other Respondents*
Expert committee	16 (42%)	9 (27%)
Individual doctor[a]	11 (29%)	15 (45%)
Parents	10 (26%)	7 (21%)
Total	38	33

[a]This group is different from those listed as saying the decision was "up to doctor" in previous tables. That label applied to those who said doctors already had the right to make such decisions, without indicating whether or not they thought doctors *should* have such authority. The category "individual doctor" refers to those who *favored* giving doctors this power, regardless of what they saw as the actual existing authority.

Many published quotations specifically rejected any parental involvement, especially the involvement of mothers. Some insisted that women were too irrational, too swayed by subjective feelings to make such choices logically. Others feared that women would destroy healthy infants for nonmedical reasons. Eugenicists worried that native middle-class women would take advantage of such power to contribute to race suicide, while moralists feared that unwed mothers would use infanticide to eliminate evidence of illicit sex. Such views were attributed primarily, though hardly exclusively, to male commentators.[5]

A mother's love could be as irrational as her desire to escape childrearing, and thus could be as likely to preclude objective decision making. One federal judge warned that "the parents' sense of love might blind them to the larger needs of humanity." Mrs. Bollinger reportedly wanted her baby to live, until Haiselden helped her to see this desire as "selfishness."[6] According to one of his opponents, Haiselden opposed even women doctors playing a role in such decisions because their "sympathetic" natures would preclude them from making the "sterner" choices demanded by science.[7]

Among the 33 nonphysicians quoted on the issue, less than one-quarter of both the women (3/15) and the men (4/17) favored including parents in the decision. The only visible gender difference was that all 4 men favored the "parents" making the choice, while 2 of the 3 women specified the "mother." The women whose published quotations supported medical decision makers without mentioning a role for parents included such prominent progressives and suffragists as Lillian Wald, Helen Keller, Mary Austin, Katharine Bement Davis, and Anita Block.[8]

This overwhelming support for medical power reflected the unprecedented faith in scientific experts shared by many turn-of-the-century progressives. Because the methods of science were objective, the decisions of scientists would be rational, impartial, and fair, they reasoned. They promoted the power of medical scientists, not as an "interest group" but as the only truly "disinterested" arbiters of social conflict. Helen Keller captured the essence of this far-reaching faith: "A jury of physicians considering the case of an idiot would be exact and scientific. Their findings would be free from the prejudice and inaccuracy of untrained observation."[9]

Haiselden himself sometimes suggested the decision should rest with the parents or the people rather than the profession, especially when he sought to defend his decision to publicize his actions. However, he generally urged the public to support physicians like himself against the conservative professional establishment, rather than take the decision out of expert hands altogether. He attacked Hippocratic professionalism as "2000 years behind the times," but sought public backing for what he called the "new school" of professionalism, not direct public power.[10]

A few advocates of withholding treatment who supported expert authority did feel uneasy about leaving the fate of defective newborns entirely to physicians. They suggested that the decision makers should include other kinds of professionals, such as lawyers or social workers, along with doctors.[11] But most of those quoted as backing selective treatment wanted doctors to decide, with the laity at least as supportive of medical decision making as were Haiselden's physician supporters.

Opponents of Medical Decision Making

Haiselden's actions captured national attention in large part because he was a physician. To many of his critics, the death of his infant patients was not as shocking as the fact that they had died by decision of their doctor.

Those who opposed granting physicians such powers included a few who wanted to rein in the growth of medical power generally. But the main critics were physicians and other advocates of medical professionalization who saw this particular authority as weakening rather than strengthening the profession overall. While some opposed giving anyone such vast power, most, including many doctors, simply preferred having someone else make the decisions.

Among the most extreme opponents of medical power in 1915 was the Chicago-based National League for Medical Freedom, a short-lived coalition of alternative healers, patent medicine vendors, and political libertarians. They bitterly fought every progressive-era expansion of medical power, including license laws, drug regulation, compulsory vaccination, and school health-education classes, denouncing each as a medical conspiracy to use the power of the state to invade the personal autonomy of all Americans. Not surprisingly, the League seized upon Haiselden's cases to document the horrors of unfettered medical power. They portrayed medical murder as the inevitable result of granting any state support to the profession.[12]

Less extreme critics of professionalism used Haiselden's example to argue that while medical power had its place, the progressive-era profession had overstepped its bounds. Religious believers who insisted that God alone should decree the time of death warned that giving doctors such power would be to usurp an authority no mortal should exercise. "God gave [life] and . . . God alone has power to take it away," asserted the *Catholic World*. "Doctors are not little Gods," cautioned Dr. Gertrude Kelly of New York.[13] Such language went beyond a specific criticism of Haiselden's actions, to imply that the medical profession had become both too materialist and too powerful and was claiming authority over areas of life beyond its proper place.

Most who attacked medicine as too powerful opposed permitting anyone to withhold treatment. But the critics of medical power also included several key supporters of selective euthanasia. Illinois State's Attorney Maclay Hoyne upheld the decision not to treat the Bollinger baby primarily because the parents had made the choice. Hoyne reasoned that "an adult may decline to be operated on if he sees fit . . . even though it is to his best interests that he should have the operation." In the case of a child, this same right should be exercised by the parents, Hoyne wrote, because they are the child's "natural" protectors.[14] Socialist Anita Block favored direct power by the masses, without reliance on any technocratic experts. "[T]here are many questions which have been hitherto reverently left to groups of specialists to determine, that are really *social* questions. . . . [I]t is for society, for the people as a whole, to determine what they will do with defectives," Block insisted.[15]

But most of those who rejected giving doctors this particular power claimed to be defending, not restricting, the status and power of the medical profession. One common charge was that medicine would be hurt because doctors would not be able to keep a monopoly on nontreatment decisions. Even though doctors could probably be trusted with such powers of life and death, it would be the "opening wedge" for others, especially parents, to kill babies for nonmedical reasons. "To authorize this practice will most certainly pave the way for and lead directly to its abuse," warned Pittsburgh obstetrician Walter Croll. "[M]any an unwelcome fetus will perish in the name of eugenics when its development is perfect." "If such liberty is given to the individual physician," wrote Chicago theologian Harris Rall, "there is no reason why it should not be granted to the individual parent. . . . a most dangerous leeway."[16]

Such power would also eventually corrupt some doctors and bring the whole profession into disrepute. "How easy it would be for the father or mother of an illegitimate child to persuade an unscrupulous doctor to put the child out of the way," warned attorney Jean Norris.[17]

To let doctors decide which infants should live was to vastly expand medical authority over the family. But these critics feared the result might be to increase rather than narrow the reproductive choices available to families. No one had the authority to make such choices in 1915. If doctors were permitted to do so, and if some of them chose to take parents' wishes into account, that would increase the opportunities for parents to influence a decision over which they had no legitimate control before. Medicalizing previously prohibited reproductive decisions was not a zero-sum game in which medical power could only come at the expense of family choice. Dependence on doctors could be the "opening wedge" to parental power.[18]

The concern that medical euthanasia would weaken the medical profession went deeper than just a fear it would inadvertently empower lay people. Many critics insisted that the foundation of medical professionalism and the basis of professional authority was the doctor's duty to preserve life. "The mission of doctors is not to destroy life but to save life," Abraham Jacobi declared. "Doctors do not claim the right to kill."[19] The *Catholic World* explained that the medical profession earned its power and prestige "for the sole reason that they are the protectors . . . of human life." This commitment to life was "the raison d'etre of the medical profession, and the respect and reverence which it has won among men. If its members abandon it, they, as professional men, commit suicide.[20] "The duty of the physician . . . is to conserve life, not to destroy it," insisted obstetrician William Dorland. "How long would any . . . medical man retain the confidence of the public if it became known that he terminated life when he thought it expedient to do so?"[21]

Allowing doctors to withhold treatment from newborns also threatened to undermine one of the key arguments obstetricians used in their ongoing struggle to supplant the midwives who still delivered almost half of all urban births in 1915. Obstetricians often accused midwives of aiding mothers who wished to abort or kill unwanted fetuses and infants.[22] Giving doctors the authority to let impaired babies die could blur what obstetricians saw as a crucial distinction between themselves and midwives, their supposed commitment to preserving life.

While these repeated claims that it is a doctor's duty never to kill seem clear and unambiguous, they actually could mean two very different things:

1. A doctor's duty is to actively oppose all killing.
2. If society wants some people killed, they'll either have to get someone else to do it, or else change the doctor's social contract.

Only the first version required doctors to become professionally involved in social policy, and only that version committed them to opposing selective infanticide itself. The second version was fully compatible with indifference to, or support for, eugenic euthanasia, so long as someone else took the responsibility. Of Haiselden's prominent critics, only a few nonphysicians like Jane Addams held the first view consistently enough to oppose war and other state-sponsored killing. Most of those who opposed giving doctors such authority endorsed only the second version, and many were startlingly candid about the limits of their concerns.

"The physician has no right under the laws, as they exist, to terminate the life of a new born infant. . . . There exists at the present time no process of law by which this, however desirable, can be accomplished," explained Columbia University obstetrician Edward Colie Jr. His colleague James Miller of Johns Hopkins agreed. The University of Chicago's John Webster held that "an obstetrician has not any right to kill or allow to die. . . . It would be necessary to have definite authorization from the State in regard to such a practice."[23]

The state had the right to kill those who threatened collective security, in war and in executions. And hereditary diseases might pose a similar threat. But while executioners may serve a needed social function, "under no circumstances is the medical man to assume the responsibilities or obligations of an executioner," wrote another leading obstetrician. "Our duty as medical men is first to prolong life," explained another medical professor. "The world undoubtedly would be better off if we could do away with the imbeciles, the hopelessly insane, the habitual criminals, etc., but that is not what we as medical men have the right to determine. Let society at large decide that question." Virginia obstetrics professor William Macon put it most frankly, "Our duty is to keep alive, and not to destroy life—this, if for nothing else, is to keep our hands clean, metaphorically speaking."[24]

Such blunt comments are thick with meaning. They presume a hierarchical division of labor between medicine and politics, in which killing remains a state monopoly, and doctors are not to be agents of the state. And they treat judgments about the value of life as subjective political or social questions, and therefore outside the authority of medical science.

Doctors who rejected this expansion of medical power ironically shared the same faith in scientific objectivity that led Helen Keller to propose doctor's juries for defectives. But while lay reformers such as Keller and medical crusaders such as Haiselden believed that the scientific method could be applied objectively to any social problem, these prominent physicians concluded that ethics and politics were inherently subjective and therefore beyond the professional role of an objective scientific doctor.

These remarks highlight a distinction too often overlooked by historians trying to understand the relationship between eugenics and medicine. By 1915 many doctors had concluded eugenic euthanasia was bad medicine, but that did not mean they considered it bad social policy. Those who ringingly denounced selective killing as a dangerous conflation of politics with medicine included many who were personally indifferent to or even enthusiastic about the elimination of defectives, so long as someone else took responsibility and the medical profession could "keep our hands clean." Likewise, those who attacked eugenic euthanasia as a threat to doctors' professional autonomy and scientific objectivity still may have supported eugenic selection under state or other social auspices.[25]

Eugenics and Gender Politics within Families and in Society

Eugenic euthanasia involved a gendered struggle for power, not only between male doctors and mothers, but between men and women within the family and in society at large. Many observers concluded that not treating impaired infants would affect women's power in these broader cultural arenas. But not even those most committed to women's rights could agree on whether Haiselden's crusade would aid or hinder their own cause.

In the conflict between doctors and parents, eugenicists often favored empowering male experts over mothers. But in conflicts between lay men and lay women, eugenics was often depicted as supporting the women. Eugenics could empower women by giving them authority to control male sexual behavior and to exercise their own reproductive choices in the name of objective science and better babies. Such ideas had roots in nineteenth-century arguments for "voluntary motherhood," but in the 1910s they appeared most frequently in works aimed at the increasingly female audience for mass culture.

Motion pictures repeatedly depicted eugenic reformers as forceful women who imposed restraints on male behavior. As will be detailed in chapter 7, anti-eugenic comedies often emphasized this image to ridicule the movement. But female control was also portrayed positively in pro-eugenic commercial and educational films on social hygiene. That genre blamed "bad girls" for men's moral failings, but such films also insisted that men live up to the sexual conduct demanded by scientifically informed "good girls." By 1915 eugenics was so associated with women in the mass media that *Forum* magazine felt it necessary to remind its readers that the subject was "—For Men Also."[26]

Yet neither the mass media nor the leading feminists of the 1910s could agree on how Haiselden's actions would affect the power of women within families or in society. Advocates of women's rights in this period used two different kinds of arguments, appealing on one hand to women's special moral fitness for power based on their unique instincts and experiences as potential mothers, and on the other hand claiming equality with men as a matter of objective similarity of talents and a gender-blind definition of justice.[27] Proponents of women's power used both maternalist and egalitarian assumptions to assess whether or not infant euthanasia was good for women. But their published quotations portrayed no consensus.

Haiselden's feminist critics included many proponents of maternalism, such as Jane Addams and Children's Bureau head Julia Lathrop. From their perspective, eugenic infanticide weakened society's commitment to child welfare, while the decisions of women such as Mrs. Bollinger undermined the claim that mothers were the natural guardians of children. Lathrop found it "almost unspeakable that a mother should desire the death of a child."[28] But others such as egalitarian feminist author LaReine Baker opposed eugenic infanticide while denouncing all appeals to exclusive maternal values.[29]

Backers of selective treatment used the same range of feminist principles to show that their position would empower women. Maternalists asserted that women's love for children would prevent any abuse of eugenics so long as mothers controlled the decisions. They also felt that eugenics would deepen society's commitment to better babies and thus raise the status and power of childrearing. And socialist feminists argued that the special needs of poor women required their access to both birth control and selective infanticide.[30] From an egalitarian perspective, the complex patriarch Simon Baruch pointed to support for Haiselden by many women doctors as a vindication of his view that women physicians could overcome their maternal sympathies to be as objective as a man.[31]

Furthermore, many advocates of women's power mixed both egalitarian and maternalist concepts simultaneously. Women's Party financial angel Alva Belmont felt that nontreatment decisions should be left to a committee of objective medical experts, but she urged that "in all justice and fairness" half the members should be women doctors. "Both as mothers and as citizens, women should have an equal say in any matter of a life or death decision for their children."[32]

Haiselden's crusade, like eugenics as a whole, was widely portrayed as likely to influence women's power in the family and in society. But the ensuing debate shows just how unclear many people were in the 1910s about what direction that influence would take and how to assess its value.

Specialization and the Limits of Objectivity

So long as different technical experts all followed the objective methods of science, most progressives expected that different kinds of specialists would produce complementary results. But in the debate over eugenic euthanasia this key assumption unravelled. The scientific method proved insufficient to unite either the medical profession or the progressive reformers. The resulting conflict provides an early example of an impending crisis of faith in objectivity that helps explain both the ambivalent relation between eugenics and other progressive reforms, and the debate over whether progressivism constituted a cohesive social movement.

Eugenicists like Haiselden shared a characteristic progressive faith in the power of the scientific method to objectively resolve social conflicts. Yet they denounced many of the most important health and welfare measures promoted by other progressives, blaming them for multiplying the ranks of the unfit.

And while most advocates of selective treatment favored leaving the decisions to scientific medical experts, different medical specialties endorsed vastly different conclusions, each claiming to have derived its position from its science. The findings of eugenics seemed to support withholding therapy; but pediatrics, obstetrics, and orthopedic surgery offered reasons to hope new techniques might preserve and improve the lives of impaired newborns.

In 1915 neither medical technology nor social reform had yet contributed much to preserving high-risk newborns. Infant mortality had begun to decline dramatically, beginning about 1910; however, virtually none of this improvement can be attributed to increased survival of those under a month old.

The only technical advance in caring for newborns during this era was the late-nineteenth-century invention of incubators for premature babies. Chicago doctors led the introduction of these devices into American medical practice, but even in Chicago physicians rarely used them. Well into the 1920s, incubators were primarily sideshow curiosities at fairs and exhibitions. Chicago had one of the earliest incubator–baby amusement park displays by 1905. Although Dr. Joseph De Lee established an incubator station at Chicago Lying–In Hospital in 1900, the unit closed only eight years later. Chicago eventually would house the nation's first permanent hospital premature nursery, but it did not open until 1922.[33]

While impaired newborns were no more likely to survive in 1915 than they had been for decades before, significant advances were being made in orthopedic surgery, rehabilitation, and physical therapy. From the 1870s on, these specialties had learned to improve the lives and functioning of those impaired children who survived infancy. They were the source of hope that medicine was on the verge of conquering birth defects.[34]

Many of Haiselden's critics cited the rapid progress of medical science as meaning that today's defective might be made into tomorrow's useful citizen. "Even defectives should not be allowed to die without every effort to give them a chance," suffragist Dr. Anna Howard Shaw declared. "We must remember that what has seemed incurable in one generation has often proved curable in the light of later discoveries." Others were even more upbeat about the pace of scientific progress. "If a defective life can be held intact for say three years longer," one social scientist predicted in 1915, "surgery and medicine will have advanced enough to remove all deficiencies, physical and mental."[35] Such critics shared, even exceeded, Haiselden's faith in the power of science to purge humanity of its imperfections; they disagreed about which specialty, therapeutics or eugenics, would produce and control this progress.

Haiselden blamed medical advances for "sav[ing] imbeciles at birth."[36] He contrasted "Surgery, bidding me follow the old pathway" of saving all lives, with the higher benevolence of his new specialty, "the Greater Surgery."[37] As a eugenicist and a general surgeon, Haiselden may have feared that future advances in surgical rehabilitation would elevate that specialty over his own. What specialists in orthopedics, plastic surgery, and physical therapy considered successful rehabilitation, Haiselden denounced as a vicious fraud, poisoning the human germ plasm.

> Specialists . . . are secured and the defective is trained as a dog or a parrot is trained. Physical deformities, if there are any, are smoothed away. The brain may be so weak that it can scarcely be called a brain at all, and yet . . . little tricks and graces are cleverly instilled into the empty hull until after a number of years it may pass as a normal human being. And here is the deadly danger.[38]

These conflicts between eugenics and pediatrics did not produce a complete separation by 1915. Until the Bollinger case, most eugenicists avoided criticizing efforts to lower infant mortality, and the 1915 meeting of the Association for the Study and Prevention of Infant Mortality still had an official Section on Eugenics. But Haiselden's activities both accelerated and illustrated the growing rivalry between them. At the conclusion of *The Black Stork*, Haiselden weighs a healthy infant to demonstrate its hefty fitness. The camera captured his unpracticed fumbling effort to put the head-end of the baby in the foot-end of the scale (Fig. 23), thus providing an amusing if apparently unintentional confirmation of the extent to which specialization had already distinguished the professional skills of pediatricians from those of surgeons.[39]

Published comments attributed to medical specialists and to Progressive Party supporters disproportionately opposed Haiselden's actions (as discussed in chapter 2). But these statements do not reflect any disagreement between eugenicists and progressives on the value of specialized expertise. Instead, this was a case in which one specialty challenged the authority of several other medical and social specialties, and the challenged disciplines united to defend their turf. Haiselden fought other progressives over whose specialty was most important, not over the importance of specialization.

This rivalry among specialists for jurisdiction over the problem of impaired newborns was characteristic of many similar disputes among progressives, visible as early as 1906 in the conflict among chemists, nutritionists, and bacteriologists over defining the goals of pure food and milk inspection.[40] The frequency of such conflicts has led several historians to deny that the term "progressive" had any coherent meaning.[41]

Haiselden's example suggests that progressivism may better be understood as a shared set of methodological assumptions, rather than a single set of coherent social programs. Haiselden and many other progressives shared a common faith in the methods of scientific inquiry. In social policy as in medicine, they expected specialization to be simply an efficient division of labor that would produce complementary solutions so long as each specialty followed the same objective methods. They did not anticipate the competition and fragmentation that resulted. But to the extent that conflicting values proved intrinsic to both social policy and science, shared assumptions about objective methods did not produce unity, either among physicians or among the reformers who had taken science as their model.[42]

PART II
Publicity

Mass-Media Medicine and Aesthetic Censorship

Publicity, Public Health, and Professional Power

While his refusal to treat deformed babies won a surprising degree of support, Haiselden's decision to take his cause to the mass media aroused far more opposition than his position on euthanasia did. Repeated official investigations upheld his right not to treat such infants. But on March 14, 1916, the Chicago Medical Society voted to expel him, according tó the *New York Times,* based "not on the fact that the physician did not operate on the baby, but because he permitted [the case] to be published . . . in a daily newspaper [and to be] exploited in moving picture shows."[1]

Of course, opposition to Haiselden's propaganda campaign cannot be fully separated from opposition to his not treating impaired babies. The expulsion was almost certainly motivated by more than just the publicity. Haiselden himself charged that hostility to his nontreatment decisions lay behind the Medical Society's action. Regrettably, the precise mix of motives cannot be determined, because the minutes of the Medical Society's lengthy disciplinary proceedings are no longer available.[2]

But publicity was clearly more than just a pretext for punishing Haiselden's refusal to operate. For one thing, the medical profession had long been deeply suspicious of anything that could be construed as self-promotion. Debate over the limits of self-advertising dates back to the dawn of the organized medical profession. From the invention of photography, some medical societies specifically regulated how doctors could be photographed for lay audiences.[3]

These rules against self-promotion originally were meant to prevent competition for business from disrupting professional unity and to preserve a genteel profession's disdain for the demeaning commercial practices of tradesmen. Thus many professional leaders initially suspected Haiselden was simply another upstart doctor using the press to drum up business for himself. Abraham Jacobi dismissed Haiselden with traditional scorn: "He wished to get free advertising, and he has it."[4]

As scientific advances began attracting news coverage of medical researchers and technical specialists, allegations of self-promotion also increasingly reflected the resentment felt by ordinary practitioners at the attention given this new kind of professional elite. In the years just before 1915, the Chicago Medical Society members were genuinely preoccupied with this type of publicity complaint. The Society investigated allegations of self-promotion brought by rank-and-file members against many prominent symbols of the new specialization, including the Mayo Clinic and the American College of Surgeons.[5]

But despite Haiselden's obvious eagerness for personal attention, his crusade did not easily fit these familiar forms of self-advertising. However much he may have craved the limelight, it soon became apparent he was more interested in promoting an idea than in increasing his practice. Such goals raised a different, and much more troubling issue: how much should the lay public be involved in medical controversies?

Concern about this aspect of publicity was not limited to those who criticized Haiselden's refusal to treat the babies. Even people outspoken in their support of letting defectives perish had serious qualms about publicizing such actions. "I think all monstrosities should be permitted to die," wrote one university president from New Mexico, "but I do condemn the physician for making such a public ado about the matter." Columbia University sociology chairman Franklin H. Giddings applauded the death of "molasses-minded" mental defectives, but felt it was a "question that should be considered soberly, thoughtfully and by rigorous intellectual processes. To put it up to the general public in all the emotional and imaginative setting of a photo-play is, in my judgment, an utterly wrong thing to do." In an editorial entitled "He Forgets Silence Is Golden," published a few months after the release of *The Black Stork*, the *New York Times* agreed that Haiselden had the right to decide against treating defectives, but denied his right to discuss it with the public. "If he is wise, as most doctors are, he settles the question for himself . . . and the incident does not become a subject of public discussion."[6]

Other segments of the press, however, vigorously asserted the public's right to participate in such decisions. Hearst's *Chicago American,* the first paper to report the Bollinger baby story, defended its coverage with rousing populist attacks on professional elitism. "The Exaggerated Ego of the Doctors Needs Curbing," admonished one long editorial. "What doctors shall do and shall not do in matters affecting life and death . . . IS THE PUBLIC'S CONCERN, and the public intends to have that fact understood."[7] Even some doctors agreed.[8]

Many physicians had eagerly welcomed the production of medical movies for lay audiences. The growing complexity of medical discoveries and an increasingly heterogeneous population made communication between professionals and the public both more necessary and more difficult. Motion pictures offered a way to bridge the gap. The new level of public faith in scientific expertise was in large measure a mass-media creation. By 1915, only a decade after the first movie theaters had opened, the silent screen was filled with films on every aspect of medicine, from how to bathe the baby to how to avoid venereal disease; all part of an intense campaign to disseminate the discoveries of scientific public health and to promote the power and expertise of the scientific physician. Recent research has just begun to reveal the scope and importance of these films in promoting the turn-of-the-century revolution in public health and medicine.[9]

But while such motion pictures explicitly encouraged people to seek and follow expert professional advice, the very act of appealing to the masses could also undermine professional authority and lead audiences to judge medical issues for themselves. Audiences selectively absorbed and actively reinterpreted the intended messages of early health films, as documented by psychologists John B. Watson and Karl Lashley's studies of World War I–era VD films.[10] And while cinematography could add an aura of modern technology and descriptive realism that heightened the authority of ideas presented on film, doctors and audiences might also see cinema as the epitome of visual trickery and illusion.[11] Thus the medical profession was already deeply ambivalent about health-related films by the time *The Black Stork* first opened in 1916.

The Black Stork, like many early health-education movies, was a feature-length melodrama. And like most health films, it attempted not simply to educate the public about medical facts, but to persuade people to change their personal lives and behavior. These dramatic and propagandistic features were in constant tension with the objective, scientific image medicine sought to convey. The melodramatic style, with its flamboyant histrionics, was poorly adapted to the explication of subtle scientific concepts. And the melodrama's demand for clearly labeled villains and heroes emphasized personal guilt and individual morality at a time when medical science claimed to seek amoral technical causes and cures. The motivational techniques that made effective propaganda further conflicted with the physicians' professional image (Figs. 4 and 5).[12] Haiselden's film in particular used shock, fear, and revulsion as central persuasive techniques. Thus while Haiselden's heavily publicized personal appearance in the movie certainly did violate professional taboos against medical self-advertising (Figs. 6 and 7), the controversy over his propaganda activities went far beyond such traditional concerns.[13]

There is yet another indicator that criticism of Haiselden's propaganda was based on more than simply his not treating impaired newborns. Dr. Martin Couney, a pioneer in saving sick babies, also used motion pictures as well as world's fair exhibits and a Coney Island sideshow to promote incubator therapy for preserving the lives of premature infants. Couney's promotional techniques in favor of saving impaired newborns were attacked almost as vehemently as Haiselden's opposing campaign, and for most of the same reasons.[14]

Medical Movies and the Rise of Aesthetic Censorship

While doctors divided over the medical value of the movies, the fledgling film industry was also very bitterly split over the appropriateness of medical topics for the screen. Film pioneers such as Thomas Edison initially hoped that shows presenting serious health issues would improve the image of the new medium and attract a higher class of clientele. But in response to *The Black Stork*, producers, exhibitors, and critics began to demand movies that provided entertainment, not intellectually demanding, emotionally upsetting, or aesthetically unpleasant medical topics. *The Black Stork* and similar medical films played a key role in the emergence of "aesthetic censorship," and in the construction of genre distinctions that reserved commercial film theaters for "entertainment." *The Black Stork* played an important role in the history of film as well as of eugenics.[15]

The rise of aesthetic controversy over medical films can be seen quite clearly in the critical reaction to *The Black Stork*. The *Chicago Post* reviewer called it a "powerful" picture, produced "with the touch of a master." The *Cleveland Plain Dealer* praised the film as both "enlightening" and having "a cleverly worked out plot" that gave it "more than mere clinical value." *Variety* likewise lauded the film's educational impact: "It is bound to make one stop and think— think real hard."[16] The *Exhibitor's Trade Review* declared the film "impressively forceful," "driven home with the cold steel of truth," and reassured theater owners that it was neither morally offensive nor dangerously radical.

However, while many critics praised its educational and social value, they found it aesthetically unacceptable. Despite the film's virtues, *Exhibitor's Trade Review* concluded it was "a grim form of entertainment." *Motography* agreed, noting that while "it argues its case well," and "[t]here can be no doubt of the interest," "[t]he picture is depressing and unpleasant."[17] *Wid's Film Daily* found the film an "impressive preachment" but its depiction of "repulsive" defectives made it poor entertainment.[18] Louella Parsons complained that it was "neither a pretty nor a pleasant picture," because "it shows poor, misshapen bodies of miserable little children." Rival critic Kitty Kelly called it the "most repellent picture" she had ever seen. The *Chicago Tribune* admitted the "ideas may be all right," but found the film "as pleasant to look at as a running sore." Pursuing such clinical metaphors to the limit, *Photoplay* called Lait's screenplay "so slimy that it reminds us of nothing save the residue of a capital operation."[19]

Similar aesthetic concerns also affected the print media. Surveying press coverage of the Bollinger case, *Current Opinion* noted, "Some newspapers spared readers from medical details on the ground that they were too revolting to print." Others apologized profusely for the necessity of discussing such indelicate subjects.[20]

By mid-1917 other eugenic films encountered the same aesthetic objections. The *Moving Picture World* admitted that *Married in Name Only* contained "scenes full of loveliness," "perfect" photography, and great "entertainment value," "when taken by themselves." But the beauty of these scenes was overwhelmed by the "distressing" story and the depictions of "morbid conditions" that made the picture overall "more an offense than a pleasure."[21] *Wid's* review of the eugenic film *Parentage* warned that unlike 1914 when " 'Damaged Goods' made a lot of money . . . today propaganda films that . . . tend in any way to show unnecessary objectionable or disgusting details are absolutely not wanted."[22]

Such unintended viewer revulsion was a key reason that *The Black Stork* and other films about eugenics often were banned. In turn the desire to eliminate such unpleasant medical topics from entertainment films spurred censors to go beyond policing sexual morality, to create and enforce aesthetic as well as moral standards for the new medium. "Picture devotees have no objection to swallowing their bitter pills sugar coated," explained the *Chicago Daily News*, but *The Black Stork* "should have been pounced on by the censors."[23]

Haiselden's film was repeatedly "pounced on" by censors and film industry regulators who objected to it as much on aesthetic grounds as for its sexual subject or its support for eugenic euthanasia. The powerful New York State Motion Picture Division rejected the film in April 1923 not only for its "inhuman" attitude toward infants but because of its "most unpleasant," "very distressing," "most revolting" depictions of disease.[24]

In a late-1916 private straw poll of community leaders from across the country, the film industry's voluntary accrediting body, the National Board of Review of Motion Pictures, found that 36 of its 52 respondents (70 percent) who expressed an opinion on the issue felt that *The Black Stork* should not be given board approval.[25] One-quarter of them (9) included aesthetic objections to the depiction of diseases among their complaints. They repeatedly insisted that audiences who might want to see "scenes that are abnormal" must themselves be sick, suffering from a "morbid" perversion of the aesthetic senses. These film regulators and censors shared the eugenic desire to pathologize ugliness, but they feared that displaying ugly diseases would only create diseased audiences.

Some opponents meant it literally when they insisted that film depictions of disease were sickening. *Variety* critic Jonathan Lowe worried that *The Black Stork's* vivid portraits of defectives would cause birth defects if pregnant women were allowed to see them. Others who believed that powerful emotions influenced bodily health in adults insisted that films like *The Black Stork* threatened the health of all viewers, not just the captive fetal audience.[26]

Even two opponents of compulsory censorship among the NBRMP's advisers hoped that *The Black Stork's* aesthetic offenses could be eliminated by industry self–censorship. Lawyer Charles Elkus felt that public "revulsion" at Haiselden's film would be sufficient to prevent future movies on "unpleasant . . . sex problems." Suffragist and University of Michigan English professor Mary Gray Peck warned that the film industry faced a public backlash unless it voluntarily stopped "dealing with pathological sex subjects. The industry simply doesn't see the storm that is gathering."[27]

Film historian Tom Gunning has noted that the earliest movies offered audiences an "aesthetic of astonishment" whose pleasures derived not from the contemplation of beauty but from the exhibition of marvels and the production of shocking thrills. Health and science films that featured huge enlargements of wriggling pathogenic bacteria and disease-carrying insects, and dramas that displayed human deformities, such as *The Little Cripple* (Pathé 1908), owed much of their attraction to this "anti-aesthetic."[28] Such depictions of disease made many health films particular targets of the new aesthetic censors.

The Black Stork thus helped provoke, and in turn became one of the first casualties of, a growing movement to censor films for their aesthetic content.[29] In 1918 the Pennsylvania State Board of Censors revised its official list of film "standards." The new regulations barred virtually all unpleasant aspects of medicine from the commercial screen. "Incidents having to do with eugenics" or "race suicide" were specifically prohibited, as were "pictures which deal with venereal disease, of any kind." Medical films were targeted not just for their possible sexual content but for their aesthetic and emotional effects. The new standards banned any "gruesome and unduly distressing scenes," including "surgical operations," "men dying," or depictions of the "insane."

During the 1920s, other state and national film regulators adopted and expanded the Pennslvania board's aesthetic objections to medical films. In 1930, these precedents were standardized in the first Production Code of the Motion Pictures Producers and Directors of America. This code barred "sex hygiene," "venereal diseases," and other sexual pathologies as "not proper subjects for theatrical motion pictures." In addition, the code labeled "surgical operations" one of seven "repellent subjects" that would receive special scrutiny, and it included a catchall restriction on all other "disgusting, unpleasant, though not necessarily evil, subjects" that was used to eliminate most other graphic depictions of diseases. The preamble explicitly defined the fundamental goals of censorship as the promotion of "ENTERTAINMENT" and "ART."[30]

Aesthetic censorship banned the subject of eugenics regardless of what position a film took on the issue. *Tomorrow's Children*, a 1934 melodrama attacking compulsory sterilizations, ran afoul of the censors for the same reason they opposed pro-eugenic films such as *The Black Stork*. In a three-year court battle that successfully defended their ban of *Tomorrow's Children*, the New York State censors insisted that eugenics was too "disgusting" a topic to appear in theaters reserved for amusement. "The sterilization of human beings is not a decent subject for public entertainment."[31]

Aesthetic objections to medical films not only played a key role in the evolution of film censorship but also helped define the boundaries of the classic Hollywood film. Medical films such as *The Black Stork* spurred the construction of distinctions between "entertainment" and such genres as education, propaganda, and exploitation films, and led to the physical segregation of the places where these genres could be shown. *Moving Picture World* complained about *The Black Stork* that while "the revelation of such a subject is of vital importance to humanity," it should be shown at eugenics society meetings and in medical schools. "The place to exploit it is not the moving picture theater." "[F]ilms of 'The Black Stork' order . . . should find other places," declared the *Chicago Daily News*. "The theater is a place for entertainment."[32] "Nontheatrical," the catchall term for any film whose aspirations went beyond pleasant entertainment, indicates the extent to which genre and geography coincided to keep alternatives to Hollywood in their place.[33]

Especially in the transitional years from 1915 to 1920, critics and censors sometimes distinguished between the exhibition of "real" disease victims and the use of "normal" actors to simulate illnesses or disabilities. Some of the same people who castigated *The Black Stork*'s display of Haiselden's actual impaired patients praised Henry Bergman for his artful enactment of "The Defective" in the film's vision sequences (as will be seen in chapter 8). This distinction conflated two different senses of "art"—the aesthetic and the artificial—asserting the aesthetic superiority of a skillfully crafted illusion over the act of mere documentation. It thereby distinguished "legitimate" movie art from peep shows, circuses, wax museums, medicine shows, carnivals, and similar productions that invited audiences to gape at actual freaks.

In this transitional period, even films of people with actual disabilities could sometimes pass muster if they were sufficiently entertaining and presented without ugliness or distress. Helen Keller appeared in her own film biography *Deliverance* (1919), and a series of other post–World War I films depicted the inspiring rehabilitation of wounded veterans.[34] But even these genres virtually disappeared from commercial theaters under assault from aesthetic censors in the 1920s. When it was released in 1932, Tod Browning's MGM film *Freaks* was the first film in over a decade to portray people with genuine disabilities, and it met strong critical condemnation. The *New York Times* review began by questioning "whether it should be shown at the Rialto— . . . or in, say, the Medical Centre."[35]

"Propaganda" was another genre only just being defined and gradually excluded from entertainment theaters in 1917. Both supporters and critics labeled *The Black Stork* a propaganda film but disagreed over what that term meant and whether it was a good or a bad thing. Newly invented media of mass persuasion appealed to many progressive reformers as a way to get people to follow expert technical advice without having to use direct state coercion, a means of reconciling the power of a scientific elite with the values of democracy and individualism. Progressive health educators proudly called their work "health propaganda."[36] Even the executive secretary of the NBRMP wrote in 1917, "[A]ll serious propaganda is . . . an earnest effort toward social betterment." "Is the motion picture not to be allowed to help the betterment of society?"[37]

But critics, censors and the entertainment industry claimed that audiences were growing increasingly intolerant of celluloid reformers. "The Black Stork is no entertainment; it's a preachment," wrote critic Kitty Kelly. Her objection was not that propaganda was deceptive or manipulative, but that it was rarely entertaining. She contrasted *The Black Stork* with *Enlighten Thy Daughter*, a sex-education film that opened two weeks later, writing of the latter: "It is direct propaganda, this picture, but so clothed in human story dramatically as to command interest."[38]

Some censors wanted to limit movie theaters to purely entertainment films. One adviser to the NBRMP opposed showing *The Black Stork* because it was "a distinct propaganda . . . rather than a consideration of the question in an open minded manner." According to another NBRMP adviser, the Minneapolis censorship board ruled "as a general proposition the so called educational and propaganda film for commercial use is to be condemned. . . . People go to the movies for recreation, amusement."[39]

In response to films like *The Black Stork*, film regulators used their power not only to create new aesthetic genre boundaries, but also to ban films which attacked or offended powerful institutions like the church or the medical profession. The same 1918 Pennsylvania regulations which inaugurated aesthetic censorship also prohibited "irreverent" depictions of "religious bodies" and ridicule of medical institutions.

Catholic Church opposition to euthanasia and eugenics influenced many film censors' responses to *The Black Stork*. Despite NBRMP Executive Secretary W. D. McGuire's position that the board was not obligated to follow church dictates "so long as a picture is not of a sacrilegious nature," one board adviser explained that he opposed Haiselden's film for the simple reason that "it is opposed by the church."[40] When Haiselden was invited to lecture at a performance of a pro-eugenic stage play, *The Unborn*, a personal appeal from New York's Cardinal Farley led the city license commissioner to ban the production.[41]

Censors and film industry regulators also often shared the medical profession's hostility to public discussion of medical controversies. Sociologist Franklin H. Giddings, in his role as NBRMP adviser, strongly opposed *The Black Stork* for involving the public in what should have been a sober decision by experts. One colleague worried that there was a large "class of moving picture patrons not mentally capable of grasping the significance of the subject." Others advised the NBRMP that "to present it in this manner to a popular audience would certainly tend to incite people to take the law into their own hands. . . ." "[I]f such a question is to be discussed at all, it should be in executive session by great doctors, or in the council of trained moralists and not by the public generally."[42] They felt that media self-censorship was essential to protect medical decision making from irrational public pressures, including political demands to expand the killing of defectives beyond medically acceptable limits.[43] The NBRMP condemned Haiselden's film in 1917 partly because "showing Dr. Haiselden refusing to save the baby's life might influence people to destroy the life of children whom they do not desire." The board's General Committee initially had voted 10–9 to approve *The Black Stork* if the plot were changed to make it clear that individual doctors and parents could not override the ethics of the medical profession. In the proposed revision, Haiselden would present his arguments for euthanasia but would abide by the judgment of the medical society. The baby would be treated and would grow up to become a criminal menace as predicted. Haiselden approved these changes, but they were never made.

NBRMP Executive Secretary W. D. McGuire urged his committee to judge the film for itself, and "not be governed in its decisions by the ethics of [the medical] profession." But the board concluded its 1917 consideration of *The Black Stork* by ruling the film was only fit for medical audiences. By 1928 the New York State censors rejected the film because any movie that "is against the ethics of the Medical Profession . . . can hardly conform to the statutes of the Motion Picture Division."[44]

Mass culture was a battleground on which many conflicting visions competed. Eugenic popularizers like Haiselden used film to promote their concepts of beauty and health. But such efforts evoked unintended meanings and provoked unwanted consequences, including the rise of aesthetic censorship and the marginalization of medical motion pictures.

While Haiselden's activities provoked intense debate over the proper relation between medicine and the mass media, one important concern in that relationship today was conspicuously missing from this controversy. Haiselden's lack of concern for patient confidentiality went completely uncriticized. He released the names and addresses of the patients involved in these cases, allowed reporters to interview them in the hospital, and permitted newspaper and movie cameramen to photograph the mothers, babies, and even the other siblings. Mrs. Bollinger initially requested that her identity not be published, and the *Chicago American* did keep her name out of their first story. She repeated her objections when Haiselden proposed using her name in his own publications, but she reportedly gave in after he convinced her that publicity would give meaning to her loss.[45] Even if all the mothers had agreed to the publicity

7

Eugenics on Film

Many in the movie world objected to *The Black Stork* not only because they found it unpleasant and controversial, but because they opposed eugenics. The film industry often lumped eugenicists with those they considered puritanical elitist reformers, hostile to all working-class amusements, from saloons to dance halls, not incidentally including movie houses.[1] And the eugenic movement's opposition to immigration likely alienated some of the immigrants who were rapidly coming to prominence in the film industry.

Still the silent screen was far from "silent" about eugenics. Dozens of films depicted eugenics and heredity before the rise of aesthetic censorship. Today, all but a handful have crumbled into dust, and most are completely unknown, even to specialists in cinema history. Many were one-reelers, for which there are still no adequate subject indexes. Even to discover their existence required page-by-page searches of old film trade magazines. In some cases, little can be learned about them beyond their titles. But for many, enough information has survived so that it is possible to reconstruct something of their content.

Early filmmakers quickly discovered that attacks on eugenics had great entertainment potential. The eugenic belief that rational science should outweigh passionate love as the motive for mating made eugenics a tempting target for comedic ridicule. The same conflict between science and love also made eugenics a fitting obstacle to be surmounted in romantic melodrama. "Love Conquers All" was always big box office; "Love Conquers Eugenics" fit the formula precisely.

Anti-eugenic farces began as early as 1904, with Edison's *The Strenuous Life, or Anti-Race Suicide,* when movies were still in transition from peep shows to nickelodeon theaters. President Theodore Roosevelt had recently popularized the belief that middle-class native-born Americans were committing "race suicide" by not having enough children. This four-minute-long film satirizes such calls for increased fertility by showing the shock and rage of a wealthy New York businessman as the doctor hands him each of his newly delivered quadruplets.

Later one-reel comedies, such as *Eugenics at the Bar "U" Ranch* (Selig 1914) and *Snakeville's Eugenic Marriage* (Essanay 1915), lampoon another stereotype associated with ex-cowpoke Roosevelt—the cowboy as a paragon of masculine physical fitness. The Bar U Ranch (whose name puns on eugenic snobbery) is visited by "Martha, an old maid," who is an ardent eugenicist in search of "a perfect mate among the sturdy men of the unspoiled west." When she subjects them to physical examinations, the cowboys fake all manner of disabilities to discourage her advances, until they find out she is rich, at which point the "best looking cowboy" consents to marry her.

Snakeville passes a law requiring medical approval of marriages. But when "Dr. McSwat" conducts a series of "astonishing" (and painful) examinations that cast doubt on the fitness of "Slippery Slim," Slim's fiance pummels the doctor into providing the required certificate.

Wood B. Wedd and the Microbes (Edison 1914) caricatures eugenics as an absurd effort to rationalize romance. His intended mate informs the hapless Wedd, "If you meet the eugenic test our two hearts will merge in one." As in the other comedies, much of the film is devoted to physical humor. Wedd's love subjects him to one painful and humiliating medical ordeal after another, but when she puts him in a steam bath for three hours to sterilize him (of his germs), Wedd finally abandons the quest.

Other anti-eugenic comedies included *A Case of Eugenics* (Vitagraph 1915), *The Eugenic Boy* (Thanhouser 1914), *A Foe to Race Suicide* (Kleine 1912), *Their Mutual Child* (American 1920), *The Very Idea* (Metro 1920, RKO 1929), and of course, *Eugenics Versus Love* (Beauty 1914). Not surprisingly, in *Eugenics Versus Love,* love wins. In an obvious caricature of Kellogg, the story concerns a eugenic contest sponsored by a breakfast food company located in "Battle River." The unwilling male winner successfully conspires to marry his own sweetheart rather than the female winner the judges have selected for him. (The film appeared the same year as "Love or Eugenics," a satiric song contributed to the Princeton Triangle Show by undergraduate F. Scott Fitzgerald.)[2]

In each of these comedies, eugenics is depicted as something imposed by emotionless professionals and rich fanatics, often women, in conflict with the feelings and choices of working-class men.

Anti-eugenic dramas included *The Eugenic Girl* (Selig 1914), *Are They Born or Made?* (Warner 1917), *A Daughter's Strange Inheritance* (Broadway Star-Vitagraph 1917), *A Victim of Heredity* (Kalem 1913), *The Power of Mind* (Mutual 1916), and the classic-of-its-kind, *A Disciple of Nietzsche* (Thanhouser 1915).

The Power of Mind argues that most "hereditary" influence is really caused by suggestion. A girl begins stealing when she discovers her father was a criminal, but she returns to honesty when a doctor tricks her into believing she was only adopted.

A Disciple of Nietzsche was a three-reel melodrama written by Paul Lonergan and featuring well-known actress Florence LaBadie. The title character, an American professor, quotes with approval long passages attributed to the German philosopher, such as: "[C]harity merely converts the unfit—who, in the course of nature, would soon die out . . . —into parasites—who live on indefinitely, a nuisance and a burden to their betters." When his daughter, a settlement house volunteer, attempts to aid a young girl of the slums, the professor pronounces the girl "one of the unfit" and drives her from his home. But supported by the love of a foreman in her factory, the girl overcomes her disadvantages, and in a dramatic reversal, rescues the professor's daughter from an impending slide into criminality, against which the daughter's wealth and breeding had been no protection. "Nietzsche has lost one disciple," the professor announces. "Never more will I despise the weak."[3]

In most of these dramas, love triumphs over eugenics when the healing power of true devotion cures a young girl of her inherited tendencies toward evil. But the power of love apparently only affected female genes. None of these films tried to claim that love could overcome a man's hereditary defects.

Most eugenicists strenuously denied the validity of the conflict between eugenics and love on which all these films depended. Michael Guyer called it an "utter misconception" and proclaimed "The Best Eugenic Marriage Also a Love Match." Haiselden insisted that eugenics sought to improve love, not destroy it, by freeing it from unscientific delusions. But even a few eugenics advocates accepted the mass-media depictions. Based on an extensive survey of satirical images, the eugenics columnist in Kellogg's *Good Health* magazine found "it is Cupid who suffers most at the hands of Eugenics," and admitted "the cartoonists are largely right in their interpretation of the spirit of Eugenics."[4]

Immediately after the Bollinger case, several filmmakers rushed to attack Haiselden's actions. Within a month of the baby's death, Pathé films released a fourteen-episode serial, *The Red Circle*. Like the other anti-eugenic dramas, this film portrayed a woman whose inherited criminal tendencies were overcome by a loving environment. Although the series had been planned before the Bollinger case, ads for the film seized on the resulting publicity to ask in bold headlines whether Dr. Haiselden would have been justified in allowing such a baby to die.[5]

In *The Regeneration of Margaret* (Essanay 1916), a Chicago-made film clearly based on the Bollinger debate, a handicapped newborn girl is abandoned to die by one doctor, but a second doctor saves her life and raises her as his daughter. She grows up to become a nurse. When the doctor who refused to treat her becomes paralyzed in his old age, she taunts him to carry out his own beliefs against saving defectives, and to kill himself.[6]

As eugenic legislation gained ground in the 1920s, those few anti-eugenic films that continued to be produced despite the growing censorship became increasingly shrill and melodramatic, a trend that culminated in the 1934 feature *Tomorrow's Children*. This Bryan Foy and Crane Wilbur production attacked the 1927 Supreme Court ruling that upheld compulsory sterilizations.[7]

The film depicts the harrowing ordeal of a young woman sentenced to be neutered because her parents and siblings are unemployed drunks and defectives. The various eugenicists—a physician, a judge, and several social workers—all are portrayed as vicious, corrupt, narrow-minded, or incompetent. And one of the key protagonists, a Catholic priest, delivers a sermon denouncing all sterilization as immoral. But the film's conclusion undercuts this sweeping indictment. Instead, Foy and Wilbur provide a last-minute revelation that the girl was only the stepchild of defectives, a resolution that echoes Miriam's reprieve in *The Black Stork*. Rather than arguing that forcing anyone to be sterilized is wrong, the ending settles for the narrower point that, while many defectives deserve to be sterilized, unacceptable mistakes will be made and some "innocents" will get hurt. Perhaps this conclusion was intended to appear more "even-handed" in an (unsuccessful) effort to avoid censorship; perhaps it seemed more effective to attack eugenics for its side effects rather than its basic premises. More likely it was an example of the filmmakers' sacrificing the power of their message to achieve a happy ending that would leave audiences feeling good.[8]

Several dramas did argue in support of hereditary determinism. *Heredity* (Biograph 1912), *Heredity* (Broadway Star 1915), *Inherited Sin* (Universal 1915), *The Power of Heredity* (Rex 1913), and *The Second Generation* (Pathé 1914) all featured characters whose inherited diseases and criminality proved resistant to the benefits of love and good environments, or whose hereditary good traits survived unfavorable surroundings. In *The Second Generation*, a young man, actually the fourth generation of hereditary lunatics, thinks he can be saved by the love of a good woman, but the family doctor convinces him not to marry. His resolve to obey the doctor comes just in time, as the family disease begins to manifest itself, and he is hauled away to an asylum shortly thereafter.

In the 1915 *Heredity*, a criminal's daughter grows up vicious despite having been adopted by a wealthy loving family, while a normal girl remains honest and productive even though she is adopted by a poor family who put her to work in a dress factory at age fourteen. *The Power of Heredity* achieved some originality by discussing the inheritance of class without linking it to crime or disease. The daughter of poor parents is adopted in infancy by a rich family, but drawn by her inherited class tastes, she falls in love with the butler.

While antihereditarian dramas were often billed as attacks on "eugenics," these prohereditarian films rarely advocated any specific eugenic measures and almost never used the word "eugenics" in their advertising. They simply popularized the pessimistic side of the nature–nurture argument.[9]

Both pro- and antihereditarian films were produced by all types and sizes of film companies in the 1910s, from major studios like

Edison, Pathé, and Biograph, to highly regarded smaller firms like Thanhouser or Selig. Most made only one film on the subject; only four made more than one. Selig and Thanhouser each made two anti-eugenic films, one comedy and one drama apiece. And producers were not always ideologically consistent. Both Broadway Star-Vitagraph and Pathé made both pro- and antihereditarian pictures.

D. W. Griffith dramatized the evolutionary triumph of brains over brawn in *Man's Genesis* (1912). And Griffith made one of the few commercial melodramas to be billed as an explicitly "eugenic" film, *The Escape* (Reliance-Majestic 1914). This picture bears several striking similarities to *The Black Stork* and conceivably could have influenced both Haiselden's film and his practice.

The story of *The Escape*, from a stage play by Paul Armstrong, traces in gruesome detail the awful consequences of human "mismating." The fictional "Joyce" family compresses into two generations all the defects and deviance found among two centuries of Jukes and Kallikaks, including prostitution, venereal disease, birth defects, alcoholism, and criminality. For nearly two hours, audiences witnessed a parade of horrors, such as a drunken father crushing his own baby and a lunatic strangling a cat. A prologue assembled by Dr. Daniel Carson Goodman precedes the drama. It recapitulates the familiar eugenic contrast between care in breeding livestock and lack of attention to human selection.

Yet despite this preliminary emphasis on breeding and selection, the plot of *The Escape* emphasizes the triumph of science and love over bad heredity. The physician-hero cures the lunatic cat-strangler with an operation and redeems the lunatic's sister from a life of sin by marrying her. Although *The Escape* was promoted as the first major pro-eugenic film, "eugenics" did not mean prohibiting procreation by the children of defective parents, but instead meant using love (for women) and surgery (for men) to overcome the effects of poor parenting.[10]

Both pro- and anti-hereditarian films generally shared Weismann's sharp distinction between environment and heredity. They simply disagreed about which force was the stronger. But *The Escape*'s concept of heredity was more ambiguous. *Moving Picture World* saw Griffith as arguing that environment was separate from and more powerful than heredity. But the *New York Dramatic Mirror* read the film as advocating the Lamarckian view that heredity itself can be altered by the environment.[11]

The heavily promoted, critically acclaimed *Parentage* (Hobart

Henley 1917) also was seen as strongly "eugenic." It contrasted the families raised by good and by bad parents. Good parenting was an inseparable combination of heredity and environment, including "prenatal influence," "the environment of the home," and premarital medical exams.[12] In this film as in Griffith's, "eugenics" meant good parenting, not just good genes.

Even educational films billed as pro-eugenic often dealt exclusively with good parenting, not good mating. The Eugenic Film Company's sole production, *Birth* (1917), provided information on neonatal care, apparently without ever discussing biological heredity.[13]

At least three commercial dramas did call for selective marriage restriction on eugenic grounds. Majestic's 1914 two-reel drama *For Those Unborn* features star Blanche Sweet as a consumptive who turns down two suitors rather than risk passing her disease to another generation. Her sacrifice is rewarded however when she discovers she doesn't really have the disease, and she marries the one man who had waited for her.[14]

Married in Name Only, a six-reel melodrama released in 1917, was billed as a "powerful eugenic argument." Producer and co-writer Ivan Abramson specialized in making artistically ambitious films on sexual hygiene and other social problems, such as *Enlighten Thy Daughter*, a 1917 plea for sex education, and *The Sex Lure*, banned in New York the same year.[15] In *Married in Name Only*, the author of a eugenics book discovers on his way to the altar that he has a family history of insanity. Rather than face the disgrace of a canceled wedding, the couple agree to a platonic marriage. After many tense ordeals testing their resolve, their sacrifice and self-control are rewarded when the husband learns he was adopted. In *The Black Stork*, the same device of an unsuspected adoption is used to reward Tom and Miriam, who had refused to marry because they believed Miriam had inherited epilepsy.[16]

This series of unlikely reprieves was almost inevitable, because none of these films could envision an acceptable social role for those judged permanently unfit to marry. The only alternatives were institutionalization *(The Second Generation)* or death *(The Black Stork)*. There was no other place in the social imagination of eugenics for those permanently denied a family. Thus most films opted for a last-minute discovery of a mistaken diagnosis. Critics preferred happy endings. And it was cinematically inconceivable that anyone with the self-control to actually comply with eugenically prescribed celibacy could really be a threat to society. That a life of such virtue could go unrewarded would be to violate the basic moral order of melodrama.

Eugenics was a particularly publicity conscious movement. Eugenic organizations sponsored exhibitions, stage pageants, "better baby contests," and similar activities, including slide and filmstrip presentations such as the eight-part "Race Decline and Race Regeneration," distributed by Dr. Weston A. Price of the Cleveland Dental Research Laboratories.[17] But while most other health-related associations sponsored scores of motion pictures in the 1910s, American eugenics organizations do not seem to have produced any movies about eugenics prior to the late 1930s.

The only American eugenics association known to have made any movies in this period was the Race Betterment Foundation of Battle Creek, Michigan, whose founding president Dr. John Harvey Kellogg was an early advocate of film propaganda. The foundation-sponsored First National Conference on Race Betterment in 1914 included health-related movies at every session, and a representative of Pathé Films even served as an official conference delegate. Yet, of nineteen different movies and slide-sets shown at the conference, only one specifically mentioned eugenics, and then only in the context of venereal disease.[18] At the 1928 Race Betterment Conference, an official of the Motion Picture Producers and Distributors of America served on the "Central Committee." Thirteen health films were shown that year, three of which had been produced by Kellogg. But again not one of the thirteen mentioned eugenics in the titles, and none dealt with issues such as sterilization and selective immigration exclusion, which were central topics of the conference papers.[19]

The National Health Council *Film List*, an annual catalogue of health motion pictures that by 1928 included over 100 pages and nearly 1,000 titles, did not even have a subject-heading for "eugenics." It listed several movies made by the Race Betterment Foundation, but none of them dealt specifically with eugenics, and no other eugenic organizations were represented at all. Almost no references to film could be found in The *Bulletin of the Eugenics Record Office, Eugenical News,* and *Journal of Heredity* in this era; the few exceptions dealt with general reproductive physiology.[20]

The lack of officially sponsored eugenics films is particularly striking in comparison to the extensive film efforts of the closely related social hygiene movement. The earliest film to specifically attack venereal disease was the commercially produced melodrama

Damaged Goods (American 1914, 1915), based on a French stage play by Eugene Brieux that had recently been produced in New York by Frederic Robinson. Social hygiene associations endorsed and used this film. And with entry of the United States into World War I, the American Social Hygiene Association (ASHA) joined with the army and Public Health Service to produce their own series of VD-education films. The first was simply a graphic depiction of clinical lesions, meant to accompany a live lecturer.[21] But this was soon followed by the full-length feature dramas, *Fit to Fight* (1918) for men and *The End of the Road* (1919) for women.[22] A third feature, *Cleared for Action* (1919), was produced for the navy and shown in Chicago in 1919, but apparently was never distributed nationally.[23] The war also stimulated production of at least eight commercially made VD feature films, several of which enjoyed varying degrees of social hygiene association and public health agency sponsorship.[24]

After the war when these films were generally banned from commercial theaters, the social hygiene association and public health officials shifted their film efforts to community groups and schools. The U.S. Public Health Service produced the *Science of Life* series (Bray 1922), while the ASHA released at least eight additional film titles in the 1920s, such as *The Gift of Life* (1920) and *Social Hygiene for Women* (1920), both of which included recycled footage from the wartime films.[25]

In addition, commercial filmmakers of the 1920s continued to reuse the war-era VD films. Samuel Cummins, a private filmmaker who had worked with the New York City Health Department on a 1919 VD film, *Some Wild Oats,* bought all the government social hygiene films in the early 1920s. Cummins reused this footage in an unsuccessful attempt to get his 1920s VD films, such as *T.N.T—The Naked Truth* (1924), into commercial theaters. The banning of this film by Newark, New Jersey, police censor William Brennan played an important role in defining the line between "entertainment" and "exploitation" genres and marked the first exposure to the civil liberties issues in film censorship for Brennan's son, future Supreme Court Justice William J. Brennan Jr.[26]

Many of these films mentioned eugenics. They labeled congenital syphilis as "hereditary," and several, including *S.O.S.: A Message to Humanity* (Sunshine 1917) and *Damaged Goods,* used the word "eugenics" in their promotion.[27] *The Science of Life* included eugenics in three reels on personal and social hygiene. Students were taught that many talents and many failings were inherited, and were urged to check the pedigrees of their intended mates.[28] But except for *The Science of Life*, no social hygiene films dealt with any other aspect of eugenics besides congenital infection, and none was endorsed by any eugenic organizations.

The lack of motion picture production by American eugenicists also contrasts with the activities of their British counterparts. The British Eugenics Society began making movies in 1924. By the end of 1925, they owned two copies of a film produced for them by Mrs. Neville Rolfe, in addition to sponsoring showings of a one-reel film called *Heredity*, made by a British anti-venereal-disease association. In the mid-1930s they produced several editions of *From Generation to Generation*.[29] But in America, it was not until 1936, when eugenic chief publicist Harry Laughlin imported a copy of the Nazi Party film *Erbkrank*, that the Eugenics Record Office first even considered the possibility of making a similar motion picture themselves.[30]

In addition to the social hygiene movement, other health educators included eugenic themes in films about maternal health, birth control, evolution, and temperance. However, the surviving information about most of them is too sketchy to determine their content. *Motherhood, The Backbone of the Nation*, a seven-reel maternal health film produced in 1917 by the Association of Collegiate Alumnae and the California Baby Hygiene Committee, devoted its entire final reel to the problem of "The Defective Child." It detailed the costs of caring for such children, but the surviving script fragments do not indicate what if anything the film advocated doing about them. A ten-part Bray Productions series called *Better Babies* distributed in 1921 included one film entitled *Every Baby's Birthright*.[31]

The Evolution of Man was produced by Dr. Raymond Ditmars in 1922, and Red Seal Pictures released *Evolution* the following year.[32] Pioneer naturalist-cinematographer George E. Stone announced the impending release of a four-reel film called *Heredity* in December 1920, but I could find no evidence that the picture was ever shown nor what it was intended to contain. Stone's previous film, *The Living World* (1920), included a Lamarckian explanation of heredity and evolution but did not mention eugenics.[33]

Films used eugenic arguments both to attack and to defend birth control. *Race Suicide* (Joseph Farnham 1916) urges the middle classes to avoid contraception and produce more children. Its multireel paean to motherhood through the ages culminates with the tragedy of a modern husband who puts his career ahead of his wife's desire for babies until it is too late.[34]

The much-debated works of pioneer Universal director Lois Weber, *Where Are My Children?* (1916) and *The Hand That Rocks the*

Cradle (1917), offer eugenic arguments in favor of contraception. These widely misunderstood films support birth control but oppose abortion. Their primary point is that birth control provides a safe way for women to avoid dangerous and immoral abortions. But Weber's films also depict a eugenic need to control lower-class fertility.[35] One crude imitation of her work, the Chicago-produced *The Law of Population, or Birth Control* (1917), emphasizes the negative eugenic argument for birth control much more heavily, with considerable Malthusian overtones.[36]

Birth control crusader Margaret Sanger, just released from jail, appeared in the semiautobiographical film *Birth Control* (Message Photo-Play 1917). While the film emphasized Sanger's special concern for the health of poor women, not enough is known about it to say whether it also included her growing support for eugenics.[37]

Newsreels also reported on eugenics, though I have not been able to determine how many such stories appeared in the 1910s and 1920s, much less what they said. But the Mutual newsreel covered Frederic Robinson's 1915 campaign for eugenic birth control.[38]

Several temperance films specifically included the claim that alcohol produced birth defects by damaging the germ plasm. *Alcohol, The Poison of Humanity* (Eclair 1911), a three-reel film "dedicated to" the Women's Christian Temperance Union, illustrates the "hereditary influence" of drink. *Safeguarding the Nation* (Carter 1922), a five-reel educational film, used its final reel to illustrate "the menace to future generations from alcohol." It portrays defective guinea pigs whose parents had been exposed to alcohol fumes and equates them with deformed human children of alcoholic ancestry. But the film advocates strict enforcement of prohibition and individual control over "self-indulgence," not selective breeding, as the solution. One educational journal criticized the film for not including the research of leading eugenicists such as Davenport and Saleeby. This reluctance to identify with eugenics probably reflected the producer's successful efforts to obtain endorsements from anti-Darwinian religious prohibitionists such as William Jennings Bryan and the leaders of the Methodist Episcopal Church.[39]

Euthanasia, too, played a key role in several early films, both comedies and melodramas. In 1905 William Osler posited chloroforming everyone at age sixty. Biograph immediately satirized the proposal on screen in *Oslerizing Papa* (1905). A more serious melodrama about mercy killing was released only a few months before *The Black Stork*. Titled *Doctor Neighbor*, this five-reel Universal-Red Feather production had the working subtitle, "A Law for the Defective."[40] Doctor Neighbor loves his ward Hazel, but she marries a young district attorney instead. Distraught when her husband loses interest in her, she wrecks her car, suffering a severe spinal injury. The doctor and his nurse take care of her, but she begs them to end the agony of her physical and mental impairments. When the doctor refuses, the nurse gives a fatal dose of morphine. The saintly physician not only tries to take the rap for the nurse, but gives up his own life to save that of the prosecutor in the case, Hazel's estranged husband. The nurse is convicted, serves a jail term, and is released.

Motion Picture News saw the film as a "very strong" "plea that it is not right to prolong a human life if that life is so distorted and mangled as to prevent its normal restoration." The reviewer noted that "without the shadow of a doubt" the plot would have seemed "more natural" if the doctor had given the fatal dose himself, "but this would have undoubtedly created an uproar" among "the medical profession [and] a wrathy censor board." Since the film features "long scenes" of Hazel "with her spine twisted and fractured" and thus "is not a cheerful picture," the reviewer speculated that the producers could not afford further provoking the censors by antagonizing the medical profession.[41]

Another film, *Has Man the Right to Kill?*, was scheduled for release by American Standard on the day before *The Black Stork*'s Midwest premiere. In this picture, the physician protagonist gives in to the pleadings of his terminally ill friend, and administers a fatal dose. After much soul-searching by all concerned, the governor pardons him but on the grounds that the drug was intended to relieve pain, not to kill.

In 1920, the Fox feature *What Would You Do?* presented an even more sympathetic endorsement of assisted suicide. Curtis Brainerd, who is having an affair with his brother's wife, suffers agonizing paralysis following a riding accident. When he begs for death, his wife Claudia leaves a loaded gun by his bed, and he kills himself. She is accused of murder by Curtis's brother, but she silences him by telling him of his brother's betrayal. Claudia not only goes free but is happily reunited with her first husband, who returns a wealthy man after having been long missing and presumed dead.[42]

Haiselden himself made several brief film appearances before *The Black Stork*. During the Bollinger and later cases, the doctor and his dying patients appeared in at least three national newsreels. Universal's *Animated Weekly* called Haiselden the "Apostle of Humanitarian Creed to Eliminate Needless Misery" and reported that his position "gathers eminent supporters among prominent physicians." The film shows the mother of the dying infant, and presents one of Haiselden's adopted daughters "as an example of what he believes children should be."[43]

Eugenics and euthanasia were not novelties to the movie-goers of 1917. Despite the precedents, though, no American film of the 1910s or 1920s came close to matching *The Black Stork* for its graphic promotion of eugenic euthanasia.

8

The Black Stork

The Movie

The Black Stork was the most explicit depiction of negative eugenics to reach the silent screen. Yet even though the film was shown across the country in various editions under several titles from 1916 to perhaps as late as 1942, no copies were known to exist until I rediscovered and preserved the only viewable print of the 1927 revision and subsequently located an unprojectable paper print of the 1916 original.[1]

The original version opens with a prologue that depicts defectives as a repulsive, dangerous, and costly menace to society. The film dramatizes a centuries-old argument for selective human mating, visually contrasting care in breeding livestock (Fig. 8) with neglect of human health and eugenics (Fig. 9). Through statistic-filled titles and striking visual juxta-

143

positions, these scenes combine an argument for making the success of livestock breeding a model for human selection, with a critique of the government for spending more money on veterinary than on human health, and an equation of human defectives with subhuman beasts.[2]

The main story follows, contrasting the lives of two couples. Claude has an unnamed "hereditary" disease, the result of his grandfather's affair with a "vile filthy" slave. (Fig. 10, from the 1927 version, shows the slave having been replaced with an "unclean" white servant girl.) Despite a stern warning from Dr. Dickey (Fig. 11)—played by Dr. Haiselden—Claude marries his sweetheart Anne. On the other hand, Miriam, who believes her mother to have had hereditary epilepsy, refuses to marry her boyfriend Tom (Fig. 12). In the attempt to dissuade Claude from marrying Anne, Dr. Dickey shows them and the audience a variety of his mentally and physically defective patients (Fig. 13), beginning with a deformed and crippled black child (Fig. 14).

The fruit of Claude and Anne's ill-advised union (Fig. 15) is a severely defective baby (Fig. 16) who will die if not operated upon. Dr. Dickey's nurse offers him his surgical gown (Fig. 17), but he refuses to put it on, explaining, "There are times when saving a life is a greater crime than taking one." This decision provokes an angry bedside confrontation with two representatives of the local medical society (Fig. 18), shown wearing old-fashioned frock morning coats in contrast to Dr. Dickey's more modern dress.

Anne is uncertain what to do, until she receives from God a vision of the baby's future—a childhood of misery and rejection (Fig. 19) and an adult life of poverty and crime, passed on to a brood of defective offspring, an outcome the film seems to blame on Catholic opposition to both birth control and eugenic sterilization (Fig. 20). Her defective son's feeble mind finally snaps under the burden of his deformities. He shoots to death the doctor who had operated to save him in infancy, the doctor who had "condemned me to live" (Fig. 21).[3]

Horrified by this premonition, Anne agrees to withhold treatment, and the infant's tiny soul leaps into the arms of a waiting Jesus (Fig. 22).[4] Congress responds to the controversy by passing a national premarital inspection law. Meanwhile, Miriam's prudent restraint is rewarded when she discovers that it was only her stepmother who had epilepsy. With her new clean pedigree, she marries Tom, and they produce a very fat and happy baby (Figs. 23 and 24).

Many aspects of *The Black Stork* lent themselves to multiple

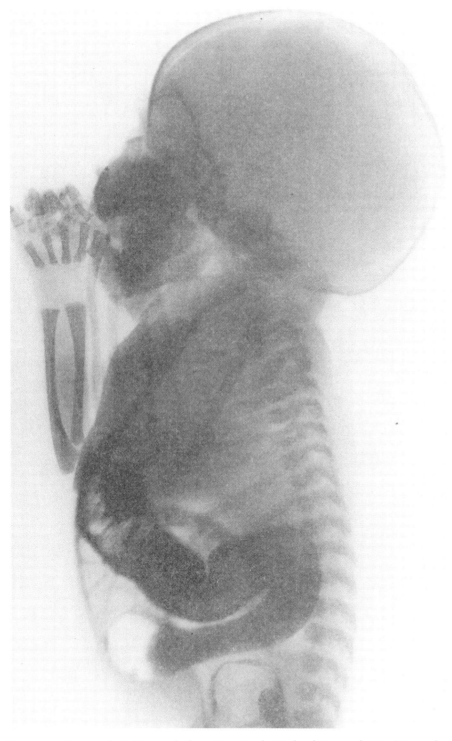

Figure 1. X-ray of Bollinger baby. *New York Medical Journal* 102 (December 4, 1915) 1133.

IS, FEASTS
EGISLATORS
T BY L. V. L.

n Reckless Spending of
's Money on Personal
ns Urged in Report.

...rities in the expense ac-
...the last Illinois general assem-
...ing upon the danger point,
...charged in a special bulletin
...erday by the Legislative Vo-

...ts make specific charges as
...waste of state funds and sug-
...remedy that there shall be re-
...ield-ruling officers for senate
...as adequate bookkeeping sys-
...orously itemized expense ac-
...gislators who draw down from
...n excess of their lawful sal-

...ning Details Bared.

...double of what happened
...in Springfield are carried in
...m, which follows in part.

He's Going to Let Her Baby Die;
This Woman Says "It's for Best."

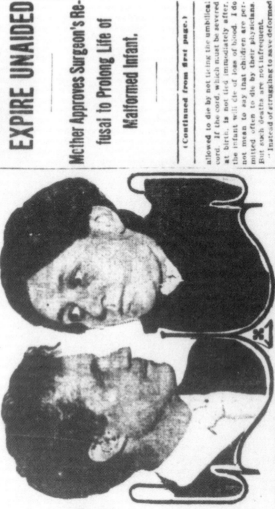

DR. H. F. HAISELDEN   MRS. ANNA BOLLINGER

DOES HUMANITY DEMAND THE
SAVING OF DEFECTIVE BABIES?

DOCTOR TO LET
DEFECTIVE BABY
EXPIRE UNAIDED

Mother Approves Surgeon's Re-
fusal to Prolong Life of
Malformed Infant.

(Continued from first page.)

allowed to die by not tieing the umbilical
cord. If the cord, which must be severed
at birth, is not tied immediately after,
the infant will die of loss of blood. I do
not mean to say that children are permitted often to die by their physicians.
But such deaths are not infrequent.

"Instead of struggling to save deformed
children and those marked plainly for
insanity and uselessness," the surgeon
cont nued, "physicians should have only
the nt. I have taught over this problem for years.

"There are no defectives among the
Japanese. The surgeons of Nippon often
fail to tie the umbilical cord. As a result, the Japanese are a wonderfully vig-

---

Figure 2. Newspaper photo of Dr. Haiselden and Mrs. Bollinger. *Chicago Tribune,*

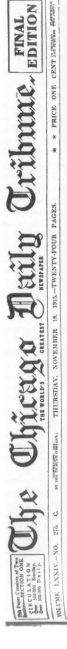

Figure 3. Page one banner headline; Bollinger case is more prominent than stories on World War I. *Chicago Tribune*, November 18, 1915, p. 1.

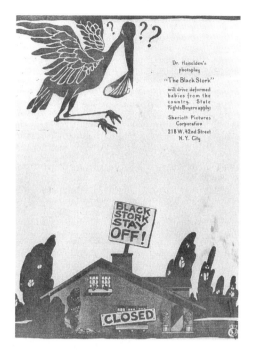

Figure 4. Sensationalized film ad. *Exhibitors' Trade Review,* March 10, 1917, p. 935.

Figure 5. Sensationalized film ad. *Motography,* April 14, 1917, ad p. 2.

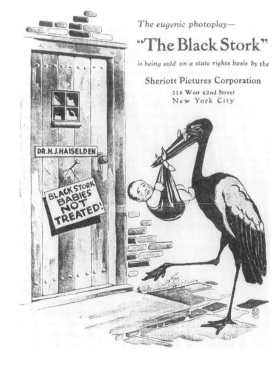

Figure 6. Ad featuring Haiselden as "star." *Chicago Herald,* April 1, 1917, p. 7.

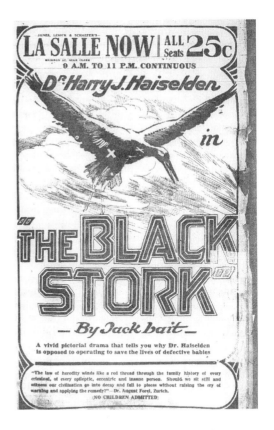

Figure 7. Ad describing Haiselden as "World Famous Surgeon." *Chicago Tribune,* April 2, 1917, p. 19.

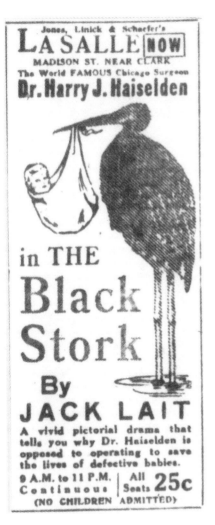

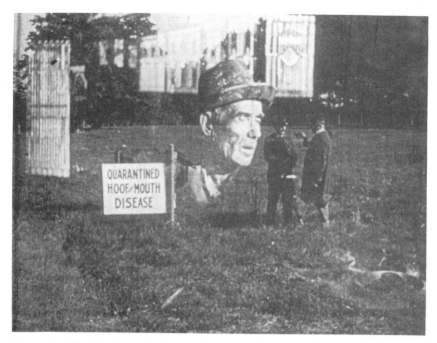

Figure 8. *The Black Stork:* Care of cattle, neglect of derelict. University of Michigan Historical Health Film Collection, used with permission of John E. Allen.

Figure 9. *The Black Stork:* Care of cattle, neglect of derelict. University of Michigan Historical Health Film Collection, used with permission of John E. Allen.

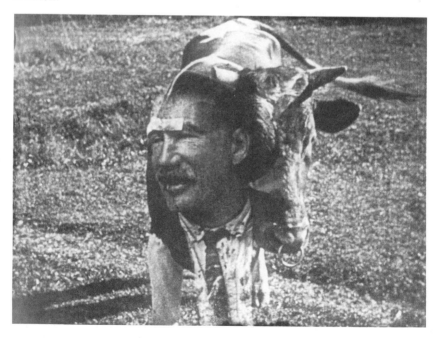

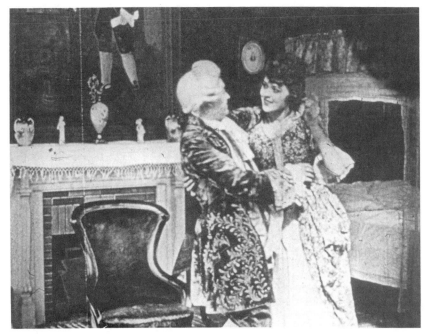

Figure 10. *Are You Fit to Marry?:* Claude's grandfather's sin. University of Michigan Historical Health Film Collection, used with permission of John E. Allen.

Figure 11. *The Black Stork:* Doctor warns Claude not to marry. University of Michigan Historical Health Film Collection, used with permission of John E. Allen.

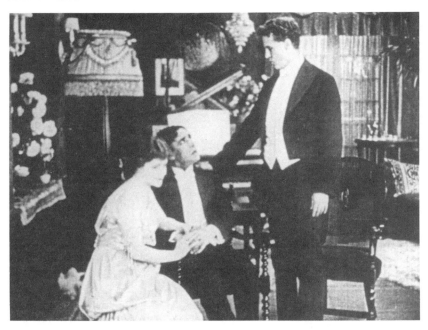

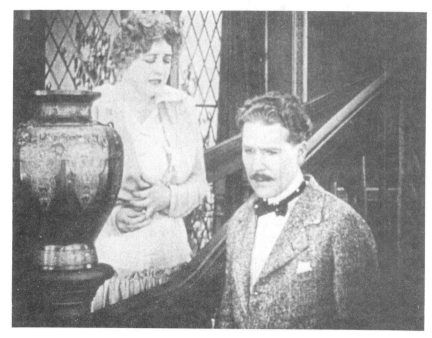

Figure 12. *The Black Stork:* Miriam refuses marriage. University of Michigan Historical Health Film Collection, used with permission of John E. Allen.

Figure 13. *The Black Stork:* Doctor demonstrates "defective" patient. University of Michigan Historical Health Film Collection, used with permission of John E. Allen.

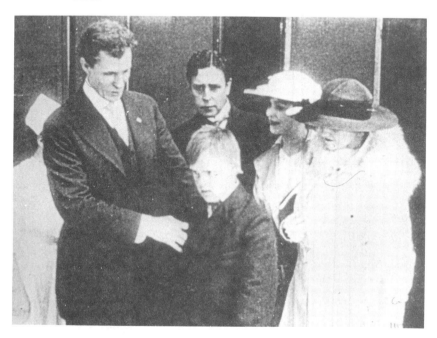

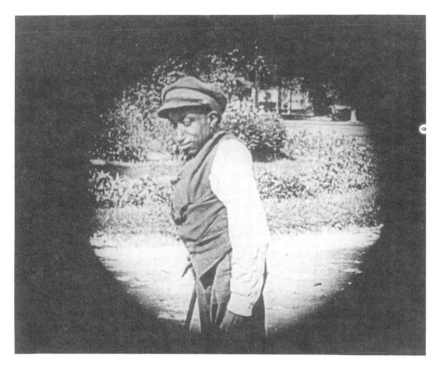

Figure 14. *The Black Stork:* Crippled black child. University of Michigan Historical Health Film Collection, used with permission of John E. Allen.

Figure 15. *The Black Stork:* Claude and Anne's baby. University of Michigan Historical Health Film Collection, used with permission of John E. Allen.

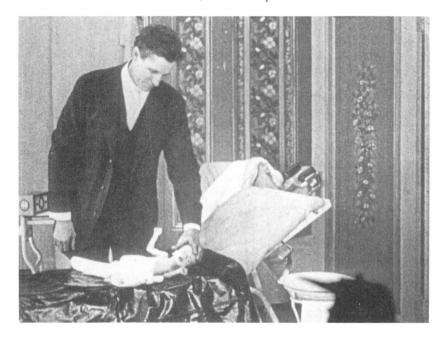

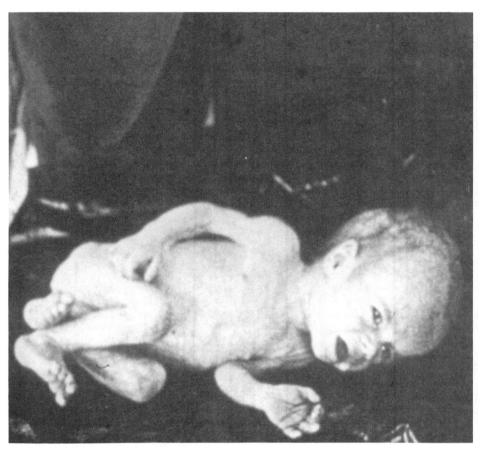

Figure 16. *The Black Stork:* Close-up of Claude and Anne's baby. University of Michigan Historical Health Film Collection, used with permission of John E. Allen.

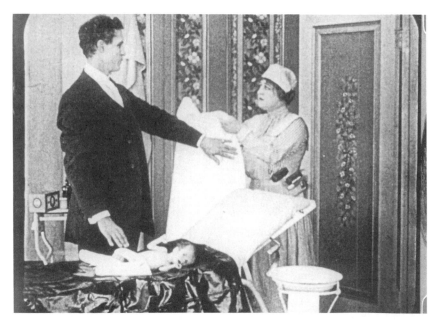

Figure 17. *The Black Stork:* Doctor refuses to operate. University of Michigan Historical Health Film Collection, used with permission of John E. Allen.

Figure 18. *The Black Stork:* Doctor confronts the medical society. University of Michigan Historical Health Film Collection, used with permission of John E. Allen.

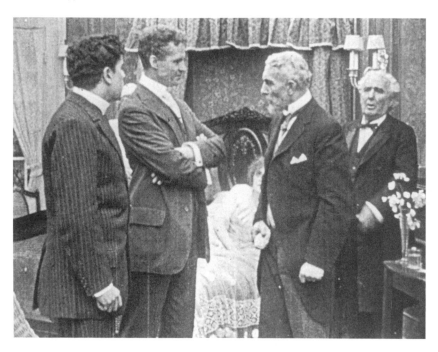

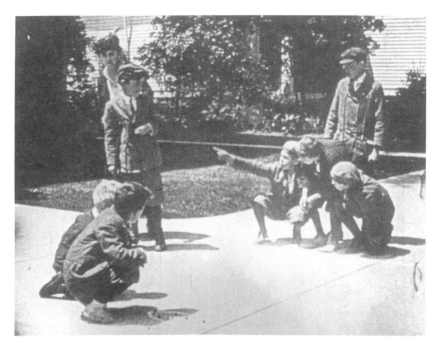

Figure 19. *The Black Stork:* Vision—childhood rejection. University of Michigan Historical Health Film Collection, used with permission of John E. Allen.

Figure 20. *The Black Stork:* Vision—breeding more "defectives." University of Michigan Historical Health Film Collection, used with permission of John E. Allen.

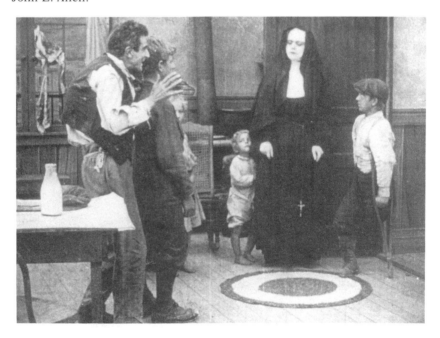

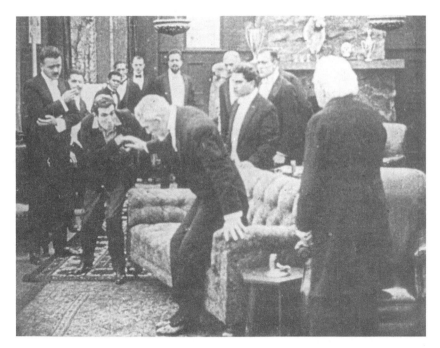

Figure 21. *The Black Stork:* Vision—shooting the doctor who saved him. University of Michigan Historical Health Film Collection, used with permission of John E. Allen.

Figure 22. *The Black Stork:* Baby's soul welcomed by Jesus. University of Michigan Historical Health Film Collection, used with permission of John E. Allen.

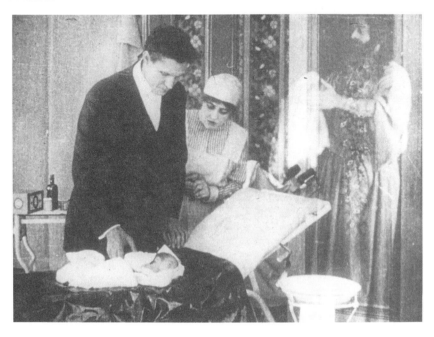

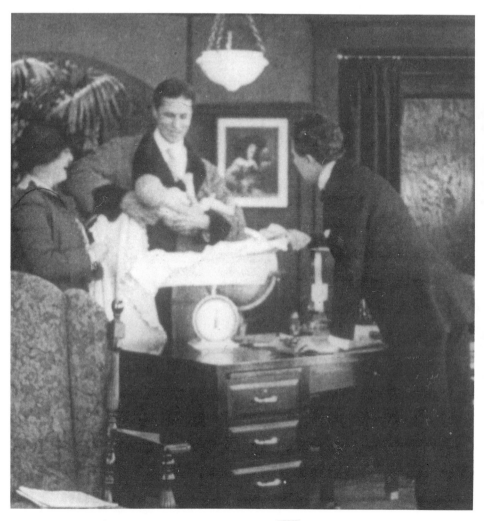

Figure 23. *The Black Stork:* Doctor fumbles baby. University of Michigan Historical Health Film Collection, used with permission of John E. Allen.

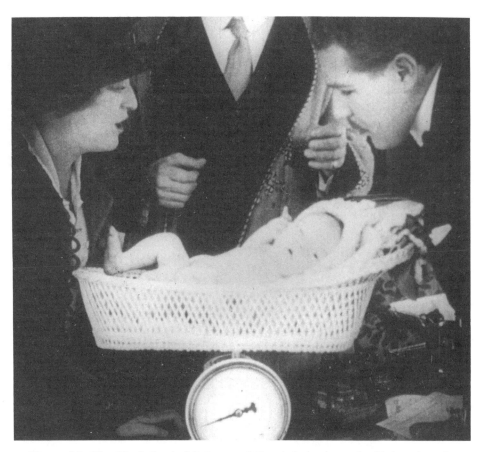

Figure 24. *The Black Stork:* Miriam and Tom's baby in scale. University of Michigan Historical Health Film Collection, used with permission of John E. Allen.

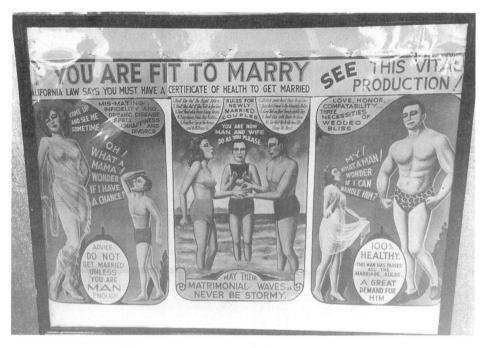

Figure 25. Russell Lee, motion picture billboard, Yuma, Arizona, February 1942. Library of Congress #USF/33/13256-M3.

conflicting interpretations. For example, the film mirrors Haiselden's own ambivalent emotions in its depictions of defectives. Anne's horrifying vision of her future grandchildren and the prologue's assortment of social deviants portray a repulsive and menacing army of subhumans. In the 1927 version, a long panorama presents the Chicago State Hospital grounds, on whose parklike campus the patients loll idly under the trees while poor normal children are shown starving in the slums.

But when Haiselden introduces individual real patients, their brave hopes and shy smiles at the camera convey an immediately appealing humanity. And Henry Bergman, who played Claude and Anne's adult son, depicted the "defective" as a tragic, even noble figure. Laboriously and meticulously dressing his bent body for a formal party, or vainly struggling to mimic a poster of a football hero in action, even shyly flirting with a derelict woman on a park bench, Bergman made his character appealingly human despite the titles that consigned him to an "abyss of abnormality" filled with "criminal desires." Critics who otherwise despised the film praised Bergman's performance for its depth and humanity.[5] Bergman's creation was pitied but not easily hated.

Haiselden's autobiography tells the story of a wealthy mother who disguised her son's defects and successfully presented him as normal at a society ball.[6] But when *The Black Stork* translates that incident to the screen, the charade fails. Bergman's character is recognized as a defective and shunned. An incident originally used to illustrate the terrifying menace of disguised defectives could now be read as pathetic, even tragic.

Depictions of sexuality were particularly open to multiple meanings that allowed audiences to view *The Black Stork*'s defectives as more human than Haiselden may have intended. The doctor displays a sixteen-year-old mentally retarded girl who smiles flirtatiously at the camera, one hand provocatively on her hip. Haiselden, whose belief in the fecundity of defectives reflected a common eugenic horror at the supposedly uninhibited sexuality of the feebleminded, probably meant the shot to be frightening. But those who did not already share his fears might find the gesture more appealing than appalling. She also could be seen as reacting to the camera by trying to imitate the seductive stance of a female film star. On this reading, her pose would parallel the pathetic dreams of athletic glory voiced by a "hopeless cripple" boy Haiselden presents along with her.[7]

The Black Stork's depictions of class were similarly subject to multiple interpretations. Claude's taint originates with a working-class woman who gives a venereal disease to a wealthy man. The scene echoes a theme first introduced in *Damaged Goods*. Recent critics have read this aspect of *Damaged Goods* as reinforcing conservative class ideologies,[8] and the same implications certainly can be found in Haiselden's film. But these modern critics don't realize that this reading is precisely the opposite of what both films' socialist backers intended: Both films dwelt more on the sins of the rich than on the dangers of the poor. Socialists like Frederic Robinson, a key promoter of both films; Upton Sinclair, who novelized *Damaged Goods;* and George Bernard Shaw, who wrote a lengthy preface to the play, each interpreted these scenes as blaming venereal disease on poverty and the class system, ignorance and traditional morality, not on the poor. According to Shaw, *Damaged Goods* did not blame the poor prostitute. "The husband alone is culpable." But Shaw cautions, all such efforts to moralize about disease are "a hideous mistake," because the play shows "Most of the victims . . . are entirely innocent persons." "I will not here go into the vexed question of whether the peasant . . . or the squire . . . is the more cleanly and hygienic, though my experience . . . makes me incline to the side of the peasant. What is beyond all question is that each seems disgusting to the other."[9]

Did these films blame poor women, rich men, or the structure of society? No one reading of the class implications of these films is necessarily "right." This multiplicity of meanings reveals not just the general problem of textual ambiguity but a very specific problem in early-twentieth-century health propaganda films. *The Black Stork* and *Damaged Goods* used melodrama to popularize the impersonal laws of science that supposedly constituted both biology and socialism. But melodrama can only portray such large abstract forces by personalizing them, representing them as individual heroes and villains. The silent screen's reliance on physical pantomime also made it harder to convey that the individuals were supposed to represent impersonal abstractions. Most important, these technical limits of the medium reinforced key ambiguities in the progressive health message. The constraints of silent melodrama amplified the internal contradiction in the progressives' faith that science could be both impersonally objective and a source of moral imperatives.

Following *The Black Stork*'s prologue, each of the main figures in the plot is introduced in a series of shots designed to reveal the central features of their characters. Claude first appears reading a book labeled "Ibsen's Ghosts," shivering with fear and despair, and piling logs on the fire while those around him loosen their collars from the heat. Looming over the hearth is a huge suit of armor.

Ibsen's stage drama, depicting a victim of congenital syphilis, had been introduced to movie audiences only a year earlier. The reference both establishes Claude as a man terrified of his diseased ancestry and lays claim to serious cultural value for the film itself. The armor signals both Claude's "wealth and position" and the continued presence of the distant past, a skeleton that won't stay in the closet but that haunts the hearth.

Anne is introduced lounging on a sofa, eating bonbons, reading a magazine, and gazing fondly at a framed photo of Claude. Upper-class feminine passivity and civilized leisure combine with romantic infatuation. Her friend Miriam represents activity and nature. Miriam first appears at the window behind Anne, rapturously embracing a caged bird, thrilling to the wind in the trees, an ample-bosomed, nurturant, vital earth mother.[10]

Claude proposes to Anne at the climax of a long and heavy-handed scene in which she plays love songs to him on the piano, oblivious to his writhing in an agony of conflicting fear and desire. Those who took the scene at face value found the action ridiculous: "They behave so abnormally," critic Kitty Kelly complained.[11]

But read symbolically, the action makes sense. In progressive-era America, the piano was second only to the hearth as an icon of family life and middle-class domesticity. Yet the piano had its raunchy side too, in the ragtime of the red-light districts and nickelodeon movie houses.[12] When Anne plays for Claude, she envisions love and home; but for him the music conjures the ghost of his diseased grandfather, warning him never to marry. That specter appears to Claude three times, each time transforming what Anne sees as an emblem of domesticity into an object of horror: first the piano, then the hearth, and finally the bedroom.[13]

The ghost is identified as Claude's grandfather. Allowing an ample thirty years per generation would make him a figure from 1856. Yet he appears in powdered wig and brocade greatcoat and conducts his seduction in a canopied four-poster, more a character from a Hogarth print of the 1750s than a man of the mid-nineteenth century. Portraying the source of the evil in colonial and even feudal (the armor) garb builds on a series of interrelated images not confined to any linear sense of chronology. Rather, these images evoke both the early Republican horror of aristocratic decadence and Nathaniel Hawthorne's vision of colonial America, haunted both by a

superstitious belief in the supernatural and by the reality of supernatural evil. They also draw on a newer association between colonial days and contaminated heredity established by the highly publicized colonial-era pedigrees of such families as the "Jukes" and
"Kallikaks."

Claude remains by Anne's side as she agonizes over the birth of
their defective baby, but throughout her lengthy vision of the child's
future, Claude is entirely absent.[14] When the adult defective seeks
his revenge, he considers killing first his mother, then Dr. Dickey,
before settling on the doctor who saved him as an infant. Yet the
person supposedly most to blame for his deformities—his father,
Claude—is never even mentioned as a possible target. When the defective leans over his sleeping mother, preparing to shoot her, she is
alone in the couple's double bed.

The cause of Claude's disappearance is never explained. Perhaps
he succumbed to his hereditary disease; perhaps Anne realized that
he deceived her and has tossed him out; maybe he ran away from
the burden and the guilt. But the lesson of Claude's absence seems
clear: Women need knowledge, not just innocent purity, to protect
themselves against hereditarily tainted men. If they don't know how
to defend themselves, they will be left to bear the consequences
themselves. The first sentence of the 1916 version explicitly warns
against such "criminal ignorance." *The Black Stork* thus anticipated
a stock theme of such films as *Fit to Fight* (1918) and *The End of the
Road* (1919), in which "innocent" characters of both sexes get venereal disease through lack of scientific knowledge, not just through
immorality.[15]

Claude's unexplained vanishing act also parallels the puzzling
1896 disappearance of Haiselden's own father from the Chicago records and the conspicuous silence about his father in his autobiography. Perhaps Haiselden had personal as well as professional experience in mind when he warned women to learn to take care of
themselves.

Although Haiselden's film justifies itself by arguing that women
need to know about eugenic and sexual dangers, Dr. Dickey does not
practice what Dr. Haiselden preaches. Instead, the on-screen doctor
follows the traditional practice of protecting female innocence and
male confidentiality by maintaining the "conspiracy of silence" that
leaves Anne ignorant of her impending disaster. When Dr. Dickey
discovers Claude and Anne embracing on the piano bench, he attempts to dissuade Claude with a series of head signals, fish-eyed
stares, and similar nonverbal warnings, from behind Anne's back.
When that doesn't work, he takes Claude outside for a lecture. But

despite the danger, he never explicitly warns Anne about Claude's condition.

Claude's disappearance also clears the field for a head-to-head contest between motherly love and heredity to see which will shape the baby's future. In direct contrast to anti-hereditarian films such as *A Disciple of Nietzsche*, the defective's downfall demonstrates that even the purest maternal affection is no match for his inborn defects.

However, *The Black Stork* does not deny that environment can influence heredity. Positive surroundings can't cure bad breeding, but a negative environment can make things much worse. Though Claude and Anne's baby was born crippled, it's only after he leaves his mother's loving home for a hostile, rejecting world that his physical handicaps lead to crime and insanity.

Reissuing this 1916 film in 1927 posed a number of problems, not the least of which was the obviously dated costumes and settings. To disguise the age of the original, the new producers revised the prologue and added an epilogue, featuring several clearly contemporary characters. These new scenes prominently display an impressive 1927 Buick Sport Touring Car, and the characters sport assertively trendy clothing.[16]

As the prologue begins, Jack announces his intention to marry Alice, the daughter of "Professor Robert Worth, eminent writer and authority on heredity." The professor, however, refuses to give his assent unless Jack undergoes "a thorough physical examination." To convince him of the need for such "humiliation," Professor Worth delivers a lecture consisting largely of scenes from the original prologue, though without the heavy-handed and obsolete statistics, and with somewhat less-inflammatory wording than in Haiselden's original titles. Where the 1916 version stormed that "defectives are housed in palaces costing fortunes" the new edition stated, "There are millions spent in caring for these defectives." The original outrageously misleading claim that the army rejected "97 men out of 100 applicants . . . because of bodily defects," was deleted, as were some of Haiselden's most florid titles, such as the one that equated kissing with spitting.

When the lecture fails to convince the rather obtuse Jack, Professor Worth tells him "a true story of a boyhood chum of mine, and the sad consequences of his marriage." The dramatic portion of the original film is then inserted as a long flashback with only a few significant alterations.

Although most of the 1916 swimming scenes were retained, all but a split second of nudity was cut, and the shots were dispersed throughout the movie. The link between physicality and purity remains visible, but the main function of the swimming scenes has become to provide visually attractive and/or comedic relief from the film's more distressing examples of degeneracy.

The 1927 version also dropped all but a glimpse of the long 1916 subplot in which a consumptive chauffeur fathers a defective child. Although there are no records documenting the reasons for this change, one that might well have been made on purely cinematic grounds, the cut eliminates any reference to tuberculosis being hereditary.

In the 1916 version Tom is identified as Claude's "secretary," but by 1927 he has risen to Claude's "partner," even though he is still shown taking dictation and following orders. Between the two dates, the job of secretary had become so feminized that to use the word for a man would likely have provoked ridicule.

By 1927 the white servant has been substituted for the black slave. And Haiselden's optimistic conclusion, in which his actions are vindicated by congressional passage of eugenic marriage legislation, was also scrapped. Otherwise virtually all of the 1916 footage was retained intact.

In the brief new epilogue, Jack is convinced by Professor Worth's story, reinforced by his reading of "Hutchinson on Heredity" and a newspaper warning: "Fit to marry?—Not if you know or suspect yourself to have a 'social' disease." He takes and passes his premarital exam and announces to Alice, "Yes, we're fit to marry."

These changes, though requiring extensive additions, appear limited to updating the film cinematically, not politically or medically. For example, eugenic successes in shaping the 1924 immigration law and the 1927 Supreme Court decision upholding eugenic sterilizations could easily have been substituted for the marriage law sequence that was cut from Haiselden's finale. Such a change could have been made simply by adding new intertitles to the old action. But no such alterations were made. Despite the great changes in eugenics by 1927, the new *Are You Fit to Marry?* remained in substance the same as Haiselden's 1916 original.

Making and Distributing *The Black Stork*

In addition to Haiselden, *The Black Stork* cast featured Hamilton Revelle (Claude), Elsie Esmond (Anne), Jane Fearnly or Fearnley (Miriam), Allan Murnane (Tom), Henry Bergman ("The Monster"),

Edgar Davenport and George Moss (leaders of the "doctors' club"), Leroy Baxter (Anne's consumptive chauffeur), and Elsie Baxter (a gardener's daughter who elopes with Anne's chauffeur).[17]

All were professional film and theater performers, most having played significant supporting roles in from three to fourteen identifiable feature films released prior to 1917. Revelle, Bergman, and Davenport were the most experienced players. Attentive stage and movie fans might well have recognized them, though none was an important star. And all but Revelle were nearing the end of their movie acting careers; only he is known to have appeared in films after 1920.[18]

One movie trade magazine also included a John T. Miltern in its cast listing. Perhaps this was John Miltern, a popular stage melodrama villain, whose first major movie role was in a 1916 Pathé production. But if this Miltern did appear in *The Black Stork*, he got surprisingly little notice for such a well-known actor, even as a novice in film.[19]

Star billing in *The Black Stork* was clearly reserved for Haiselden himself. At the height of the Bollinger case publicity, his name was probably as widely known as almost any film actor's. His critics alleged that he received $25,000 to appear in the film, a salary comparable with that of all but a few top movie performers.[20] Haiselden probably did not regret the absence of big-name actors to upstage him or demand top billing. At any rate, in the releasing company's trade publicity, Haiselden was billed as "THE STAR," and in the newspaper advertisements, he was the only cast member to get name billing.[21]

The next most prominent person involved in making the film was the scriptwriter, Jack Lait. A popular thirty-three-year-old Chicago muckraking reporter whose short stories appeared regularly in national magazines, Lait had two years experience writing stage and film scripts by 1916. He later achieved notoriety as coauthor of the scandal-mongering *USA Confidential* series of books and editor of the tabloid New York *Daily Mirror*. His succinct comment on the Bollinger baby: "Let it die," and his follow-up column exposing the miserable existence of " 'Hopeless' Babes Who Were 'Saved' on View in State Hospital" appeared in Hearst's *Chicago Herald* within a week of the baby's birth. Lait was the only person beside Haiselden whose name appeared in the *Black Stork* newspaper ads; he was the only individual involved with the original film to be given a screen credit in the 1927 version.[22]

Haiselden announced plans to make a feature film about the

case less than a month after the Bollinger baby's death.[23] Production apparently began at the Rothacker Film Manufacturing Company's studio, conveniently located only a few blocks from the German-American Hospital, and the NBRMP regarded the film as a Rothacker production.[24] However, by June 10, 1916, the work shifted to the Wharton, Inc., studios in Ithaca, New York. Haiselden himself went to Ithaca several times, including a trip in September 1916 for a preview and editing. There is no evidence that any of his scenes were actually shot in Ithaca, and many of the film's exteriors are clearly Chicago locations.[25]

Neither Rothacker nor Wharton was a major film producer, but they were hardly inconsequential by 1916 standards. Wharton produced *The Black Stork* under contract to Hearst's newly created International Film Service, and William Randolph Hearst himself visited the Ithaca studio during the final assembly of the film. Both Wharton and International were closely tied to the giant Pathé company, and there were rumors that Wharton had been purchased outright by Hearst. Wharton produced several major dramatic serials for Hearst and Pathé, including the infamous anti-Japanese film, *Patria*, and the classic Pearl White cliff-hangers, *Perils of Pauline* (1913) and *Exploits of Elaine* (1915). A leading trade publication even mistakenly listed *The Black Stork* as an International Film Service production. The Whartons did not see that error as an accident; they promptly accused Hearst of deliberately stealing credit for their work.[26]

Hearst enterprises played a crucial though shadowy role in making Harry Haiselden a household name. Haiselden first revealed the Bollinger case to Florence Patton, a friend who worked for Hearst's *Chicago American*, thus allowing that paper to break the story with an exclusive scoop. From November 23 through the end of 1915, the paper published a daily installment of Haiselden's serialized autobiographical account of the case, usually as a front-page feature. This revealing, book-length narrative also was reprinted in other Hearst papers, including the *Boston American*. The Hearst-owned *New York American* gave Haiselden more extensive and more favorable coverage than any other major daily in that city, and Hearst medical correspondent Woods Hutchinson showered Haiselden with repeated accolades. Jack Lait wrote *The Black Stork* while employed as a columnist for Hearst's *Chicago Herald*, and Pathé produced one of the first newsreels to cover the Bollinger case.[27]

The issue certainly lent itself to the type of sensational "yellow journalism" at which the Hearst organization excelled. Haiselden's

German-American connections and his concerns about Japanese power might have played some role as well, since at the time Hearst and Wharton were using fear of the "yellow peril" to divert America from declaring war on Germany. And, despite Hearst's own far-from-conventional personal life, he supported antiprostitution and other health-related moral reforms.

Yet the precise nature and extent of the Hearst–Haiselden connection remains unclear. The two men do not seem to have had any direct correspondence with each other, and Hearst had some good reasons for avoiding any personal endorsement of Haiselden's crusade. For one thing, despite his reputation for ruthlessness, Hearst could be quite sentimental about disabilities. As a young man, he had written to his father, "I have begun to have a strange fondness for our little paper [the *San Francisco Examiner*]—a tenderness like unto that which a mother feels for a puny or deformed offspring. I should hate to see it die after it has battled so long and so nobly for its existence." [28] And a marked speech defect was reportedly one of the things Hearst found captivating about Marion Davies, the actress with whom he began a lifelong infatuation in 1916. Perhaps more important, Catholic hostility to Haiselden made identification with him impolitic at a time when Hearst was building an alliance with New York's Irish-dominated Tammany political machine to install John Hylan as mayor in the 1916 election. Hearst's in-laws and several close advisers were also committed Catholics. [29]

Furthermore, promotion of *The Black Stork* almost certainly suffered from the growing hostility between Hearst and the Whartons. A few weeks before the film's midwest release, the Ithaca producers severed their connection with Hearst, following repeated complaints that they were not receiving sufficient credit for their productions. By 1919 their dispute wound up in court. [30]

Hearst could be relentless in using his newspapers to promote films he backed, but when *The Black Stork* opened in Chicago, the *Herald*'s Louella Parsons panned it in a brief two-inch review, even though the paper carried several quarter-page ads for the film. [31] By April 1917 Hearst clearly was no longer actively backing Haiselden or his movie.

Haiselden's original producer, Rothacker Film, was the first and largest maker of "industrial films," advertising and training movies sponsored by major manufacturers and businesses. Founded in 1909 by a partnership that included future Universal Studios mogul Carl Laemmle, the company had just begun to branch out into entertainment films following a mid-1916 reorganization. The studio was headed by Watterson Rothacker, who also ran one of the largest movie developing labs of the silent film era. At its peak in 1920, Rothacker released over a dozen entertainment features, although by 1922 they returned to making industrial and educational films exclusively.[32]

Although they were not New York or Hollywood, Chicago and Ithaca were not yet the cinematic backwaters they would become when the movie industry stampeded west after World War I. Ithaca provided scenic rural settings conveniently located between the New York–New Jersey cradle of American cinema and Chicago. In 1916 Chicago was still the "third coast" for film, home to pioneering giants such as Selig and Essanay, half a dozen smaller studios, and the important trade publications *Photoplay* and *Motography*. Wharton, Inc., founder Theodore Wharton began his film career with Thomas Edison in New York, but arrived in Ithaca in 1912 as a location producer for Chicago-based Essanay.[33]

The 1927 version of Haiselden's film was produced by Quality Amusement Corporation. W. H. Strafford wrote and directed the new prologue and epilogue. Quality Amusement may have specialized in updating and rereleasing older films; the only movie on which they held a copyright was a Thomas H. Ince western, which they copyrighted a year after Ince had died. Their office was located in downtown Chicago, literally around the corner from the theater where *The Black Stork* had opened a decade earlier.[34]

The Black Stork inaugurated the conversion from live stage to movie theater of what had been Chicago's LaSalle Opera House. The LaSalle, on West Madison one block south of City Hall, was run by Jones, Linick, & Schaefer, whose chain of downtown movie houses, including the Orpheum, Studebaker, and Colonial, made them the leading film exhibitors in the Loop. Chicago's downtown theaters would soon be eclipsed by the new streetcar suburb movie palaces of Balaban & Katz, but in 1917 Jones, Linick, & Schaefer was the big time. While their other theaters played standard entertainment fare, the LaSalle may have been intended to specialize in more provocative subjects, at least at the start. *The Black Stork* was followed by *Enlighten Thy Daughter*, a well-reviewed dramatic argument for sex education.[35]

In Cleveland and Cincinnati, *The Black Stork* opened at the Orpheum and Alhambra respectively, theaters whose names conjured the aura of exotic opulence sought by the typical first-class 1917 cinemas. But by 1919 Haiselden's film was being booked into less-glamorous-sounding venues, such as Baltimore's Little Pickwick and Blue Mouse.[36]

In towns where local censors frowned on sex or controversy, and in rural areas far from established film distribution networks, *The Black Stork* also may have had a long run among the many traveling "road shows." Such touring film exhibitors combined various forms of early-twentieth-century mass culture, from the traditional medicine show to the new mobile film-projector trucks used by state and local health departments to bring officially sponsored health education movies to rural audiences. Road shows were profitable and popular into the 1940s, but their films could be shown many hundreds of times without leaving any permanent record.

Film collector John E. Allen Sr. began his career as a teenaged assistant to one such touring show in the Rochester, New York, area during the late 1920s. In a 1973 interview, he described to me the conditions under which his and many other road shows brought films such as *The Black Stork* to audiences in the 1920s and 1930s. Since the advertising was usually much more lurid than the films themselves, an important rule of thumb was to "get all the paper down before the crowd came out," so the departing audience would not be able to compare the posters with what they had seen on the screen. Most advertising was word-of-mouth or via telephone pole fliers rather than in the newspapers. These techniques, intended in part to avoid attracting the attention of censors and license inspectors, made the road shows almost invisible to historians as well.

The show on which he worked was run by "Doc Watkins," who specialized in bringing films on birth control, venereal disease, and eugenics to farm women from upstate New York to the deep South. After the showings, "Doc" held private consultations in a tent. Mr. Allen never learned whether "Doc" had any kind of degree. But the market for such films must have been good, since he claimed to send "several hundred dollars a week to a birth control lobbyist in Washington."[37]

The right to distribute *The Black Stork* to theaters was sold on a state-by-state basis. Such "state-rights" distribution was commonly used, especially for the products of smaller studios not affiliated with a national exchange and for films considered controversial enough to require different specially cut local versions to pass the patchwork of local film censors. For example, D. W. Griffith's 1914 eugenics film, *The Escape*, was a state-rights release, the first time a Griffith production had been distributed in that manner.

H. E. Smith of Detroit apparently bought rights to Haiselden's film the day it was first copyrighted. And by the end of 1916, R. H. Hadfield, who had worked with Wharton on the production, established the "Black Stork Company" as the Chicago-based distributor. From January 1917, all sales of state-rights were handled by Sheriott Pictures, a large company with offices in both Chicago and New York, but Sheriott went out of business within a few months, and all unsold franchises reverted to Hadfield. Later distributors included H. J. Brooks of South Bend, Indiana (1923), Bland Brothers of Chicago (1927), and three New York City organizations: Judel Film Company (1925), Famous Italian Pictures (1928), and Piccadilly Film Company (1928).[38]

State-rights purchasers were not necessarily small-time operators. Sheriott sold the Illinois rights to Clarence Joseph Bulliet, the highly regarded publicist for distinguished stage actor Robert B. Mantell; however, most of the others who bought this film were apparently quite obscure.[39]

Initially, the picture promised great commercial success. "This should certainly get the money," the influential trade paper *Wid's Film Daily* advised prospective exhibitors. Bulliet reportedly purchased the Illinois rights for $35,000, a record price up to that time. Many feature films cost less than that to produce. Less than three years earlier, the Illinois rights to Griffith's eugenics film brought in only $8,000. When Lewis J. Selznick paid $35,000 for New York rights to another 1917 film, the sex education feature *Enlighten Thy Daughter*, the sum was considered so extraordinary that he purchased two-page spreads in the trade magazines to announce the price.

But such publicly trumpeted prices cannot be taken at face value. Bulliet's son, who was nine years old in 1917, told me he has long been skeptical about the $35,000 price tag reportedly paid for Haiselden's film. As he remembers it, his father was manager of Sheriott's Chicago office, and he suspects the sale may actually have been a private internal transfer with the announced price chosen purely for publicity.[40]

Smith of Detroit reportedly paid $20,000 for Ohio rights to *The Black Stork* one week before Bulliet's record-setting purchase. He pledged that the film would not be shown for less than the standard feature admission price of twenty-five cents, and that price was maintained throughout two-week runs in Chicago and Cleveland. After only three days, however, the Cincinnati exhibitor lowered the admission to fifteen cents for the remainder of a two-week booking, perhaps an indication of poor attendance.[41]

Distributors such as Bulliet were attracted to a film like *The Black Stork* not only because they hoped to make money on that film, but because they were trying to expand the audience for motion pictures in general. Bulliet claimed to have done careful market research indicating that the film would draw large numbers of middle-class women to the theaters, and building an audience among this segment of the population was a prime goal of movie exhibitors at that time.[42]

While the opinions of *The Black Stork* held by many local community leaders and film censors are remarkably well recorded, it is not possible to reconstruct anything like a full record of when and where it was shown. Because distribution was so decentralized and because the film remained in circulation for so long, only those specific showings that attracted notice in the trade magazines or news media could be identified.

The first recorded showing of *The Black Stork* was the private screening Wharton put on for Haiselden and a party from Chicago on September 24, 1916. The public premiere was announced for Ithaca in mid-October 1916. The film debuted in New York City for the NBRMP, November 24 and 27, 1916. A seven-reel version that Haiselden incorrectly claimed had been revised to meet the board's criticisms was copyrighted December 8, 1916. This was the paper print I have called the "original" film. The usually tough Chicago Film Censorship Board apparently approved the film after a series of cuts requested on November 22, 1916, and March 31, 1917, had been made. The resulting five-reel version was previewed February 13, 1917, for Chicago film critics. On March 9 a six-reel edition reportedly was shown during a debate on eugenics in the Ohio Legislature. A similar showing for Illinois legislators had been announced a few days earlier. The five-reel version was also screened in New York City February 23, 1917, by the NBRMP.[43]

Although the board refused to approve it, this edition opened two-week commercial runs in Chicago, Cincinnati, and Cleveland on April 1, 1917. In each city, Haiselden himself accompanied the film, delivering in-person lectures at one or more showings. Later efforts to exhibit the film included Houston and Indiana before September 1917.[44]

On January 31, 1918, a six-reel version retitled *Are You Fit to Marry?* finally won approval from the NBRMP, although there is no evidence the cuts they had previously demanded had been made. Additional cuts were requested May 24, 1918. These changes were made, and *Are You Fit to Marry?* opened a three-day run in Baltimore on January 13, 1919, deceptively promoted as a new film "never before seen by the human eye." Haiselden reportedly once again lectured in person at the Baltimore theater. Meanwhile the Chicago censors apparently reapproved the film twice, on April 16, 1918, and June 5, 1925.

The New York State Board of Censors turned down applications from distributors in South Bend, Indiana (April 4, 1923), and New York City (November 9, 1928); the latter was for a seven-reel edition supposedly produced in 1925. The Quality Amusement reissue of 1927, the only surviving projectable print, ran seven reels, including the new prologue and ending. It won an adults-only permit from the Chicago censors on December 3, 1927, and February 7, 1928. This was probably the same film turned down by the Pennsylvania censors on January 7, 1928. The last-known showing may have been recorded by Farm Security Administration photographer Russell Lee, who documented a billboard advertising a film reportedly called *Are You Fit to Marry* in Yuma, Arizona, in February 1942 (Fig. 25).[45]

Despite its eventual long history of showings, the initial thirteen-month delay in winning NBRMP approval and the hostility of key state censors in the 1920s apparently kept the film out of many first-run houses outside the midwest. Even there the film did not get the attention it might have received had it not opened two days before America's entry into World War I.

9

Medicine, Media, and Memory

From Haiselden's death in 1919 to the present, controversies over eugenic euthanasia and medical refusal to treat impaired newborns periodically appeared and disappeared from the American mass media. Each time the public rediscovered these issues, the memory of Haiselden's crusade became dimmer. With each revival of interest, these subjects were increasingly portrayed as unprecedented novelties of modern science.

Each new wave of attention was shaped by the particular political and medical circumstances of its own time. Yet key underlying assumptions first illuminated in the debate over the Bollinger baby and *The Black Stork* continued to shape public and professional discourse long after Haiselden and his cases had been forgotten. Both the differences and the similarities to Haiselden's era remain important to understanding medicine, genetics, and euthanasia today.

From Haiselden to Hitler: Infanticide, Eugenics, and Euthanasia, 1919–1945

American eugenicists achieved their greatest political successes in the 1920s, with legislation imposing selective ethnic restrictions on immigration and judicial approval of compulsory sterilization. In contrast, supporters of euthanasia won no comparable victories. Indeed, many historians claim discussion of mercy killing almost disappeared from American public life in the 1920s.[1]

As support for euthanasia appeared to wane, many American eugenicists retreated, at least temporarily, from the links Haiselden had forged between the two causes. For example, Irving Fisher, who had opposed eugenic euthanasia before the Bollinger case but had then backed Haiselden, started to distance himself again by 1917. Fisher now reiterated that "eugenics does not require the old Spartan practise of infanticide," although his cautiously ambiguous statement leaves unclear whether he disavowed all infanticide or only compulsory infanticide.[2] Even Dr. William J. Robinson, one of Haiselden's most vigorous supporters in 1915–16, wrote in 1917 that "no eugenic considerations will induce us to adopt Spartan-like methods and to neglect or kill off the weak and puny. . . . Every child that is born . . . is entitled to the very best of care."[3]

Although eugenics was politically successful and euthanasia was not, both issues virtually disappeared from American feature films in the 1920s and 1930s. The growth of state and industry censorship codified a rigid genre structure in which most controversial or unpleasant medical subjects were banished from "entertainment" theaters to classrooms, road shows, and other marginal locations. While the American Film Institute's index of feature films lists six titles on eugenics and thirty-eight on other aspects of heredity between 1915 and 1920, for 1921–30 it includes only one eugenics film and four on heredity.[4]

The lull in public discussion of euthanasia and the separation of that issue from eugenics both proved only temporary, however. By the mid-1930s, American newspapers and magazines resumed extensive coverage of mercy killing, and by the late 1930s, both topics returned to the screen. The 1936 Paramount musical comedy *College Holiday*, with Jack Benny, George Burns, and Gracie Allen, used eugenics as the pretext for screwball farce. By contrast, the 1939 educational film *Heredity* taught eugenics as established science.

Four theatrical films presented euthanasia as a central theme between 1934 and 1940, although unlike the pre-1921 films, none was allowed to explicitly endorse the practice. Joseph Breen, administrator of the Motion Picture Association's new Production Code, ruled that mercy killing was murder. He denied approval to any picture that put the subject in a positive light or in which a mercy killer was allowed to go unpunished. For example, Breen twice rejected the 1936 film that 20th Century Fox originally titled *The Mercy Killer.* It won approval only after the title was changed to *Crimes of Dr. Forbes* and the ending was altered to have the patient die of an accidental drug overdose rather than intentional euthanasia.[5]

The resurgence of interest in euthanasia paralleled its renewed connection with eugenics. Several key leaders of the Euthanasia Society of America, organized in 1938, were at least as committed to killing defectives on eugenic grounds as they were to relieving the sufferings of terminal illness. One prominent founder, New York neurologist Dr. Foster Kennedy, favored legalizing euthanasia *only* for impaired newborns; he opposed mercy killing of sick but genetically normal adults.[6]

In 1937 one respected magazine opinion survey reported that a majority of those with a view on euthanasia supported it for "defective infants" but not for the "incurably ill." And a majority of these infanticide supporters felt the decision should be made by a "medical board" without requiring family permission.[7]

The Illinois Homeopathic Medical Association lobbied for euthanasia of "imbeciles" and others in 1931.[8] William W. Gregg wrote in 1934 that "in the case of human monstrosities the attending physician . . . sees to it that such mistakes of nature do not live." He cited the stand by the Illinois homeopaths as evidence the practice would soon be legalized.[9] In the early 1930s the Congress of the British Royal Sanitary Institute also debated a proposal from two leading doctors who advocated the killing of "human mental monstrosities."[10] In a widely publicized incident of 1935, an anonymous British physician admitted to having killed five incurable patients, including at least one newborn "clearly doomed to imbecility."[11]

Several leading eugenicists likewise resumed attacks on doctors who saved defective infants. University of Michigan pathologist Aldred Scott Warthin wrote in 1930, "It is certain that modern preventive medicine . . . is causing an increase in the number of the unfit who survive to maturity." "What is the use in saving them," he queried, when "there are too many people living now without whom the world would be much better off!"[12]

These incidents recapitulated many themes first publicly aired in Haiselden's crusade two decades earlier. And at least a few participants continued to cite Haiselden's precedent. One medical author in 1933 described the basic outline of a Bollinger-type case in hypothetic terms. He then revealed that "such cases are on medical record," but did not refer to any specific examples.[13] Newspapers did occasionally mention Haiselden by name in connection with specific later cases; the *New York Times* did so in 1924 as did the *Chicago Tribune* in 1938.[14] A 1935 article in the *American Mercury* used Haiselden's example to illustrate the martyrdom awaiting doctors who challenged religious opposition to mercy killing.[15]

But surprisingly few 1930s articles on such cases even hinted that the issue had a history. Even the 1927 version of *Are You Fit to Marry?* deleted the original screen credit to Dr. Haiselden and tried to frame the story in a contemporary setting. The few articles mentioned above are the only examples discovered so far in which Haiselden was even alluded to during the 1930s.

While it is hard to prove why something didn't happen, a number of explanations for this relative amnesia seem plausible. For one thing, Haiselden had been a deliberate loner, a self-proclaimed provocateur who chose to operate outside the research institutes and congresses of organized eugenics. He dramatically demonstrated how a single person's actions can illuminate and reconfigure the conceptual boundaries of an issue. But without an ongoing institution committed to perpetuating his crusade, memory of his actions barely survived his own short life span.

In addition, media coverage of this subject fits the cyclical attention span and the preoccupation with novelty that journalism critics today allege to be characteristic of American public depictions of all complex unresolved problems.

However, Haiselden did not simply fade from memory; he appears to have been deliberately erased. Haiselden was forgotten in part because powerful forces in medicine and the media determined that he should not be discussed. Professional opposition to publicizing this issue and the film industry's refusal to allow theatrical depictions of unpleasant medical subjects curtailed coverage of Haiselden's activities even in his own lifetime,[16] and the continued operation of these forces repressed any further discussion once he had ceased to generate new cases.

Furthermore, by the 1930s, when the issues he had raised were again permitted into public discourse, both sides in the debate had good tactical reasons not to resurrect Haiselden's example. Opponents of eugenic euthanasia had little to gain by reminding the public that there had been precedent for such actions and that Haiselden had enjoyed extensive public support. Supporters would not benefit by acknowledging their links to an individual whose publicity-seeking had alienated both doctors and the media.

When American discussion of eugenic euthanasia resumed in the 1930s, comparative examples were drawn not from recent American history but from contemporary Germany. Americans had begun to associate eugenic killing with German Social Darwinism and the philosophy of Nietzsche by the 1910s. During World War I, a diverse mix of antiwar socialists, Mendelian geneticists, religious traditionalists, and Anglophile interventionists used such associations to portray the "rape of Belgium" and other wartime atrocities as direct results of German eugenics. Democratic socialist biologist O. C. Glaser called extermination of the unfit the "Hun" method of eugenics.[17] One 1915 commentator equated the Bollinger case with eugenic-inspired German war crimes, reminding Haiselden, "This is hardly the year to call for more Schrecklichkeit [horribleness] toward babies."[18]

While American eugenicists of the 1920s temporarily distanced themselves from euthanasia, German eugenicists retained the link. In 1920 jurist Karl Binding and psychiatrist Alfred Hoche wrote a widely publicized volume that called for killing the mentally and physically defective. Two years later Ernst Mann called for killing cripples at birth; the proposal was formally presented before the Reichstag.[19]

And while American filmmakers shunned the issue, German cinema devoted increasing attention to eugenics in the 1920s, with films such as *The Curse of Heredity* (Der Fluch der Vererbung), *Man, The Right of the Unborn, Survival of the Fittest,* and *Inherited Instincts* (Verebte Instinkte). Weimar social hygiene films also emphasized eugenics, in such productions as *The Hygiene of Marriage* and *The Enemy in the Blood* (Fiend im Blut). A number of these titles were shown in the United States during the 1920s, where they constituted virtually the only films available on eugenics apart from *Are You Fit to Marry?*[20] The association of eugenics movies with foreign films was probably reflected in the fact that by 1928 even Haiselden's picture was being distributed by two companies whose names implied they specialized in foreign movies—Piccadilly Films and Famous Italian Pictures.[21]

German and American eugenics retained close ties through the 1920s and 1930s. German race hygienists regarded the United States as a leader in applying eugenic theory to public policy, and they carefully followed American immigration, sterilization, and similar laws.[22]

By the 1930s racial hygiene, eugenics, and euthanasia played a complex but central role in the evolution of Nazi ideology and in the legitimation of Nazi genocide. Depicting their intended victims as carriers of racial "diseases" constituted a key feature of Nazi propaganda and justified the power of the Nazi state as necessary to protect the public health from such contamination. Programs for killing incurably ill institutional patients, such as the operation code-named "T-4" that secretly gassed over 100,000 disabled Germans, pioneered the machinery and trained the medical personnel who were then transferred to run the death camps for the "racially diseased."[23]

Motion pictures, many only recently rediscovered in East German archives, were essential to the Nazi effort to label their targets as sick, and to promote killing as the cure. Two early Nazi Party productions, *Erbkrank* [Hereditary Disease] (1934) and *Was du ererbt* [What You Inherit] (1935), feature crude photography of repulsive-looking institutionalized handicapped and mentally ill patients. *Erbkrank*'s silent intertitles provide these cases with individual price tags for their annual care. The film sought to foster disgust, resentment, and hatred, but did not yet advocate any specific policies to discharge these emotions.[24]

Two more-polished sound films, *Opfer der Vergangenheit* [Victims of the Past] (1937) and *Alles Leben ist Kampf* [All Life Is Struggle] (1940), contain similar footage of asylum patients, but these productions go on to urge compulsory sterilization as the solution. *Das Erbe* [The Inheritance], a film about the making of a eugenics educational film, first introduced German audiences to the idea of euthanasia for the unfit. And killing the physically and mentally impaired is the primary message of three films produced specifically to combat public opposition to the T-4 program. *Dasein ohne Leben* [Existence Without Life] (1939), *Geisteskrank* [Mentally Ill] (1939), and *Ich Klage An* [I Accuse] (1941) were distributed on direct orders of S.S. Chief Heinrich Himmler. The first and third focus on voluntary mercy killing, while the second apparently urged killing all incurables.[25]

While many American scientists distanced themselves from what was known of German eugenics in the 1930s, key leaders of the American eugenics and euthanasia organizations, such as Charles Davenport, Harry Laughlin, and Foster Kennedy, enthusiastically endorsed the Nazi eugenic program and its promotion of euthanasia. As late as 1942, Kennedy's only criticism was that the Nazis went too far in trying to sterilize all the feebleminded. "In their higher grades they are greatly needed for the simpler forms of work."[26]

American supporters particularly admired the Nazi film efforts. The New Jersey Sterilization League, an important eugenic advocacy group, translated and helped distribute a Nazi film they called *The Fatal Chain of Hereditary Disease* (1938).[27] After seeing *Erbkrank* in 1936, Laughlin urged American eugenicists to copy it. The next year, the newly organized Pioneer Fund, of which Laughlin was a founder, made one of its first projects an effort to distribute *Erbkrank* and other Nazi eugenics films to American schools and churches. Laughlin showed *Erbkrank* at the Carnegie Institution in Washington, D.C., and distributed advertising fliers to over 3000 high school biology teachers nationwide. At least twenty-eight had booked the film by 1938.[28]

American supporters deliberately soft-pedalled or denied the harsher aspects of these films. For example, *Erbkrank* declares, "Jewish liberal thinking forced millions of healthy volk-nationals into need and squalor—while the unfit were overly coddled." The film states unequivocally, "The Jewish people has a particularly high percentage of mentally ill," and it illustrates the point with a disgusting-looking asylum patient labeled "Fifty-five-year-old Jew—deceitful—rabble-rouser." The movie also portrays "an idiotic black bastard from the Rhineland," an area occupied by French African troops after World War I. Yet Laughlin's promotional literature repeatedly assured American audiences, "there is no racial propaganda of any sort in the picture," insisting three times in one paragraph that the film applied its objective scientific lessons "regardless of race."[29]

The long history of interaction between American and German eugenics provides a crucial context for the striking parallels between Haiselden's crusade and the Nazi campaign for eugenic killing two decades later. Haiselden's destruction of what he called "lives of no value"[30] helped promote concepts and catch-phrases that became central to the legitimation of genocide. Thus part of Haiselden's historical importance derives from the light his actions shed on the way in which ideas and images later used by the Nazis first took shape.

The Black Stork in particular contains direct parallels with several Nazi productions, including *Erbkrank* and *Alles Leben ist Kampf*. All three films feature stark visual contrasts between loathsome expensive defectives and poor but healthy working people. As the camera cuts from institutional patients to poor farmers and urban workers, the films explain:

> Our defectives are housed in palaces costing fortunes while our unfortunate normal children live like maggots in filthy hovels where the death rate is high.
>
> *The Black Stork*

> Where palaces are built for the offspring of drunkards, criminals, and imbeciles, while the worker and peasant must put up with miserable huts, such a nation approaches its end with giant steps. . . . [Under the old order] healthy families were housed in half-fallen-down huts and cramped back houses. But for lunatics who were totally indifferent to their surroundings, palaces were built.[31]
>
> *Erbkrank*

> The past system built palaces for idiots and the criminally insane. While poor but healthy men had to live in falling-down hovels.
>
> *Alles Leben ist Kampf*[32]

However, I could find no evidence that Haiselden's cases or his crusade played any direct role in influencing the course of German genocide. Apparently neither Weimar nor Nazi eugenicists knew anything specifically about Haiselden or his film, nor did they mention that an American doctor had refused to treat defective infants.[33]

Nor can I find any evidence that Haiselden's words or ideas were directly shaped by earlier German sources that might also have influenced Nazi thinking. Haiselden had been educated in a German-American school and ran a largely German hospital, so he may well have learned about the monist opposition to saving impaired newborns. And Sigmund Engel's Socialist-Darwinist call for eugenic infanticide was translated in 1912 by Eden Paul, a close colleague of Haiselden supporters William and Frederic Robinson. However, Haiselden never cited any German precedents in his propaganda, nor did he acknowledge any German influence on his ideas.

The only likely link between Haiselden and Hitler is indirect, through Madison Grant's *Passing of the Great Race*. Grant's book was translated into German in 1925 and soon became a staple of Nazi race theory. Hitler reportedly called the book his "bible." The architects of genocide attempted to follow Grant's strategy of gradually expanding their targets, beginning with "defective infants" and culminating in "worthless race types."[34] If, as seems probable,

Grant had Haiselden's example fresh in his mind when he wrote that section, Haiselden's crusade may well have had a secondhand impact on the development of Nazi eugenic strategy.[35]

Additional research conceivably could turn up evidence that Haiselden was directly influenced by early German race theorists, and/or that Nazi race hygienists drew directly on Haiselden's examples. But the parallels between them do not depend for their significance on such direct links of intellectual ancestry. Rather, the similarities are important because they illuminate how Nazism built upon internationally shared eugenic concepts and images. For example, their common contrast between "palace" and "hovel" had already provided an evocative metaphor for class conflict even before Haiselden used it.[36] And class-based resentment of public spending on asylums dated to the mid-nineteenth-century origins of those institutions. The year before the Bollinger case, John Harvey Kellogg complained that institutional pampering created an "aristocracy of lunatics."[37]

From the specific language of their film propaganda to their broadest assumptions about the moral duty to eugenic science, both Haiselden and Nazism shared a common early-twentieth-century vocabulary. Recognition that genocide drew upon ideas that were developed outside of Nazism and beyond the borders of Germany cannot legitimately be used to diffuse historical responsibility for the uniquely horrible application of these concepts by specific individual Nazis and by the Nazi state and society. Conversely, Haiselden's anticipation of themes central to Nazi ideology does not make him the historical or moral equivalent of a Nazi. His actions seem to have played at most a peripheral and indirect role in the evolution of genocide.

But if Haiselden's ideas did not cause the holocaust, both grew in similar soil. His story does illuminate some of the specific forces, large and small, that made it possible for Nazism to claim the intellectual and moral authority of twentieth-century medical science.

Baby Doe, Doctor Death, and the Human Genome Project: Comparing Haiselden's America with the Present

Baby Doe

When the selective refusal to treat impaired babies emerged once again in public debate during the 1970s, Harry Haiselden had been long forgotten. The history of infanticide by lay people—parents, midwives, and governments, dating back to ancient Greece—was widely discussed in these debates. But the role played by past American physicians in such decisions is now virtually unknown.

Doctors reported not treating impaired newborns at Boston Children's Hospital in 1947, Johns Hopkins in 1969, and elsewhere, but the practice attracted little professional notice and almost no media attention until 1973. In that year, Raymond Duff and A.G.M. Campbell of Yale and John Lorber in Britain published descriptions of selective treatment in two leading medical journals. A U.S. Senate committee held hearings on the issue the following year. And in Maine a state court ordered surgeons to operate on a reparable lethal digestive tract defect in a blind and allegedly brain-damaged baby, though both the parents and the doctors had agreed to withhold surgical treatment.

A 1977 straw poll showed physicians much more willing to withhold therapy than in Haiselden's day, but sharp specialty differences still remained. Nearly 80 percent of pediatric surgeons, but only about half of general pediatricians, said they would agree to a parental request not to treat a Down syndrome baby for a correctable lethal bowel defect.[38]

With the cases of "Baby Doe" in Bloomington, Indiana, in 1982 and "Baby Jane Doe" in Stony Brook, New York, a year later, the issue once again erupted into the kind of front-page mass-media coverage not seen since Haiselden's era seven decades earlier. President Ronald Reagan's outspoken Surgeon General C. Everett Koop, a pediatric surgeon, had long equated selective nontreatment with abortion. He denounced both as violations of medical ethics. In March 1983 the Department of Health and Human Services issued a series of sweeping regulations to prevent hospitals from selectively withholding treatment. The agency claimed authority to issue such rules under a 1973 law banning federal discrimination against the handicapped.[39]

In the resulting glare of publicity, other similar cases came to light. In a 1977 to 1983 University of Oklahoma study, thirty-three infants with spina bifida were left untreated. At the opposite extreme, a 1983 book detailed the case of "Baby Andrew" Stinson, a premature infant whose painful death in 1977 had been prolonged by heroic medical treatment despite the parents' objections.[40]

The controversy reached the U.S. Supreme Court. Their June 9, 1986 ruling in *Bowen* v. *American Hospital Association* invalidated the strict federal restrictions.[41] The Court held that the 1973 law did not give the federal government authority to force hospitals to treat or report an infant whose parents had refused to permit treatment.

Meanwhile, in 1984 Congress defined "child neglect" to include the withholding of "medically indicated" lifesaving treatment from disabled infants, except for those who were irreversibly comatose, those who were going to die soon anyhow, and those for whom treatment was both "virtually futile" and "inhumane."[42] This law generally has been seen as favoring treatment of almost all savable newborns.[43] However, enforcement was left to each state's child protection agency, and vast discretion was granted to the medical profession and individual doctors. The act specifically stated that it did not authorize any government body to "establish standards prescribing specific medical treatments for specific conditions."[44] And the determination of which treatments are lifesaving, which are futile, and which are inhumane was explicitly left to "the treating physician's . . . reasonable medical judgment."

Futile, effective, and inhumane are not purely objective terms on which medical science can agree.[45] Thus the *Bowen* decision and the child abuse amendments did not end the controversy over selective nontreatment. Many current disputes arise when at least one parent disagrees with a doctor's judgment that treatment is not indicated. As of 1994, state and federal courts continued to wrestle with such cases, sometimes allowing treatment to be withheld, as in the 1993 Flint, Michigan, case of anencephalic "Baby Terry"; other times ordering doctors to provide treatment, as in the similar 1992–94 case of "Baby K" in Fairfax, Virginia.[46]

The initial Baby Doe debates overtly focused only on what was best for the infants. However, following a much-publicized 1990 study on the costs of treating premature babies, and several recent proposals to use anencephalic newborns as organ donors,[47] considerations of social utility have reemerged, particularly when the issues are raised in the context of national health care reform. In addition, while the Baby Doe cases dealt with surgical treatment for relatively rare life-threatening intestinal or spinal defects, current attention is centered on the less dramatic but far more common dilemmas posed by the treatment of severely premature infants.

And perhaps for the first time since *The Black Stork*, selective nontreatment of impaired infants has returned to the movie screen. The best-known recent film on the subject, *Who Should Survive?* (Joseph P. Kennedy Jr. Foundation 1972), documents the decision not to treat a Down syndrome baby's intestinal blockage. A similar, more recent example is *Born Dying* (Norman Baxley and Associates

1985). A 1983 segment of the controversial television show *Quincy*, titled "For Love of Joshua," opposed withholding treatment from a baby with Down syndrome. Surgeon General Koop, like his boss, was a master of mass communications. In his memoirs, Koop claims he first gained the notice of the Reagan administration for *Whatever Happened to the Human Race?*, a series of five films he helped produce to dramatize opposition to abortion and infant euthanasia.[48]

The sudden flood of media attention since 1982 cannot be explained entirely by the novelty of the first Baby Doe cases. At the same time that Baby Jane Doe filled the nightly newscasts, forty-eight similar cases were reported to the Department of Health and Human Services, but only one local newspaper, New York's *Newsday*, bothered to report on them.[49] As in Haiselden's era, changes in the level and focus of reporting did not depend on the actual number or newness of such cases, but on changing conceptions of whether the media should publicize medical uncertainties, and changing constructions of these cases' broader cultural and political significance.[50]

In the Baby Doe debates, both the mass media and most academic studies presented the issue as unprecedented. Thus in 1983, the President's Commission for the Study of Ethical Problems in Medicine attributed the controversy entirely to "new medical capabilities," and claimed that the debate "began . . . in the early 1970s."[51]

Certainly new technologies, from neonatal intensive care units to prenatal genetic screening, have drastically altered the context and dimensions of the issues. Decades of debate over abortion, civil rights, and feminism have also changed the contemporary cultural setting. Yet to assume that the issues have never been faced before and that they are simply products of new technology not only distorts the past but prevents examining the extent to which things have or haven't changed since the days of Harry Haiselden.

Doctor Death

While the Baby Doe debates were characterized by historical amnesia, current controversies over "medically assisted suicide" and human genetics research have been conducted in the looming shadow of the past. Both topics evoke extensive comparisons with Nazi genocide, and both have produced varying degrees of attention to earlier American precedents as well.

Voluntary euthanasia of pain-ravaged adults gained renewed attention from ethicists, doctors, and patient advocates in the early 1970s. This interest reflected increased emphasis on personal autonomy in health care, promoted in part by a new profession of bioethics; an explosion in the expense of medical treatment; and a growing dread that modern technology extended life without restoring health, and at the cost of great suffering.[52] Academic debate over euthanasia grew following such pivotal court cases as those of Karen Quinlan, Elizabeth Bouvia, and Nancy Cruzan.

But while academics and lawyers debated, Derek Humphry's Hemlock Society published *Final Exit*, a self-help suicide manual designed to enable individuals to skip the theory and get on with the practice.[53] And in June 1990, Michigan pathologist Dr. Jack Kevorkian gained the title "Doctor Death" when he began publicly to assist patients who wished to kill themselves.

Initial media coverage of Kevorkian focused on the novelty of his "suicide machine." As in the Baby Doe cases, the preoccupation with new machinery threatened to preempt any historical awareness. But aided by a court order impounding the unimpressively low-tech "machine," reporters eventually shifted focus from the allegedly novel equipment to the broader issue of "doctor-assisted suicide" and its links to the history of euthanasia.[54]

To the extent that Haiselden is remembered at all today, it is the euthanasia movement that occasionally still invokes his name as an early pioneer of the cause.[55] And there are important substantive and stylistic similarities between Haiselden and modern euthanasia advocates, especially Kevorkian, even though Kevorkian does not recall ever hearing about Haiselden. Like Haiselden, Kevorkian practices a propaganda of the deed. Both of them forced people to take sides by acting on formerly abstract theories and by doing publicly what others have done only in private. Both cast themselves as lone provocateurs, critical of less-action-oriented organizations. But both shifted the parameters of debate, making these formerly extreme organizations seem closer to the mainstream. Both were highly conscious of the importance of mass-media coverage, and both have been criticized as much for their publicity-seeking as for their actions.[56]

Human Genetics

Dramatic advances in molecular genetics, particularly the ability to isolate, replicate, and decode small segments of genetic material, have revolutionized the study of human heredity within the past two decades. Four different kinds of new medical knowledge have resulted from this work:

1. Location of a small but rapidly growing number of specific genes that play a role in causing specific diseases.
2. Development of diagnostic screening tests for some of these genes.
3. Creation of a massive project to map the location and spell out the chemical code of each human gene (the "human genome project").
4. Testing of experimental treatments for specific genetic diseases through the use of replacement gene products or replacement genes.

Development of the human genome project in particular has proceeded with considerable attention to the past. In funding the effort, Congress mandated that a significant fraction of the budget be devoted to the ethical, legal, and historical implications of human genetic research.

Past and Present

To what extent do current human genetics, euthanasia, and the treatment of impaired infants differ from past practices? Many ethicists, scientists, and historians emphasize significant differences. Though they generally discuss genetic research and euthanasia as separate issues, their grounds for distinguishing between past and present are quite similar for each. In both cases, they point to three main distinctions.

First, the strong contemporary commitment to individual autonomy in medical decision making supposedly marks a sharp break from the days of Haiselden or Hitler. This commitment to free choice, embodied in the modern doctrine of "informed consent," was first codified in response to the Nuremberg revelations of Nazi medical murder. On this view, past abuses resulted from compulsory measures for the collective good, defined and imposed by the state. So long as individual parents and patients are free to choose whether and how to use medical knowledge, many believe that modern genetics and modern euthanasia will each promote humane health care without the danger of repeating the past. From this perspective, the major ethical problem in modern human genetics is not preventing its imposition on the unwilling but assuring that its expensive benefits are fairly distributed to all who want them. Likewise, laws that deny patients access to euthanasia, not the practice itself, are seen as unethical violations of autonomy.

Thoughtful advocates of this position recognize that not only government actions, but poverty, pain, and ignorance can also interfere with free individual choice. And most acknowledge that in cases such as sex-selection or the preservation of valuable genetic diversity, society's collective interests might legitimately require regulating some individual preferences, at least until "market" forces can produce a corrective change in individual values. But these are seen as manageable problems, so long as the fundamental commitment to autonomy remains intact.[57]

A second frequently asserted difference from the past is that history has shown the dangers of mixing science and ideology. This doctrine holds that, if contemporary medicine is rigorously isolated from social and political influences, euthanasia can be limited to those with objectively hopeless diagnoses, and genetic therapies confined to people with objectively defined diseases. So long as the indications for genetic medicine or euthanasia are kept as objective as those for any other medical procedure, these practices need not be any more troubling than treating an infection.[58]

Third, modern medicine is widely seen as being better able to deliver on its promises than it was in the past. Past eugenics, it is alleged, was bad science not only because it was value-laden, but because it was based on poor data, sloppy reasoning, and inadequate technical information. Eugenic techniques of the first half of this century were totally inadequate to accomplish eugenic goals. Since the vast majority of recessive disease genes are carried by healthy heterozygotes, and since every person probably carries several such genes, for the techniques of the past to have eliminated genetic diseases would have required eliminating the human species. Similarly, past euthanasia was plagued by vast uncertainties of medical prognosis, especially for newborns. Today, such technical shortcomings seem on the verge of being vanquished, by the advances in molecular biology.

These differences are significant and profoundly important. Yet in comparing Haiselden's era with the 1930s and with the present, this study also finds important and disturbing continuities. First, while the professed commitment to individual autonomy is more explicit and elaborated today than ever before, such ideas are not nearly as new as they seem. A therapeutic rationale for honoring many patient choices and an ideological allergy to state-dictated medicine were both firm components of American medical professionalism before the advent of eugenics. One of the strongest judicial affirmations of the right to refuse treatment came in 1914.[59] But given the rapid and unprecedented rise of deference to professional expertise in the progressive era, these commitments proved severely inadequate. Even now, despite unprecedented support for personal autonomy, many studies indicate that this commitment is honored more in theory than in daily medical practice.[60]

Furthermore, many of the structural and cultural pressures that limited individual freedom in Haiselden's era remain important today. As Haiselden's socialist supporters repeatedly pointed out, a poor family struggling to make ends meet does not have the same freedom to choose to raise a disabled child as a wealthy family does. And if eliminating those with defects became the social norm, families who would like to choose otherwise would be subjected to enormous social pressures, as the cultural toleration for human differences contracted. This was part of the logic behind Madison Grant and William McKim's proposals for the gradual expansion of eugenic targets. If everyone else on the basketball team gets a gene implant for producing extra growth hormone, what does it mean to say that a player who objects to the procedure has the right to refuse? The absence of government coercion does not guarantee real individual choice. Effective freedom would require elimination of entrenched cultural and structural barriers, not simply refraining from interfering with individual decisions.[61] Thus, although the current commitment to individual choice is an important and valuable difference from earlier coercive state goals in health care, it is neither new enough nor meaningful enough to fully immunize modern medicine from the problems of the past.

Second, although current genetics has produced much more specific and detailed scientific information than past eugenicists ever had available, as in Haiselden's day, the perception that genetic knowledge has outpaced social and cultural knowledge may lead to vastly exaggerated expectations for the utility of this information. If faith in the power of heredity and genetic science outstrips understanding of the limits of their ability to predestine human affairs, it could once again make potentially valuable social changes seem inefficient or impossible. Such a gap between knowledge and expectations can occur despite, and perhaps even because of, how far current genetic knowledge seems to have advanced.[62]

Further, if the techniques of genetic engineering ever do fulfill current expectations, it might actually be possible to eliminate unwanted genes without eliminating the people who currently carry them. Such techniques carried to the logical extreme could make possible genocide without homicide, the bloodless extermination of unwanted characteristics. Thus the greater ability of modern genetics to achieve its goals is only a reassuring difference from the past if it is used for better goals.

It is in regard to goals that this study finds the most important continuities between past and present. First, the specific values that converted past eugenics into a rationale for genocide are still alive and killing. The ethnic bloodbath in the former Yugoslavia is only the most visible example of the resurgence of overtly racist nationalism, throughout formerly communist Europe, in both parts of reunited Germany, and among the nationalist parties of western Europe, including the recent governmental role of the "neo"-Fascists in Italy. And from Los Angeles to Crown Heights, racial murder is not a thing of the past in the United States either.

The effort to keep current genetics and euthanasia "objective" is in part a well-meaning recognition of the continued danger from such lethal values. But comparison with Haiselden's era indicates this attempt to keep science value-free may be recreating one of the most dangerous aspects of early eugenics. Racism became part of eugenics in Haiselden's time, not just because racism was prevalent in his culture, but because progressives shared a faith in the objective truth and hence the moral force of their own beliefs. The present concept of objectivity as "value-neutrality" differs significantly from Haiselden's belief that objectivity was a method for discovering morally binding "true values."[63] But both kinds of objectivization allow cultural values to masquerade as objective truths.

Past eugenic racism was based on values most thoughtful people today consider anathema. The problem, however, was not that eugenics *had* values, but that it had *bad* values. Like it or not, defining genetic health and disease can never be a purely objective technical question, because defining sickness and health always requires an evaluative judgment. Even if all observers agree on the existence and consequences of a particular human difference, they are not likely to call that difference a "disease" unless they also agree that it is a "bad" thing to have. Thus trying to make any medical science "value-free" can never succeed; explicit or implicit values will always be needed. Pretending that medicine can be purely objective only repeats the most flawed aspect of Haiselden's eugenics. It permits subjective values to claim the moral authority of scientific truth, while delegitimating the kinds of political and ethical scrutiny that alone can enable a culture to debate and evaluate these value judgments intelligently.

Of course, simply to admit that distinguishing good and bad genes requires an ethical decision does not guarantee that present decisions will later be judged correct. But it need not always be an admission of futility or a recipe for gridlock either.[64] The many human differences that are almost universally recognized as diseases are accorded that status because of an implicit value consensus. For example, even though it is a value judgment, few today would question that dying prematurely and in great pain is bad.

While human genetics can never be purely objective, perhaps modern science will make the methods of gene therapy as routine as other medical treatments and the definition of genetic disease no more value-laden than any other branch of pathology. But in Haiselden's day and in Nazi Germany, what was done "in the name of eugenics" was also done in the name of infection control and surgery.[65] Even if genetic therapy were to become no more ethically problematic than antibiotics, that similarity should not be a lullaby for genetics, but an alarm clock for the rest of medicine.

Appendix: Individuals Involved in the Controversy

The tables as well as many of the generalizations in chapter 2 are based on the following list of individuals who took a position either on the treatment of impaired infants or on mass-media coverage of the issue in response to the activities of Dr. Haiselden.

Citations are to the first source in which I encountered the views of the individual,* though many quotes were widely reprinted in other publications. Multiple citations are listed only when a source located later contained opinions substantively different from those in the first. "See Index" indicates the individual's views are discussed in the text. Unless otherwise noted, a reference to the NBRMP indicates a response to that board's unpublished survey. With the exception of that survey, the

---

* See Notes for abbreviations of sources.

sources listed here may not have accurately recorded the views of the specific individuals represented as holding them. See chapter 2 for a discussion of the utility and the limitations of such evidence.

Individuals directly involved in the production or distribution of Haiselden's film are also listed here, based on the inference that they supported at least some mass-media depictions of the subject. However, no opinions about the treatment of impaired newborns can be attributed to someone based solely on his or her involvement with the film, and no such implications have been drawn.

Abbe, Robert, M.D.: *CA* 11/27/15
Abt, Isaac, M.D.: *CH* 11/17/15; *CA* 7/25/17
Ackermann, Paul, M.D.: *NYT* 11/16/17
Adair, Fred Lyman, M.D.: *MRR* Feb. 1916
Adams, J. Lee, M.D.: *WP* 11/18/17 p. 10
Adams, Mrs. W. R.: *Omaha News,* in NBRMP
Addams, Jane: *NYT* 11/18/15
Adler, Felix: NBRMP
Alexander, Rev. John L.: NBRMP
Alexander, Selma, M.D.: *NYAm* 11/18/15 p. 6
Anderson, Rev. Augustine Hugo Wells: *CH* 11/17/15
Anderson, Carl, M.D.: *CA* 11/16/17
Arnold, Victor Page: *CH* 11/17/15
Arnow, Irwin, M.D.: *CH* 11/18/15
Arthur, Clara B.: *DN* 11/18/15
Austin, Mary Hunter: *NYAm* 11/23/15 p. 10
Bacon, Charles Sumner, M.D.: *MRR* Feb. 1916
Ballou, W. H.: *NYAm* 11/19/15
Barclay, M. R., M.D.: *NYT* 11/16/17
Barker, Lewellys, M.D.: *NYT* 11/18/15; *CN* 11/17/15
Barnett, Irving, M.D.: *CA* 12/23/15
Baruch, Simon, M.D.: *NYS* 11/21/15 vii:1
Batchelder, Ernest A.: NBRMP
Baughman, Greer, M.D.: *MRR* Feb. 1916
Baxter, Elsie: LC paperprint
Baxter, Leroy: LC paperprint
Bean, Rev. Waldemar: NBRMP
Beard, Charles A.: *NYT* 11/18/15
Belknap, Eugene W., M.D.: *MRR* Feb. 1916
Bell, Clark: *NYT* 11/18/15

Bell, John Norval, M.D.: *MRR* Feb. 1916

Bellamy, George A.: NBRMP

Belmont, Mrs. Oliver Hazard Perry (Alva Erskine Smith Vanderbilt): *NYT* 11/20/15

Benson, Reuel Allen, M.D.: *NYS* 11/18/15 p. 3

Berger, Frank J., M.D.: *NYT* 11/16/17

Bergman, Henry: LC paperprint

Berwick, Edward: *Independent* 1/3/16

Biel, Marion H.: *CN* 11/17/15

Birss, Mrs. F. J.: *Omaha News,* in NBRMP

Blaisdell, George: *MPW* 2/24/17 p. 121

Block, Anita C.: *MRR* Feb. 1916, p. 122

Block, Siegfried, M.D.: *NYAm* 11/18/15

Blount, Anna, M.D.: *CN* 11/17/15

Bogart, Leon M., M.D.: *CE* 7/24/17

Boissevain, Inez Milholland: *CH* 11/18/15

Bollinger, Allen: *CT* 11/17/15

Bollinger, Anna: *CT* 11/17/15

Bowe, Augustine J.: *NYT* 11/18/15

Bowen, William Sinclair, M.D.: *MRR* Feb. 1916

Boynton, Rev. Nehemiah: *NYAm* 11/18/15

Branely, Margaret: *WP* 11/25/15 p. 3

Briggs, Frank H.: *MPN* 2/24/17 p. 1244

Briggs, L. Vernon, M.D.: *CH* 11/18/15

Britton, Gertrude Howe: *NYT* 11/17/15

Brock, Walter B.: *Independent* 1/3/16

Brody, I.: NYSA-MPD

Brooks, H.J.: NYSA-MPD

Brotherton, Mrs. Wilbur: *DN* 11/18/15

Brown, J. R., M.D.: *CT* 11/19/15

Brown, Rev. William Adams: NBRMP

Brylawski, Aaron: *MPN* 2/24/17 p. 1244

Bulliet, Clarence Joseph: *Motography* 3/24/17

Bullock, Georgia: *Call* 12/3/15 p. 8

Burke, Rhoda: *WP* 11/19/15 p. 2

Burton, Rev. Marion LeRoy: NBRMP

Butler, Glentworth Reeve, M.D.: *NYS* 11/18/15 p. 3

Cabot, Hugh, M.D.: See Index.

Cabot, Richard Clarke, M.D.: See Index.

Carroll, Rev.: *New World* 12/24/15

Carter, Thomas Albert, M.D.: *NYT* 11/16/17

Chadwick, Florence, M.D.: *DN* 11/18/15

Chislett, Howard Roy, M.D.: *NYT* 11/19/15
Christian, Andreas Forest, M.D.: *CH* 11/18/15
Christie, B. W., M.D.: NBRMP
Clapham, Edward G.: *Independent* 1/3/16
Clark, John Bates: NBRMP
Clark, John Edward, M.D.: *DN* 11/17/15
Cocks, Rev. Orrin G.: NBRMP
Cocroft, Susanna: *CH* 11/18/15
Coe, Helen L. (?): NBRMP
Cohn, Rabbi Frederick: NBRMP
Coles, Stricker, M.D.: *MRR* Feb. 1916
Colie, Edward M. Jr., M.D.: *MRR* Feb. 1916
Conybeare, S. E.: *MPN* 2/24/17 p. 1244
Cooley, Mrs. Harlan Ward (Nellie Wooster): *CT* 11/17/15
Copeland, Royal, M.D.: *WP* 11/18/15
Coulter, Ernest K.: *CN* 11/17/15
Covill, W. M.: NBRMP
Crawford, Mary M., M.D.: *NYAm* 11/19/15
Crile, Mrs. George Washington: NBRMP
Croll, Walter Lewis, M.D.: *MRR* Feb. 1916
Cross, Edwin, M.D.: *NYT* 11/16/17
Crothers, Thomas Davison, M.D.: *NYT* 11/18/15
Culbertson, Carey, M.D.: *MRR* Feb. 1916
Cunningham, Joseph L., M.D.: *CA* 11/16/17
Cutter, Irving S., M.D.: *Omaha News*, in NBRMP
Darcey, James F.: *DFP* 11/23/15
Darrow, Clarence: *WP* 11/18/15
Davenport, Charles B.: *Independent* 1/3/16
Davenport, Edgar: LC paperprint
David, R. A., M.D.: *CA* 11/16/17
Davis, Katharine Bement: *WP* 11/18/15; *Call* 11/18/15
Day, Mrs. Frank L.: *DN* 11/18/15
De Birmingham, Jose, M.D.: *NYAm* 11/30/15
De Forest, Robert W.: NBRMP
De Lee, Joseph Bolivar, M.D.: *MRR* Feb. 1916
Deacon, Frank, M.D.: *CH* 3/15/16
Dean, Jonathan M.: NBRMP
Dennett, Mary Ware: *CN* 11/17/15
Deters, Clement: *New World* 11/19/15
Dewitt, Leslie Higley Stark, M.D.: *MRR* Feb. 1916
Dorland, William Alexander Newman, M.D.: *MRR* Feb. 1916
Downes, William A., M.D.: *Call* 11/26/15

Drake, C. Saint Clair, M.D.: *NYT* 12/10/15
Dudley, Rev. George Fiske: *WP* 11/18/17
Edgar, James Clifton, M.D.: *MRR* Feb. 1916
Edsall, Frank H., M.D.: *DN* 11/22/15
Edson, Andrew W.: NBRMP
Edwards, R. H.: NBRMP
Eisner, Edward: *Call* 11/28/15
Eliot, Rev. William G. Jr.: NBRMP
Elkus, Charles DeY.: NBRMP
Ellis, Robert Hale, M.D.: *MRR* Feb. 1916
Esmond, Elsie: LC Paperprint
Fallows, Rev. Samuel: *NYT* 11/18/15
Faltermayer, Jacob, M.D.: *CT* 12/8/15
Farington, Grace Safford: *MPN* 2/24/17 p. 1244
Farley, Rev.: *NYAm* 11/30/15
Fearnly, Jane: LC Paperprint
Feinberg, Israel, M.D.: *NYT* 11/27/15; *DFP* 11/28/15; *Call* 11/28/15
Feser, Raymond Leonard, M.D.: *CH* 7/24/17
Fischer, Louis, M.D.: *NYT* 11/18/15
Fisher, Irving: See index.
Fisher, John, M.D.: *CE* 7/24/17; *NYT* 11/16/17
Fitzgerald, R. S., M.D.: *MRR* Feb. 1916
Fitzsimmons, Rev.: *NYT* 11/18/15
Fogdall, Rev. Sorenus P.: *Independent* 1/3/16
Forrester, Joseph, M.D.: *NYT* 11/16/17
Foster, Eugene C.: NBRMP
Foster, Festus: NBRMP
Fowler, Russell Story, M.D.: *NYS* 11/18/15 p. 3
France, Antoinette: *CN* 11/17/15
Freed, Beulah: *CA* 11/27/15
Freer, Otto Tiger, M.D.: *CH* 3/15/16
Fry, Henry Davidson, M.D.: *MRR* Feb. 1916
Gannon, J. A., M.D.: *WP* 11/18/17 p. 10
Gibbons, James Cardinal: *CT* 11/20/15 p. 8; *Baltimore Catholic Review* 11/19/15
Gibney, Virgil Pendleton, M.D.: *NYT* 11/18/15
Giddings, Franklin H.: *Independent* 1/3/16, for treatment; NBRMP, for film
Gilchrist, John H.: public action reported in NBRMP
Gill, O. M., M.D.: *DN* 11/18/15
Gilman, Robbins: NBRMP
Girvin, John H., M.D.: *MRR* Feb. 1916

Glaser, Otto Charles: *Good Health* 52 (1917): 571
Golden, John F., M.D.: *NYT* 11/19/15
Goldsmith, Evelyn M.: *NYT* 11/26/15 p. 8
Goldsmith, Julius, M.D.: *NYT* 11/25/15
Gorton, David Allyn, M.D.: *NYAm* 11/23/15
Graham, Mrs. W. T.: *Omaha News*, in NBRMP
Gregory, Menas Sarkis [T?]., M.D.: *NYAm* 11/19/15
Grimshaw: *CA* 12/28/15 magazine page
Griswold, Don M., M.D.: *DN* 11/18/15
Guenther, Theodore C., M.D.: *NYT* 11/16/17
Guernsey, Florence: *CH* 11/18/15
Hadfield, R. H.: *IDJ* 2/3/17
Haiselden, Harry J., M.D.: See Index.
Halbert, L. A.: NBRMP
Hamilton, Alice, M.D.: *Survey* 12/4/15 pp. 265–66
Hamilton, R. Andrew: NBRMP
Hamilton-Muncie, Elizabeth, M.D.: *CN* 11/17/15
Harding, H. T., M.D.: *WP* 11/18/17 p. 10
Harmon, Frank, M.D.: *CT* 11/18/15
Harris, Genevieve: *Motography* 2/24/17
Harris, Sara: *NYAm* 11/18/15
Healey: *WP* 11/18/15 p. 6
Heaps: *WP* 11/18/15 p. 6
Heffernan, Mrs. William S.: *CN* 11/17/15
Heineck, Aime Paul, M.D.: *CH* 3/15/16
Hektoen, Ludwig, M.D.: *NYT* 11/19/15
Hirst, Barton Cooke, M.D.: *MRR* Feb. 1916
Hitt, Isaac R.: *WP* 11/18/17 P. 10
Hodzima, Pauline: *NYS* 11/13/17
Hodzima, Stephen: *NYS* 11/13/17
Hoffman, Peter M.: *NYT* 11/18/15
Hollander, W. K.: *CN* 4/6/17
Hollison, J. H., M.D.: *CH* 7/25/17
Holmes, Rudolph Wieser, M.D.: *MRR* Feb. 1916
Holt, L. Emmett, M.D.: *NYT* 11/25–27/15
Hopkins, Caroline, M.D.: *CA* 12/23/15
Howell, J. C., M.D.: *Independent* 1/3/16
Hoyne, Archibald, M.D.: *CN* 11/15/17
Hoyne, Maclay: See Index.
Hulbert: *DN* 11/17/15
Humiston, Charles E., M.D.: *CA* 11/13/17
Hutchinson, Woods, M.D.: *NYAm* 11/18/15 p. 6

Hynes, Thomas Vincent, M.D.: *MRR* Feb. 1916
Irwin, Rev. Mabel: *NYAm* 11/25/15 p. 14
Irwin, May: *Call* 11/29/15
Jacobi, Abraham, M.D.: *NYS* 11/18/15 p. 3
Jacobs, S. Nicholas, M.D.: *Call* 12/15/15
James, Walter Belknap, M.D.: *NYAm*, 11/22/15 p. 6
Janeway, Henry Harrington, M.D.: *NYS* 11/1915 p. 14
Jenks, Rev. Edwin Hart: NBRMP
Jenks, Nathan, M.D.: *MRR* Feb. 1916
Johnson, Alexander: *Independent* 1/3/16
Johnson, J. J.: *MPN* 2/24/17 p. 1244
Johnson, Julian: *Photoplay* June 1917, p. 155
Jourdan, A.E.W., M.D.: *CE* 7/24/17; *NYT* 11/16/17
Kan, Louis J., M.D.: *CE* 7/24/17; *NYT* 11/16/17
Kayser, Paul: *Independent* 1/3/16
Keating, F. W., M.D.: *NYS* 11/18/15 p. 3
Keeley, James: *CH* 11/18/15 p. 6
Keller, Helen: *TNR* 12/18/15
Kellogg, John Harvey, M.D.: *Good Health* 51 (1916): 7–9
Kelly, Gertrude B., M.D.: *CH* 11/18/15
Kelly, Kitty: *CE* 4/4/17
Kendall, Sarah, M.D.(?): NBRMP
Kimball, Reuel B., M.D.: *CA* 11/27/15
Kincaid, John H., M.D.: *NYT* 11/16/17
Kingsbury, John Adams: *NYS* 11/21/15 vii:8
Knight, M. M.: *Independent* 1/3/16
Knox, James Hall Mason Jr., M.D.: *NYS* 11/18/15 p. 3
Koehler, Gustav, M.D.: *CT* 11/19/15; *NYT* 11/16/17
Kolman, Rose: *NYAm* 11/25/15 p. 11
Krasnow, Henry R., M.D.: *CH* 7/25/17
Kremicier, A.: NYSA-MPD
Kuhn, Leroy Philip, M.D.: *CE* 7/24/17
La Fetra, Linnaeus Edford, M.D.: *NYS* 11/19/15 p. 14
Ladova, Rosalie: *CN* 11/17/15 p. 3
Lait, Jack: See Index.
Lathrop, Julia: *CT* 11/18/15
Laurenson, Rev. R. S.: *WP* 11/18/17 p. 10
Lavelle, Rev.: *NYAm* 11/18/15
Lawrence, Josephine: *CN* 11/17/15 p. 3
Lawrence, Oma Moody: *Motography* 3/3/17 p. 1462
Lee, Edward Wallace, M.D.: *NYS* 11/19/15 p. 14
Levine, Michael: *CA* 7/30/17 p. 3

Levy, Maude B.: NBRMP
Lewis, Henry F., M.D.: *NYT* 11/19/15; *CT* 12/15/15
Lindsay, Samuel McCune: *NYT* 11/18/15
Lindsey, Benjamin Barr: *CH* 11/18/15 p. 4
Lipshulch, George U., M.D.: *NYT* 11/18/15
Litzenberg, Jennings C., M.D.: *MRR* Feb. 1916
Lord, John Prentiss, M.D.: NBRMP
Lowe, Joshua "Jolo": *Variety* 3/2/17
Lucey, Patrick Joseph: *NYT* 12/24/15; 2/7/16
Lusk, E. E., M.D.: *Independent* 1/3/16
Macneille, Raymond: *NYT* 11/18/15
Macon, William Douglas, M.D.: *MRR* Feb. 1916
Macy, Valentine Everit: NBRMP
Mahoney, Francis X., M.D.: *BG* 11/18/15 p. 5
Mann, Matthew Derbyshire, M.D.: *MRR* Feb. 1916
Manning, U. G.: NBRMP
Manton, Walter Porter, M.D.: *DN* 11/24/15
Mattys: *NYAm* 7/25/17 p. 2
Mazur, M. E.: public role noted in NBRMP
McCorkle, John A., M.D.: *NYAm* 11/19/15 p. 6
McCulloch, Catherine Waugh: *CN* 11/17/15 p. 3
McElroy, Rev. Benjamin Lincoln: *Independent* 1/3/16
McGuire, W. D. Jr.: NBRMP
McNally, W. D. (W. H. McNamara?): *WP* 11/19/15; *NYS* 11/20/15
Meier, D. Edward, M.D.: *CE* 7/24/17
Melody, Rev. J. W.: *New World* 11/26/15
Merritt, W. B.: *MPN* 2/24/17 p. 1244
Meter, Eva: *NYT* 7/25/17
Meter, Mrs. Samuel: *DN* 7/24/17
Meter, William: *NYT* 7/25/17
Miller, James Raglan, M.D.: *MRR* Feb. 1916
Milne, Peter: *MPN* 2/24/17 p. 1256
Miltern, John T.: *MPN* 3/3/17 p. 1349
Mindlin, Michael: *Call* 12/7/15
Moje, Herman A., M.D.: *CA* 12/23/15
Monash, David, M.D.: *MRR* Feb. 1916
Moore, Rev. Willis A.: *DN* 11/18/15
Morris, Robert Tuttle, M.D.: *NYAm* 11/23/15 p. 10
Moses, Ernest C.: *CT* 11/17/15
Moss, Frank: *NYAm* 11/19/15
Moss, George: LC paperprint
Moyer, Harold Nicholas, M.D.: *NYT* 11/18/15; *CH* 11/21/15

Murnane, Allan: LC paperprint
Murphy, John B., M.D.: *CT* 11/19/15
Myers, Rev. Johnston: *CA* 7/25/17
Nammack, Charles E., M.D.: *NYAm* 11/19/15
Nammack, William H., M.D.: *NYAm* 11/27/15
Neil, Henry: *Call* 12/12/15
Newman, Henry J. E., M.D.: *MRR* Feb. 1916
Norris, Jean: *NYAm* 11/19/15 p. 6
Norris, Kathleen: *Call* 11/28/15
Northrup, William Perry, M.D.: *NYAm* 11/22/15 p. 6
O'Neill, A. Augustus, M.D.: *CA* 11/13/17
Ohl, Mrs. Lewis (Ada): *Call* 11/27/15
Paddock, Charles Evart, M.D.: *MRR* Feb. 1916
Paddock, M. E.: NBRMP
Page, Edward Day: NBRMP
Paine, Alonzo Kingman, M.D.: *MRR* Feb. 1916
Painter, Harry McMahon, M.D.: *MRR* Feb. 1916
Palmer, Mrs. A. M.: *NYAm* 11/19/15
Park, William H., M.D.: *NYAm* 11/19/15
Parker, Beulah (Poynter?): *Call* 11/18/15 and 11/28/15
Parkes, Charles Herbert, M.D.: *CA* 12/23/15
Parsons, Louella: *CH* 4/2/17 p. 11
Pearl, Raymond: *Independent* 1/3/16
Peck, Mary Gray: NBRMP
Percy, W. L.: NBRMP
Perkins, L. B.: *WP* 11/18/17 p. 10
Peters, Rev. John Punnett: NBRMP
Peterson, Reuben, M.D.: *MRR* Feb. 1916
Phillips, Rev. Louis K.: *CN* 11/17/15 p. 3
Pierce, Mrs. Norval (Drucilla Wahl): *CT* 11/17/15
Polak, John O., M.D.: *MRR* Feb. 1916
Polk, William M., M.D.: *NYAm* 11/22/15 p. 6
Price, William H., M.D.: *DN* 11/18/15
Pritchard, William B., M.D.: *NYS* 11/18/15 p. 3
Quackenbos, John D., M.D.: *NYT* 11/18/15
Rader, Rev. Paul: *CN* 11/17/15 p. 3
Rall, Rev. Harris Franklin: NBRMP
Ramsey, W. R., M.D.: *WP* 11/18/15
Rankin, Arthur B., M.D.: *NYT* 11/19/15
Rausch, William Carl Jr., M.D.: *MRR* Feb. 1916
Reddin, Willie May: *Independent* 1/3/16
Reiffert, Edith: *NYAm* 11/19/15

Reinhardt, Henry G. W., M.D.: *Washington Star* 11/18/15
Reisner, Rev. Christian Fichthorne: *NYS* 11/22/15 p. 6
Revelle, Arthur Hamilton [Engstrom]: LC paperprint
Reynolds, James Bronson: NBRMP
Rhodus, Charlotte: *CN* 11/17/15 p. 3
Rice, Eri Perry, M.D.: *CA* 12/23/15
Richards, Charles Daniel: *CH* 11/20/15 p. 2
Riordan, P. D., M.D.: *NYAm* 11/19/15 p. 6
Roberts, Carl Glennis, M.D.: *CH* 7/24/17
Roberts, Frank H. H.: *Independent* 1/3/16
Roberts, Joseph E.: *NYT* 11/25/15
Robertson, John Dill, M.D.: *NYT* 11/20/15
Robinson, Frederic H.: *CA* 11/24/15; *Call* 11/23/15
Robinson, William J., M.D.: *Call* 11/28/15
Roe, Clifford: *WP* 11/18/15 p. 6
Rosenberg, Maurice, M.D.: *NYT* 11/25/15
Rubovits, William H., M.D.: *MRR* Feb. 1916
Russell, H. Everett, M.D.: *NYS* 11/19/15 p. 14
Rutherford, Clarendon (Clarence?), M.D.: *CT* 12/8/15; *CE* 7/24/17;
    NYT 11/16/17
Sachs, Theodore B., M.D.: *CA* 12/23/15
Sargent, Franklin H.: NBRMP
Saunders, Rev. Benjamin Walker: *Independent* 1/3/16
Savage, Cora: *NYAm* 11/19/15
Schlesinger, Mrs. Bert: NBRMP
Schowalter, Max J. (J. Max?), M.D.: *CE* 7/24/17
Schreiber, Karl L., M.D.(?): NBRMP
Schupmann, Albert, M.D.: *NYT* 11/16/17
Schupmann, Martin August, M.D.: *NYT* 11/16/17
Schwartz, Anna: *WP* 11/19/15 p. 2
Scott, George A. H.: *DFP* 11/17/15
Seligman, Isaac N.: NBRMP
Senior, F. S., M.D.: *NYAm* 11/22/15 p. 6
Serviss, Climena, M.D.: *CH* 11/17/15 p. 4
Shaw, Rev. Anna Howard, M.D.: *NYS* 11/18/15
Shippen, Rev. Eugene R.: *DN* 11/17/15
Smith, George Jay: NBRMP
Smith, H. E.: *Exhibitors' Trade Review* 3/17/17
Smith, Munroe: *NYS* 11/18/15 p. 3; *NYT* 11/18/15
Smith, Oscar J.: *NYT* 11/18/15
Smith, P.: *Independent* 1/3/16
Somers, Andrew Bartholomew, M.D.: *MRR* Feb. 1916

Southard, Elmer Ernest, M.D.: *CH* 11/18/15 p. 4

Spalding, Heman, M.D.: *CN* 11/15/17

Speidel, Edward, M.D.: *MRR* Feb. 1916

Sproc, Charles, M.D.: *CH* 7/25/17

Stanke: *NYT* 1/28/18

Stechmann, F. W., M.D.: *NYAm* 11/18/15; *CH* 11/18/15 p. 4

Steele, Daniel Atkinson King, M.D.: *NYT* 11/19/15

Steinhoff, Ferdinand Heinrich, M.D.: *CA* 12/23/15

Stevens, Mary Thompson, M.D.: *DN* 11/17/15

Stokes, Rose Harriet Pastor: *NYAm* 11/24/15 p. 8

Stone, Herbert Marion, M.D.: *MRR* Feb. 1916

Strafford, W. H.: *Are You Fit to Marry?*

Strange, Nat S. [Stronge?]: public role from NBRMP

Streeter(?), Albert: NBRMP

Sturgess, T. F.: NBRMP

Sullivan, Michael F.: *NYAm* 11/23/15 p. 7

Sumney, H. C.: NBRMP

Swope, Horace M.: NBRMP

Swormstedt, L. B.: *CT* 11/18/15

Talliaferro, Sidney S.: *WP* 11/18/17 p. 10

Tancock, Rev. James A.: NBRMP

Taylor, Rev. A. W.: NBRMP

Taylor, F. M.: NBRMP

Test, Frederick Cleveland, M.D.: *CN* 11/17/15 p. 3

Thomas, Rev. C. F.: *BG* 11/20/15 p. 2

"Tinee, Mae": *CT* 4/2/17

Tower, William Lawrence: *CT* 12/11/15

Turman, A. E., M.D.: *MRR* Feb. 1916

Ure, Mrs. William G: *Omaha News* in NBRMP

Van Leuven-Browne, Blanche: *DN* 11/18/15

Van Peyma, Peter, M.D.: *MRR* Feb. 1916

Vance, Rev. Joseph A.: *DN* 11/17/15

Vaughan, Phillips C., M.D.: *CH* 7/24/17

Vaughan, Victor C., M.D.: *DFP* 11/18/15

Verden, Charles: *CN* 11/18/15 p. 3

Vittum, Harriet: *CH* 11/17/15

Von Colditz, Grambow Thomsen, M.D.: *CT* 11/17/15

Von Wagner, Johanna: *DN* 11/18/15

Wald, Lillian D.: *NYAm* 11/18/15; *Independent* 1/3/16

Walsh, Catherine: *NYT* 11/20/15

Walsh, James Joseph, M.D.: *Independent* 1/3/16

Walsh, Jeremiah Henry, M.D.: *CT* 12/15/15

Warner, H. E.: *Independent* 1/3/16
Washburn, George Hamlin, M.D.: *MRR* Feb. 1916
Way, Henry J., M.D.: *CT* 12/15/15
Webster, John Clarence, M.D.: *MRR* Feb. 1916
Weiskopf, H. C., M.D.: *CH* 7/24/17
Weitzel, Edward: *MPW* 2/24/17 p. 1244
Welz, Walter E., M.D.: *MRR* Feb. 1916
Werder, Julius: *CT* 12/8/15
Wharton, Leopold: See Index.
Wharton, Theodore: See Index.
Wilder, Loren, M.D.: *CA* 12/23/15
Wile, Ira S., M.D.: *NYT* 11/18/15
Wiley, Harvey W., M.D.: *CN* 11/18/15 p. 3
Williams, Carrington, M.D.: *NYS* 11/19/15 p. 14
Williams, Frankwood E., M.D.: *CH* 11/18/15 p. 4
Williams, Talcott: NBRMP
Winthrop, Egerton Leigh Jr: NBRMP
Wolf, Louis H., M.D.: *CH* 7/25/17
Wood, Mrs. Court F.: *CT* 11/18/15
Woodward, W. C., M.D.: *CT* 11/18/15
Wynekoop, Charles Ira, M.D.: *DN* 11/17/15 p. 3
Young, Rev. S. Edward: *NYAm* 11/19/15
Younger, Charles Benjamin, M.D.: *CH* 11/17/15
Zahn, Ruby M.: *DN* 11/18/15
Zilberman, Belle Neuman: *NYAm* 11/21/15
Zimmerman, Rev. A. H.: *WP* 11/18/17 p. 10

Notes *

Abbreviations

AFI	American Film Institute
BA	Boston American
BG	Boston Globe
CA	Chicago American
Call	New York Call
CE	Chicago Examiner
CH	Chicago Herald
CN	Chicago Daily News
CT	Chicago Tribune
DAB	Dictionary of American Biography
DFP	Detroit Free Press
DN	Detroit News
ExTrR	Exhibitors' Trade Review

* Unless stated otherwise, all newspaper articles cited begin on page 1.

IDJ	*Ithaca Daily Journal*
JHMAS	*Journal of the History of Medicine and Allied Sciences*
LC-MBRS	Library of Congress Motion Picture, Broadcasting, and Recorded Sound Division, Washington, D.C.
MRR	*Medical Review of Reviews*
MPN	*Motion Picture News*
MPW	*Moving Picture World*
MOMA	Museum of Modern Art, New York
NBRMP	National Board of Review of Motion Pictures Papers, New York Public Library, Controversial Film Correspondence
New World	*Chicago New World*
NLM-HMD	National Library of Medicine, History of Medicine Division, Bethesda, Maryland
NYAm	*New York American*
NYDM	*New York Dramatic Mirror*
NYS	*New York Sun*
NYSA-MPD	Motion Picture Division Scripts, New York State Archives, Albany
NYT	*New York Times*
OED	*Oxford English Dictionary*
TNR	*New Republic*
UM-HHFC	University of Michigan Historical Health Film Collection
WP	*Washington Post*
WWW	*Who Was Who in America*

Chapter 1

1. *New York Medical Journal* 102 (December 4, 1915), 1132–34; the X-ray was taken seventy-two hours after oral administration of a bismuth solution. Walter B. Cannon of Harvard pioneered this method for examining the bowel in 1896–97, using bismuth subnitrate as the contrast medium. Saul Benison, A. Clifford Barger, and Elin L. Wolfe, *Walter B. Cannon: The Life and Times of a Young Scientist* (Cambridge, Mass.: Harvard University Press, 1987), pp. 53–56. *CA*, November 27, 1915.

Instructions for creating an artificial anus are found in the Talmud. Duret of Brest is credited with having performed the first successful lower quadrant colostomy to correct an imperforate anus, in 1793. But while the procedure itself is not complex, it remained very risky until the late-nineteenth-century adoption of antisepsis. Even in 1915 death from infection was not unlikely. Owen Wangensteen and Sarah Wangensteen, *The Rise of Surgery* (Minneapolis: University of Minnesota Press, 1978), p. 120; Albert S. Lyons and R. Joseph Petrucelli, *Medicine: An Illustrated History* (New York: Abrams, 1978), p. 72.

For details not available elsewhere, see *CA*, November 26, 1915.

2. Many of these cases were covered extensively in the news media. For an overview of each, see the following. Bollinger: *New York Medical Journal*

102 (December 4, 1915): 1132. Meter: *NYT* July 25, 1917, p. 11; *CA* July 24, 1917, afternoon ed.; *MRR* 23 (October 1917): 697–98. Werder: *CA* December 8, 1915, afternoon ed. Grimshaw: *CA* December 28, 1915, magazine page; *Call* December 13, 1915. Hodzima: *CA* November 13, 1917; *NYS* November 13, 1917; *NYT* November 16, 1917, p. 4; *CH* November 20, 1917. Stanke: *NYT* January 28, 1918, p. 6. For cases before 1915, see *CA* November 23, 1915, p. 3.

3. The Roberts baby's spine was intact to the lumbar vertebrae. If the defect had been repaired successfully, she could have lived as a paralytic, but the high risk of infection from the untreated defect had to be weighed against the high risk of infection from the treatment. See newspapers for November 25–December 3, 1915, esp. *NYT* November 25, 1915; *CH* November 25, 1915; *WP* November 25, 1915, p. 3; *NYAm* November 25, 1915. For the St. Louis quote, *DFP* November 23, 1915, p. 9.

4. *NYT* March 3, 1916, p. 20; *Call* December 4, 1915. For similar pleas from other despairing parents and children themselves, in a total of eight separate additional cases, see *DN* November 22, 1915; *WP* November 19, 1915, and November 23, 1915, p. 4; *Independent* January 3, 1916, p. 25; *Call* November 23, 1915, p. 1, November 27, 1915, p. 5. For support from parents of healthy children, see *NYS* November 20, 1915.

5. Haiselden's account began in the *CA*, November 23, 1915, p. 3, and ran daily through December 30, 1915. For interviews and other photos of Mrs. Bollinger, see *WP* November 19, 1915, p. 2; Fig. 2 is from *CT* November 17, 1915, p. 7. For photos and addresses of later patients, see *CA* and *NYS* November 13, 1917 (Hodzima). Fig. 3 is from *CT* November 18, 1915.

For Haiselden's courting and flattering of the press, see *CA* December 16, 1915, magazine page. For his public lectures, see *NYAm* November 30, 1915; *CT* April 9–14, 1917, p. 15; *Cleveland Plain Dealer* April 2, 1917, p. 4; *ExTrR*, January 25, 1919, p. 640; *MPN* April 28, 1917, p. 2675.

Newspapers were examined for November 12–December 30, 1915; February 5–7 and March 14–16, 1916 (Bollinger, Roberts, Werder, and Grimshaw cases); July 22–27 and November 12–20, 1917 (Meter and Hodzima cases); January 25–30, 1918 (Stanke case); and June 18–20, 1919 (obituaries). For a full list of papers examined, see the Bibliography.

6. I found and arranged for restoration of the only viewable print of the 1927 version from the collection of John E. Allen, Park Ridge, N.J. It is available for on-site research use at the University of Michigan Historical Health Film Collection. An unprojectable paper print of the 1916 version is at the LC-MBRS, #LU-9978, Box 109. For a full list of all known showings, see chap. 8 below.

7. Wald: *Independent* January 3, 1916, p. 25; Lindsey: *CH* November 18, 1915; Darrow: *WP* November 18, 1915; Beard: *NYT* November 18, 1915, p. 4. Darrow later repudiated eugenics in "The Eugenics Cult," *American Mercury* 8 (June 1926): 129–37.

8. *Independent* January 3, 1916, p. 23.

9. Keller in *TNR*, December 18, 1915, pp. 173–74, and *Call* November 26, 1915. Haiselden's critics initially cited her case to prove the value of handicapped lives, e.g., *WP* November 18, 1915, p. 6; *NYS* November 18, 1915, but Keller strongly supported Haiselden. So did at least one

other handicapped advocate for the disabled, see *DN* November 18, 1915, p. 25.

Cardinal Gibbons relied on the distinction between ordinary and extraordinary measures, holding that surgical intervention went beyond what is ordinarily required, *CT* November 20, 1915, p. 8, quoting *Baltimore Catholic Review*, November 19, 1915. For similar views of an obstetrician at Catholic Georgetown University, see *MRR* 22 (February 1916): 99. For further discussion, see chap. 4 below.

10. *CN* November 17, 1915; *NYAm* November 19, 1915; *NYT* November 18, 1915.

11. *NYS* November 21, 1915, pt. VII, p. 1; *CT* November 19, 1915; *MRR* 22 (February 1916): 100; *WP* November 18, 1917, p. 10; *NYS* November 19, 1915, p. 14. For similar comments of nurse Lillian Wald, see *Independent* January 3, 1916, p. 25. For other less specific but uncontroverted claims that secret nontreatment of defectives had long been commonplace, see *DN* November 20 and 24, 1915; *NYT* November 18, 1915, p. 4. Patricia Spain Ward, *Simon Baruch* (Tuscaloosa: University of Alabama Press, 1994).

12. *CH* November 18, 1915, p. 6; *CT* November 18, 1915, p. 6; *CA* December 21, 1915, editorial p.; *DN* November 18, 1915, p. 4, (endorsing nontreatment but rejecting active killing); *DFP* November 20, 1915, p. 4; *NYAm* November 23, 1915, p. 22, see also November 19, 1915, p. 20. Other newspapers quoted in *Current Opinion* 60 (January 1916): 43; *TNR* November 27, 1915, pp. 85–86.

13. Cabot: *CH* November 18, 1915, p. 4; Vaughan: *DFP* November 18, 1915, p. 2; Hamilton: *Survey* December 4, 1915, pp. 265–66; Shaw: *CH* November 18, 1915, p. 4; Copeland: *WP* November 18, 1915; Adair and De Lee: *MRR* 22 (February 1916): 95, 97; Jacobi: *NYS* November 18, 1915, p. 3; Kellogg: *Good Health* 51 (1916): 7–8; Addams: *NYT* November 18, 1915; Lathrop: *CT* November 18, 1915.

14. *BG* November 19, 1915, p. 12; *WP* November 18, 1915, p. 4; *NYS* November 19, 1915, p. 6; *St. Louis Post-Dispatch* and *Chicago Evening Post* in *Current Opinion* 60 (January 1916): 43. The *Ann Arbor News* switched from support to opposition between November 17 and 18, 1915. *Survey* December 4, 1915, pp. 265–66; *NYT*, November 19, 1915, p. 10, compare to July 26, 1917, p. 10.

15. *NYT* November 20, 1915. The second postmortem found a number of additional anomalies, including the lack of a testicle, a kidney, and the coccyx, and the presence of hemorrhages in the brain and spine. *DN* November 18, 1915; *DFP* November 20, 1915; *CA* December 22, 23, and 24, 1915, magazine pages. The full text of the coroner's jury "verdict" was widely reprinted, e.g., *CH* November 20, 1915.

16. *NYT* November 18, 1915, and December 24, 1915, p. 7; *CH* December 23, 1915, p. 18. Party politics was not determinative. Hoffman was a Republican, while Lucey and Hoyne were Democrats. See "Taking Sides" in chap. 2 below.

17. *NYT* December 10, 1915, p. 16, and February 7, 1916, p. 18.

18. *NYAm* July 25, 1917; *CH* November 20, 1917.

19. Stephen Louis Kuepper, "Euthanasia in America, 1890–1960," Ph.D. diss., Rutgers University, 1981, pp. 79–80.

20. *NYT* March 15, 1916, p. 5; *Ithaca Daily Journal* September 25, 1916.

21. Except as noted, all biographical information is from the autobiography in *CA* November 23, 1915, p. 3; *CT* November 17, 1915, p. 7, and November 18, 1915, p. 2; *Physicians Blue Book,* comp. Walter R. McDonough (Chicago: William J. Lowitz, 1897), pp. 31, 73; and the following United States Census, Manuscript Returns, Kendall County Illinois: 9th Census 1870, Little Rock Township, p. 37, no. 299; 10th census 1880, Plano, p. 5, no. 31.

22. This and the preceding paragraph are based on the *Lakeside Annual Directory of the City of Chicago* (Chicago: Chicago Directory Company) 1887–1912 inclusive. Cook County records searched from 1880–1915 inclusive; Kendall County records (Plano) searched from 1877–1915 inclusive, by Cook County Clerk David Orr and Kendall County Clerk Paul Anderson, for whose help I am very grateful.

23. *CT* November 18, 1915, p. 2, and November 19, 1915, p. 5; *CA* November 23, 1915, p. 3; *CH* June 19, 1919.

24. But he thought Chicago had the worst medical education in America. Abraham Flexner, *Medical Education in the United States and Canada* (New York: Carnegie Foundation, 1910), pp. 207–209, 217–20. For a more favorable evaluation of medical Chicago, and of P&S in particular, see Patricia Spain Ward, "The Other Abraham: Flexner in Illinois," *Caduceus: Museum Quarterly for the Health Sciences* 2 (Spring 1986): 1–66; *Medicine in Transition: The Centennial of the University of Illinois College of Medicine,* ed. Edward P. Cohen (Urbana: University of Illinois Press, 1981). On the general local background, see Thomas N. Bonner, *Medicine in Chicago 1850–1950* (Madison, Wis.: American History Research Center, 1957).

25. Chicago Medical Society, *History of Medicine and Surgery and Physicians and Surgeons of Chicago* (Chicago: Biographical Publishing, 1922), pp. 336; McDonough, *Physicians Blue Book* (1897); Walter R. McDonough, *Chicago Medical Directory* (Chicago: Chicago Medical Society, 1905), p. 58; *Chicago Medical Directory* (Chicago: McDonough & Company, 1917), pp. 90, 185; *Chicago Medical Directory* (Chicago: McDonough & Company, 1919), p. 49.

26. *CA* November 23, 1915, p. 3. Haiselden recalled the book as a small work compiled by Sargent and titled *How to Get Strong and How to Remain So.* I could not locate any such volume. Perhaps Haiselden had in mind the popular *Health, Strength and Power* (New York: Caldwell, 1904), in which Sargent asserted that each person's physical and mental abilities are "largely determined by heredity," although training and exercise determine whether the individual "ever attains his ultimate . . . capacity," p. 11.

Or perhaps Haiselden confused Sargent with an earlier fitness educator, William Blaikie, whose 1879 book *How to Get Strong and How to Stay So* had been reissued in 1902 (New York: Harper & Bros., 1879, 1902). But that book makes virtually no reference to heredity, except to imply in passing that women needed to exercise so that they could pass on their acquired strength to their sons, p. 50.

27. I use this term for all those who proclaimed themselves in favor of what they called "eugenics." Rather than imposing my a priori definition to

distinguish "correct" and "mistaken" uses of the word in the past, I will examine the many competing things people at the time used the word to mean.

28. *CH* November 19, 1915, p. 3; *CH* July 27, 1916; Patrick Almond Curtis, "Eugenic Reformers, Cultural Perceptions of Dependent Populations, and the Care of the Feebleminded in Illinois, 1909–1920," Ph.D. diss., University of Illinois at Chicago, 1983, pp. 171–78. Lait, who specialized in "undercover exposés" of vice and corruption throughout his long career, may have been the "Mr. Palmer" who accompanied Haiselden. Martin Elks argues that the acceptance of high death rates in such institutions was the functional equivalent of eugenic murder, in "The Lethal Chamber," *Mental Retardation* 31 (August 1993): 201–207.

29. *CA* November 27, 1915. While many hospitals bought such machines shortly after they appeared in the late 1890s, the creation of formal X-ray departments, and the use of X rays in routine diagnosis, took much longer to catch on. Joel Howell, "Early Use of X-ray Machines and Electrocardiographs at the Pennsylvania Hospital, 1897–1927," *Journal of the American Medical Association* 255 (1986): 2320–2323; and "Machines and Medicine: Technology Transforms the American Hospital," in *The American General Hospital: Communities and Social Contexts*, ed. Diana Long and Janet Golden (Ithaca, N.Y.: Cornell University Press, 1989), pp. 109–134. On X-ray sterilization, see Paul Weindling, *Health, Race and German Politics Between National Unification and Nazism 1870–1945* (Cambridge: Cambridge University Press, 1989), p. 391. On Ochsner, see Howard Kelly and Walter Burrage, *Dictionary of American Medical Biography* (New York: D. Appleton, 1928).

30. *WP* July 25, 1917. George Rosen, "Christian Fenger: Medical Immigrant," *Bulletin of the History of Medicine* 48 (1974): 129–45; James L. Stone, "The Development of Neurological Surgery at Cook County Hospital," *Neurosurgery* 34 (January 1994): 97–102. For Haiselden's linkage of psychosurgery and eugenics, see chap. 4 below.

31. *CT* November 18, 1915, p. 2, and November 19, 1915, p. 5; *CA* November 23, 1915, p. 3; *CH* June 19, 1919.

32. Biographical information from previously cited news articles. On Mrs. Bollinger's regrets, see *CE* July 28, 1917. For Mrs. Meter, see *CT* May 8, 1938, pt. 1, p. 2; Kuepper, "Euthanasia in America," p. 83.

33. *CT* January 28, 1918, p. 12. See chapters 6 and 9.

34. *CN* June 19, 1919, p. 5.; *CT* June 20, 1919; Kuepper, "Euthanasia in America," p. 83. Other obituaries appeared June 19, 1919, in *CH* p. 1 and *NYAm* p. 6; and *NYT* June 20, 1919, p. 6. His body was returned to Chicago where he was buried July 7, *Ithaca Journal*, July 9, 1919, p. 3. Efforts to trace the Rutherfords or Haiselden's daughters beyond the mid-1920s have not been successful.

35. Chicago Medical Society, *History of Medicine and Surgery*, p. 336; *Chicago Medical Directory* (1917), pp. 90, 185; *Chicago Medical Directory* (1919), p. 49; *Polk's Chicago City Directory 1928–29*, vol. 1, (Chicago: Polk, 1928), p. 774; Chicago telephone directories Summer 1930, Summer 1932, and 1960–61. Sites visited November 5, 1988.

36. The *NYT* recalled Haiselden in connection with a similar case in

1924; thereafter, he was never mentioned by name, except for one article in 1950. *NYT* September 30, 1924, p. 25; January 8, 1950, sect. IV, p. 2. A few magazines mentioned Haiselden during the revival of interest in euthanasia of the 1930s; see Kuepper, "Euthanasia in America," pp. 100, 120. Kuepper's 1981 dissertation includes the only previous scholarly attention to Haiselden. See chap. 9 below.

37. *NYT* May 15, 1990, national ed., p. B6.

38. For example, Mark Haller, *Eugenics* (New Brunswick, N.J.: Rutgers University Press, 1963), p. 124; Daniel Kevles, *In the Name of Eugenics: Genetics and the Uses of Human Heredity* (Berkeley: University of California Press, 1985), ch. 4. For exceptions see Dorothy Nelkin and M. Susan Lindee, *The DNA Mystique: The Gene as a Cultural Icon* (New York: W. H. Freeman, 1995), and the works of Juan Leon and Robert Rydell.

39. I will reserve the term "popular culture" for ideas that demonstrably originated with the lay public.

40. Rudolph Vecoli, "Sterilization: A Progressive Measure?" *Wisconsin Magazine of History* 43 (Spring 1960): 190–202. Kevles refers only once to euthanasia outside Nazi Germany, *Name of Eugenics*, p. 92. On sterilization see Philip Reilly, *The Surgical Solution* (Baltimore: Johns Hopkins University Press, 1991).

Two exceptions are Russell Hollander, "Euthanasia and Mental Retardation," *Mental Retardation* 27 (April 1989): 53–61; and Elks, "The 'Lethal Chamber.' " For a contemporary comment on this issue, see Eden Paul, "Eugenics, Birth Control, and Socialism," in *Population and Birth Control* (New York: Critic & Guide, 1917), pp. 142–43.

41. Karl Pearson described his eugenics as "the 'better-not-born' doctrine," quoted in the *Proceedings* of the National Conference on Race Betterment, 1 (1914): 500.

42. If a gene for racism could be located and eradicated, such action could be considered eugenics, too. Loren Graham, "Science and Values: The Eugenics Movement in Germany and Russia in the 1920s," *American Historical Review* 82 (December 1977): 1133–64.

43. George L. Mosse evocatively called racism a "scavenger ideology," *Towards the Final Solution: A History of European Racism* (London: J. M. Dent & Sons, 1978), p. 234. The metaphor aptly captures the cultural source of eugenic values, but misses the selective process that allowed the scavengers some control over which particular prejudices would be judged "useful." Thanks to Anne Stoler for getting me thinking about this metaphor, and to the reviewers for Oxford University Press for pushing me to develop it.

44. I. Van der Sluis, "The Movement for Euthanasia," *Janus* 66 (1979): 131–72; Stephen Klaidman and Tom L. Beauchamp, "Baby Jane Doe in the Media," *Journal of Health Politics, Policy and Law* 11 (Summer 1986): 271–84.

45. *NYS* November 18, 1915. For an example of "monstrosity" as technical term, see *NYS* November 21, 1915, pt. VII, p. 1. The military term "ineffective" was also sometimes used in medicine. For specific terms, see *Oxford English Dictionary* and first *Supplement*.

46. *American Journal of Care for Cripples* 1 (1914): 37.

47. Thus they in turn have been discarded and replaced, either by further attempts to coin value-free neologisms, or, more hopefully, by words expressing positive values ("special education," "challenged"). Paul K. Longmore, "A Note on Language and the Identity of Disabled People," *American Behavioral Scientist* 28 (January/February 1985): 419–23.

Chapter 2

1. This attempt to sketch two millennia of background is of necessity a synthesis based mostly on a secondary literature whose breadth and depth are somewhat uneven. In what follows, "infanticide" will be used to include both active killing and passive abandonment, except where more precise distinctions are warranted by the sources. For non-Western examples, see chap. 3, note 62 below.

2. Plato, *Republic*, Book 5, 460; Aristotle, *Politics*, Book 7, Chap. 16, 1334B-1336A; Soranus, *Gynecology*, Book 2, trans. Owsei Temkin (Baltimore: Johns Hopkins University Press, 1956), Chap. 10, pp. 79–80; G.E.R. Lloyd, *Science, Folklore, and Ideology: Studies in the Life Sciences in Ancient Greece* (Cambridge: Cambridge University Press, 1983), p. 170; Paul Carrick, *Medical Ethics in Antiquity: Philosophical Perspectives on Abortion and Euthanasia* (Dordrecht and Boston: D. Reidel, 1985), Chap. 6.

The most comprehensive short history is Robert F. Weir, *Selective Nontreatment of Handicapped Newborns: Moral Dilemmas in Neonatal Medicine* (New York: Oxford University Press, 1984), Chap. 1. See also Darrel W. Amundsen, "Medicine and the Birth of Defective Children: Approaches of the Ancient World," and Gary B. Ferngren, "The Status of Defective Newborns from Late Antiquity to the Reformation," both in *Euthanasia and the Newborn*, Philosophy and Medicine Series, vol. 24 ed. Richard C. McMillan, H. Tristram Engelhardt Jr., and Stuart F. Spicker, (Dordrecht: D. Reidel, 1987), pp. 3–22, 47–64.

Also see Mark Golden, *Children and Childhood in Classical Athens* (Baltimore: Johns Hopkins University Press, 1990), Chap. 4; and Thomas Wiedmann, *Adults and Children in the Roman Empire* (New Haven: Yale University Press, 1990). Anne Ellis Hanson, Sally Humphreys, and Lily Kay also contributed to my understanding of the classical context.

3. It took divine intervention to prevent the sacrifice of Isaac and the abandonment of Ishmael and Hagar. The prolonged struggle to extirpate the cult of Molech reveals both the depth of official commitment and the extent of popular resistance to the campaign against ritual infanticide. Genesis 21–22; Leviticus 18.

4. On lay infanticide and abandonment in these centuries, see John Boswell, *The Kindness of Strangers: The Abandonment of Children in Western Europe from Late Antiquity to the Renaissance* (New York: Pantheon, 1989); P. C. Hoffer and N.E.H. Hull, *Murdering Mothers: Infanticide in England and New England 1558–1803* (New York: New York University Press, 1981); Maria W. Piers, *Infanticide* (New York: Norton, 1978); *History of Childhood Quarterly* 1 (Winter 1974); Weir, *Selective Nontreatment*, chap. 1; Ferngren,

"Defective Newborns." On Luther, see Weir, *Selective Nontreatment*, pp. 27–28, n. 47.

On monsters, see Katharine Park and Lorraine Daston, "Unnatural Conceptions: The Study of Monsters in 16th- and 17th-Century France and England," *Past and Present* 92 (1981): 20–54.

Several studies of current medical issues contain useful historical surveys of lay infanticide, including: *Which Babies Shall Live?* eds. Thomas H. Murray and Arthur L. Caplan (Clifton, N.J.: Humana Press, 1985); Jeff Lyon, *Playing God in the Nursery* (New York: Norton, 1984); Earl Shelp, *Born to Die?* (New York: Free Press, 1986); Helga Kuhse and Peter Singer, *Should the Baby Live?* (New York: Oxford University Press, 1985); "Special Issue: Imperiled Newborns," *Hastings Center Report* 17 (December 1987); and Stephen G. Post, "History, Infanticide, and Imperiled Newborns," *Hastings Center Report* 18 (August/September 1988): 14–17.

It is certainly reasonable to hypothesize a role for physicians in monstrous birth cases, given their roles as expert witnesses in diagnosing other unnatural phenomena. For suggestive examples see Richard Palmer, "The Church, Leprosy and Plague in Medieval and Early Modern Europe," in *The Church and Healing* ed. W. J. Sheils (Oxford: Basil Blackwell, 1982), pp. 79–99 at p. 91; Sanford J. Fox, *Science and Justice: The Massachusetts Witchcraft Trials* (Baltimore: Johns Hopkins Press, 1968), pp. 63–90. Thanks to Mary Wessling for the first example.

The most useful survey of American lay infanticide and the most detailed on explicitly medical examples is Cynthia B. Cohen, "The Treatment of Impaired Newborns in American History: Implications for Public Policy," unpublished manuscript, 1985, Department of Philosophy, Villanova University. I thank Prof. Cohen for sharing this manuscript with me.

5. Robert Burton, *The Anatomy of Melancholy* (London: George Routledge, 1931), p. 188.

6. In addition to the sources in notes above, see Catherine Damme, "Infanticide: The Worth of an Infant under Law," *Medical History* 22 (January 1978): 1–24; Mary Wessling, "Infanticide Trials and Forensic Evidence: Wurttemberg 1757–1793," in *Legal Medicine in History*, ed. Michael Clark and Catherine Crawford (Cambridge: Cambridge University Press, 1994); and George K. Behlmer, "Deadly Motherhood: Infanticide and Medical Opinion in Mid-Victorian England," *JHMAS* 34 (October 1979): 403–27.

The connection between infanticide and sexual transgression is quite ancient. Leviticus 18 condemns child sacrifice to Molech as part of a long litany of sins, all the rest of which are explicitly sexual in nature.

7. Case is in Tom Beauchamp and Laurence B. McCullough, *Medical Ethics: The Moral Responsibilities of Physicians* (Englewood Cliffs, N.J.: Prentice-Hall, 1984), pp. 1–2. See also Cohen, "Impaired Newborns," pp. 79–80. This baby's inability to draw its first breath without assistance formally qualified it as a "stillbirth," something the Bollinger case clearly was not. For the contemporary state of the art in resuscitating newborns, see John Snow, "On Asphyxia, and On the Resuscitation of Still-Born Children," *London Medical Gazette* 29 (1841): 222–27.

8. W. Bruce Fye, "Active Euthanasia: An Historical Survey of Its Conceptual Origins and Introduction to Medical Thought," *Bulletin of the His-*

tory of Medicine 52 (1979): 492–502. See also O. Ruth Russell, *Freedom to Die: Moral and Legal Aspects of Euthanasia* (New York: Human Sciences Press, 1975); Derek Humphry, *The Right to Die: Understanding Euthanasia* (New York: Harper & Row, 1986); Van der Sluis, "The Movement for Euthanasia"; C. W. Triche and S. D. Triche, *The Euthanasia Controversy 1812– 1974, A Bibliography* (Troy, N.Y.: Whitston, 1975); Kuepper, "Euthanasia in America."

9. See Martin S. Pernick, *A Calculus of Suffering: Pain, Professionalism and Anesthesia in Nineteenth Century America* (New York: Columbia University Press, 1985).

10. The usage may have begun in veterinary practice. For one early example, Laurence Turnbull, *The Advantages and Accidents of Artificial Anaesthesia*, 2d ed. (Philadelphia: P. Blakiston, 1885), p. 262.

Anthony Trollope, *The Fixed Period* (Ann Arbor, University of Michigan Press, 1990); Herbert Spencer, *Facts and Comments* (New York: D. Appleton, 1902), pp. 231–33; William Osler, "The Fixed Period," *Aequanimitas; With Other Addresses* (London: H. K. Lewis, 1906), pp. 391–411.

For a fictional discussion of whether a doctor should have saved an adult black man whose face had been badly burned, see Stephen Crane, "The Monster," in *Tales of Whilomville* (Charlottesville: University Press of Virginia, 1969).

Modern advocates of euthanasia insist the term properly applies only to voluntary death, e.g., Olive Russell, *Freedom to Die*, pp. 19–20; Derek Humphry, *Right to Die*, passim. Whatever validity that claim has today, that is not the only way the term has been used since the 1870s.

11. The literature on eugenics is vast. For an introduction to American eugenics, see Kenneth L. Ludmerer, *Genetics and American Society* (Baltimore: Johns Hopkins University Press, 1972); Haller, *Eugenics;* Philip Reilly, *Genetics, Law, and Social Policy* (Cambridge: Harvard University Press, 1977); Reilly, "The Surgical Solution: The Writings of Activist Physicians in the Early Days of Eugenical Sterilization," *Perspectives in Biology and Medicine* 26 (1983): 637–56; Barry Alan Mehler, "A History of the American Eugenics Society, 1921–1940," Ph.D. diss., University of Illinois, 1988.

To place America in world context, see Kevles, *In the Name of Eugenics; The Wellborn Science: Eugenics in Germany, France, Brazil, and Russia*, ed. Mark Adams (Oxford: Oxford University Press, 1989); Gar Allen, "Genetics, Eugenics, and Class Struggle," *Genetics* 79 (June 1975), supplement pp. 29– 45; Jan Sapp, "The Struggle for Authority in the Field of Heredity 1900– 1932: New Perspectives on the Rise of Genetics," *Journal of the History of Biology* 16 (1983): 311–42.

On "Social Darwinism," see Richard Hofstadter, *Social Darwinism in American Thought* (Philadelphia: University of Pennsylvania Press, 1944); Robert C. Bannister, *Social Darwinism: Science and Myth in Anglo-American Social Thought* (Philadelphia: Temple University Press, 1979).

On the role of eugenics in Germany, see chap. 9 below.

12. Ernst Haeckel, *The Wonders of Life* (New York: Harper & Bros., 1905), pp. 21, 114–20; Haeckel, *The History of Creation*, vol. I (New York: D. Appleton, 1876, orig. 1868), pp. 170–71; Van der Sluis, "Euthanasia," 134– 37; Daniel Gasman, *The Scientific Origins of National Socialism* (London:

MacDonald, 1971), p. 91. On Ploetz, Stephen Trombley, *The Right to Reproduce: A History of Coercive Sterilization* (London: Weidenfeld and Nicolson, 1988), p. 71. For eugenic disavowals of euthanasia see chap. 4 below.

13. Sigmund Engel, *The Elements of Child-Protection*, trans. Dr. Eden Paul (New York: Macmillan, 1912). Quotes are from pp. 257–58, except for "joint outlook" in Preface p. v; "euthanasia" in Index under "defectives" p. 272; and "ultra-Darwinian" p. 47.

14. For Goddard, see Russell, *Freedom to Die*, p. 59. For Rentoul, see Trombley, *Right to Reproduce*, p. 19.

15. Quoted by Michael Meyer in *New York Review of Books*, January 13, 1994, p. 26.

16. Simeon Baldwin, "The Natural Right to a Natural Death," *Journal of Social Science* 37 (1899): 1–17, quoted in Cohen, "Impaired Newborns," p. 87; Eugene S. Talbot, *Degeneracy* (New York: Scribner's, [1898]), pp. 3–4. Thanks to Joy Harvey for the last reference. For other U.S. proposals to kill the mentally retarded, as early as 1883, see Hollander, "Euthanasia."

17. William McKim, *Heredity and Human Progress* (New York: G. P. Putnam's Sons, 1900), pp. 188–92; G. Stanley Hall, "What is to Become of Your Baby?" *Cosmopolitan* 48 (April 1910): 661–68, esp. 663; Dorothy Ross, *G. Stanley Hall* (Chicago: University of Chicago Press, 1972), pp. 318–19. Thanks to Alice Smuts for the Hall references.

18. An exhaustive survey of the ethnohistorical literature is Edward Westermarck, *The Origin and Development of the Moral Ideas*, vol. 1 (London: Macmillan, 1906), pp. 393–413. Specifically on antiquity, see Allen G. Roper, *Ancient Eugenics* (Oxford: B. H. Blackwell, 1913).

By 1915 ancient precedents were well-enough known to be cited by both sides in the debate over Haiselden's actions. See *CT* November 18, 1915, p. 2; *DN* November 18, 1915, pp. 2, 25; *Independent* January 3, 1916, p. 26; *Journal of the American Medical Association* 65 (1915): 2025.

19. Reilly, *Surgical Solution*, pp. 37–38; Kuepper, "Euthanasia in America," p. 65; *New York Medical Journal* 100 (December 26, 1914): 1251.

20. On the Michigan plan, see Curtis, "Eugenic Reformers," pp. 69–70; *CE* May 22, 1903; *DN* May 22, 1903; on Rodgers, see *Michigan State Gazeteer* (Detroit: R. L. Polk, 1903); *DN* May 21, 1903, p. 3. For Kempster, *NYT* January 26, 1906; for Gregory, Van der Sluis, "Euthanasia," p. 135.

21. James LeRoy Smith, "Shall Degenerates Be Condemned to Death?" *Physical Culture* 21 (January 1909): 49–52.

22. For a key interpretive overview of the era, see Robert Wiebe, *The Search for Order 1877–1920* (New York: Hill & Wang, 1976). On population shifts with particular reference to Chicago, see James Grossman, *Land of Hope: Chicago, Black Southerners and the Great Migration* (Chicago: University of Chicago, 1989); John Bodnar, *The Transplanted* (Bloomington: Indiana University Press, 1985).

23. Samuel P. Hays, *The Response to Industrialism* (Chicago: University of Chicago Press, 1957); Olivier Zunz, *Making America Corporate, 1870–1920* (Chicago: University of Chicago Press, 1990); Martin Sklar, *Corporate Reconstruction of American Capitalism* (New York: Cambridge University Press, 1988); David Noble, *America by Design: Science, Technology and the Rise of Corporate Capitalism* (New York: Oxford University Press, 1977); Gary Gers-

tle, *Working Class Americanism* (New York: Cambridge University Press, 1989); Harold Faulkner, *The Quest for Social Justice* (New York: Macmillan, 1931); David Montgomery, *The Fall of the House of Labor* (New York: Cambridge University Press, 1987); Alice Kessler-Harris, *Out to Work: A History of Wage-Earning Women in the United States* (New York: Oxford University Press, 1982).

Joel Williamson, *The Crucible of Race* (New York: Oxford University Press, 1984); Ronald Takaki, *Strangers from a Different Shore: A History of Asian-Americans* (Boston: Little, Brown, 1989); David Chalmers, *Hooded Americanism*, 3d ed. (Durham: Duke University Press, 1987).

24. Daniel Rodgers, "In Search of Progressivism," *Reviews in American History* (December 1982), pp. 113–32; Richard L. McCormick, *The Party Period and Public Policy* (New York: Oxford University Press, 1986); Stephen Skowronek, *Building a New American State* (New York: Cambridge University Press, 1982); James T. Kloppenberg, *Uncertain Victory: Social Democracy and Progressivism in European and American Thought* (New York: Oxford University Press, 1986); Daniel Nelson, *Frederick W. Taylor and the Rise of Scientific Management* (Madison: University of Wisconsin Press, 1980); Wiebe, *Search for Order;* Gabriel Kolko, *Triumph of Conservatism* (Glencoe, Ill.: Free Press, 1963); Theda Skocpol, *Protecting Soldiers and Mothers: Origins of Social Policy in the United States* (Cambridge: Harvard University Press, 1992); Nancy Cott, *Grounding of Modern Feminism* (New Haven: Yale University Press, 1987); Samuel P. Hays, *Conservation and the Gospel of Efficiency* (Cambridge: Harvard University Press, 1959).

25. On orthopedic surgery, see Wangensteen and Wangensteen, *Rise of Surgery*, esp. pp. 535–40; Morris Vogel, *Invention of the Modern Hospital* (Chicago: University of Chicago Press, 1980), pp. 63–64; David LeVay, *The History of Orthopedics* (Park Ridge, N.J.: Parthenon, 1990); Arthur Keith, *Menders of the Maimed* (London: H. Frowde, 1919). On a closely related field, see Glenn Gritzer and Arnold Arluke, *The Making of Rehabilitation: A Political Economy of Medical Specialization 1890–1980* (Berkeley: University of California Press, 1985). For more on these developments, see chap. 5 below.

On physical disabilities, see Saul Benison, "An Interpretation of the Early Evolution of Care and Treatment of Crippled Children in the United States," *Birth Defects: Original Article Series*, vol. 12, no. 4 (1976): 103–115; *The Origins of Modern Treatment and Education of Physically Handicapped Children: An Anthology*, ed. William R. Phillips and Janet Rosenberg (New York: Arno, 1980); and for the post–Social Security era, Edward D. Berkowitz, *Disabled Policy: America's Programs for the Handicapped* (Cambridge: Cambridge University Press, 1987).

26. On institutions for the insane, see David Rothman, *Conscience and Convenience: The Asylum and Its Alternatives in Progressive America* (Boston: Little, Brown, 1980); Gerald Grob, *Mental Illness in American Society 1875–1940* (Princeton: Princeton University Press, 1983).

On other mental disabilities, see James W. Trent, *Inventing the Feeble Mind* (Berkeley: University of California Press, 1994); Peter L. Tyor and Leland V. Bell, *Caring for the Retarded in America: A History* (Westport, Conn.: Greenwood, 1984); Tyor, "Segregation or Surgery: The Mentally Retarded in America 1850–1920," Ph.D. diss., Northwestern University, 1972; and Russell Hollander, "Mental Retardation and American Society: The Era of Hope," *Social Service Review* (September 1986), pp. 395–420.

27. Paul de Kruif, *Microbe Hunters* (New York: Harcourt, Brace, 1926), chap. 5, sects. 2–3 capture Pasteur's sense of unlimited possibilities in the new methods. Harry Dowling, *Fighting Infection* (Cambridge: Harvard University Press, 1977); Judith Walzer Leavitt, *Brought to Bed: Childbearing in America* (New York: Oxford University Press, 1986), chap. 7.

28. Paul Starr, *The Social Transformation of American Medicine* (New York: Basic, 1982); Charles Rosenberg, *The Care of Strangers* (New York: Basic, 1987); Kenneth Ludmerer, *Learning to Heal* (New York: Basic, 1985); Martin S. Pernick, "Medical Professionalism," *Encyclopedia of Bioethics*, Vol. III (New York: Free Press, 1978), pp. 1028–1034.

29. Richard Shryock, *The National Tuberculosis Association 1904–1954* (New York: Tuberculosis Association, 1957); Michael Teller, *The Tuberculosis Movement* (Westport, Conn.: Greenwood, 1988); Grob, *Mental Illness*, chap. 6; James T. Patterson, *The Dread Disease: Cancer and Modern American Culture* (Cambridge: Harvard University Press, 1987), pp. 71–78; *Dying for Work*, ed. David Rosner and Gerald Markowitz (Bloomington: Indiana University Press, 1987).

30. Allan Brandt, *No Magic Bullet* (New York: Oxford University Press, 1987).

31. Linda Gordon, *Woman's Body, Woman's Right: A Social History of Birth Control in America* (New York: Viking, 1976); James Reed, *From Private Vice to Public Virtue: The Birth Control Movement and American Society Since 1830* (New York: Basic, 1978); David M. Kennedy, *Birth Control in America* (New Haven: Yale University Press, 1970); Ellen Chesler, *Woman of Valor: Margaret Sanger and the Birth Control Movement in America* (New York: Simon & Schuster, 1992). For more on the controversial relation between birth control and eugenics, see note 42 below.

32. Richard Meckel, *Save the Babies: American Public Health Reform and the Prevention of Infant Mortality 1850–1929* (Baltimore: Johns Hopkins University Press, 1990); Joyce Antler and Daniel M. Fox, "The Movement toward a Safe Maternity," in *Sickness and Health in America*, ed. Judith Leavitt and Ronald Numbers (Madison: University of Wisconsin Press, 1985), pp. 490–506; Thomas E. Cone, *History of American Pediatrics* (Boston: Little, Brown, 1979); Sydney Halpern, *American Pediatrics: The Social Dynamics of Professionalism 1880–1980* (Berkeley: University of California Press, 1988); *Children and Youth in America: A Documentary History*, ed. Robert H. Bremner (Cambridge: Harvard University Press, 1971), vol. II, parts 6–7; Rothman, *Conscience and Convenience;* Molly Ladd-Taylor, *Raising a Baby the Government Way* (New Brunswick: Rutgers University Press, 1986); Skocpol, *Protecting Soldiers and Mothers;* Lawrence Cremin, *Transformation of the School* (New York: Knopf, 1961); Sheila Rothman, *Woman's Proper Place* (New York: Basic, 1978); Susan Tifflin, *In Whose Best Interest? Child Welfare Reform in the Progressive Era* (Westport, Conn.: Greenwood, 1982); Alisa Klaus, *Every Child a Lion: Origins of Maternal and Infant Health Policy in the United States and France 1890–1920* (Ithaca, N.Y.: Cornell University Press, 1993); *In the Name of the Child: Health and Welfare 1880–1940*,

ed. Roger Cooter (New York: Routledge, 1992). See also chap. 5, notes 33 and 42 below.

33. For medicalization of the family as a power grab by male professionals, see Christopher Lasch, *The Culture of Narcissism* (New York: Norton, 1979); Rothman, *Woman's Proper Place*. For medical power as partly the result of women's choices, see Leavitt, *Brought to Bed*.

34. Martin S. Pernick, "The Patient's Role in Medical Decisionmaking: A Social History of Informed Consent in Medical Therapy," *Making Health Care Decisions*, Report of the President's Commission for the Study of Ethical Problems in Medicine, (Washington, D.C.: 1982), vol 3, pp. 28–32. *Jacobson v. Massachusetts*, 197 U.S. 11; *Schloendorff v. Society of New York Hospital*, 211 N.Y. 125, at 127; 105 N.E. 92.

35. Martin S. Pernick, "Progressives, Propaganda and Public Health: The Army Venereal Disease Education Films of World War I," unpublished paper, Duquesne History Forum, November 1, 1974, Pittsburgh, Penn. For more critical views of propaganda, see chap. 6 below.

36. *CA* December 30, 1915, magazine page.

37. However, Kuepper's study of euthanasia, which included newspapers I did not use from Los Angeles, San Francisco, Philadelphia, Boston, and St. Louis, mentioned only one individual whom I had not found in my sources.

For list of newspapers, see the Bibliography. Many small-town papers covered the story; for a sampling of clippings, see *MPN* February 17, 1917, p. 996. The papers from two college towns, Ann Arbor and Ithaca, covered the story by rewriting material from the national wire services, but surprisingly did not interview local people for additional comments.

On the low standards of veracity and violent competition of Chicago papers in this era, see Stephen Longstreet, *Chicago 1860–1919* (New York: David McKay, 1973), pp. 450 ff.; Ben Hecht, *A Child of the Century* (New York: Simon & Schuster, 1954), pp. 125, 151; William MacAdams, *Ben Hecht* (New York: Scribner's, 1990).

38. Compare *Medical Record* [New York], November 27, 1915, p. 925, with *NYT* November 29, 1915, pt. I, p. 10.

39. *BG*, November 18, 1915, p. 5. For Hugh, see *CH* November 18, 1915, p. 4; *BA* November 17, 1915, p. 3. For Ted, see Patricia Spain Ward, "The Medical Brothers Cabot: Of Truth and Consequence," *Harvard Medical Alumni Bulletin* 56 (Fall 1982): 30–39. On Phillip, see Hugh Cabot to Ethel [Mrs. Frank Cabot], July 21, 1918, in Patricia Ward's possession. I am very grateful to her for sharing this information. See also Chester Burns, "Richard Cabot Clarke and the Reformation of American Medical Ethics," *Bulletin of the History of Medicine* 51 (Fall 1977): 353–68.

40. At the time it was widely accepted that such polls did have some statistical validity in assessing public sentiment. See *Independent* January 3, 1916, p. 23; *NYAm* November 18, 1915, p. 6; *DN* November 18, 1915, p. 25.

41. Reilly, *Surgical Solution;* Trombley, *Right to Reproduce;* Stefan Kühl, *The Nazi Connection: Eugenics, American Racism, and German National Socialism* (New York: Oxford University Press, 1994).

42. Kevles argues that "reform" eugenics remained largely distinct

from the conservative "mainstream" movement. G. R. Searle and Greta Jones contend that, with the exception of women, the British Labour Party had rejected eugenics by 1919. Jones criticizes Kevles, Diane Paul, and Michael Freeden for overemphasizing the significance of socialist eugenics. Like Garland Allen, Jones emphasizes that eugenics was rooted in efforts to control the industrial working class, though they differ on whether business or professional interests predominated.

Others such as Stefan Kühl criticize Kevles not for overemphasizing but for oversimplifying the political diversity of early eugenics. Though he sees the movement as conservative dominated, Kühl argues that a simple "reform" versus "mainline" dichotomy overlooks the variety of distinct political groups who favored eugenics.

Conflicting views of Margaret Sanger's career recapitulate the larger debates about eugenic politics. Linda Gordon sees Sanger's adoption of eugenics as a turning point in Sanger's betrayal of her socialist, anarchist, feminist roots, and her embrace of conservative male medical authority. But for James Reed, Sanger was primarily a single-issue crusader who espoused eugenics, socialism, or conservative professionalism pragmatically to the extent they furthered birth control. Ellen Chesler also sees Sanger as consistently devoted to one cause, but sees that as women's health.

Kevles, *Name of Eugenics*, pp. 64–65, 85–90, and 169–75. On European politics, see Michael Freeden, "Eugenics and Progressive Thought: A Study in Ideological Affinity," *The Historical Journal* 22 (1979): 645–71; Greta Jones, "Eugenics and Social Policy Between the Wars," *The Historical Journal* 25 (1982): 718–28; and Jones, *Social Hygiene in 20th Century Britain* (London: Croom Helm, 1986); Graham, "Science and Values"; Adams, *Wellborn Science;* Diane Paul, "Eugenics and the Left," *Journal of the History of Ideas* 45 (1984): 561–90; G. R. Searle, *Eugenics and Politics in Britain* (Leyden: Noordhof, 1976); Trombley, *Right to Reproduce;* Ian Macnicol, "Eugenics and the Campaign for Voluntary Sterilization in Britain," *Social History of Medicine* 2 (August 1989): 147–70, esp. 148–49; Garland Allen, "Genetics, Eugenics and Class Struggle"; Robert Proctor, *Racial Hygiene: Medicine Under the Nazis* (Cambridge: Harvard University Press, 1988), pp. 22–24; Atina Grossmann, "Abortion and Economic Crisis: The 1931 Campaign Against Paragraph 218," in *When Biology Became Destiny: Women in Weimar and Nazi Germany,* ed. Renate Bridenthal, Grossmann, and Marion Kaplan (New York: Monthly Review Press, 1984), pp. 66–86; Weindling, *Health, Race and German Politics,* esp. pp. 342–68.

On U.S. eugenic politics in addition to the general histories in note 11 above, see Vecoli, "Sterilization: A Progressive Measure?"; Donald K. Pickens, *Eugenics and the Progressives* (Nashville: Vanderbilt University Press, 1968); Kühl, *Nazi Connection;* Garland Allen, "Eugenics and American Social History 1880–1950," *Genome* 31 (1989): 885–89; Greg Mitman, "Evolution as Gospel: William Patten, the Language of Democracy and the Great War," *Isis* 81 (September 1990): 446–63; Gordon, *Woman's Body*.

43. Curtis, "Eugenic Reformers," pp. 69–70; *CE* May 22, 1903.

44. *Notable American Women* (Cambridge: Harvard University Press, 1971), vol. 3, p. 528.

45. In the *Call,* Haiselden's and Bollinger's articles and link to birth

control are in November 20 and 23, 1915. Women's page editor Anita Block's views are in December 12, 1915, magazine sect., and *MRR* 22 (February 1916): 124. Frederic Robinson in *Call* November 23, 1915; William J. Robinson in *Call* November 28, 1915, magazine p. 13. *Call* attacks on hypocrisy include November 18, 1915, p. 6; November 27, 1915, cartoon p. 6; November 28, 1915, magazine sect., p. 2; and December 12, 1915, magazine sect., woman's page. Haiselden himself ridiculed those who opposed subsidized school lunches for poor children while attacking him, *CA* November 14, 1917, p. 3. See also *Independent* January 3, 1916, p. 23; *Literary Digest* December 11, 1915, p. 1386.

46. Goldman was in Chicago November 22–December 7, 1915. See *Emma Goldman Correspondence*, microfilm edition, reel 9, especially Goldman to [Margaret Sanger], December 7, 1915. For Keller, see *Call* November 26, 1915, p. 5.

47. *American Socialist* November 27, 1915, p. 2; March 25, 1916, p. 2. *Alarm*, December 1915, p. 2. See also elliptical notice in *Appeal to Reason*, November 27, 1915 [Girard, Kans.].

48. "Where the Fraser River Flows," (1912), quoted in Montgomery, *House of Labor*, p. 93.

49. Quotation is from the *Call* November 21, 1915, magazine sect., p. 16; note that this position does not rule out eugenic euthanasia in a socialist society.

One *Call* article, by mothers' pension advocate Judge Henry Neil, did reject selective nontreatment, December 12, 1915, magazine sect.

50. Headline in *New World* November 26, 1916, p. 1. *New Orleans Morning Star* in *Current Opinion* 60 (January 1916): 43. Haiselden, like most eugenicists, did argue for human selection by analogy to livestock breeding. See chap. 8 below.

"Right to life" in *New World* November 19 and 26 and December 24, 1915; kidnap attempt in *CT* November 18, 1915, p. 2; medicine theft in *CE*, November 14, 1917, p. 6, and November 15, 1917, p. 9. For other Catholic opposition, see *CT* November 21, 1915; *Survey* December 4, 1915, p. 227; *Catholic World* 102 (December 1915): 421–24.

For Haiselden's view of Catholic church, see *CT* December 15, 1915. Block: *MRR* 22 (February 1916): 123.

51. For more on the opposition of various specialties, see chap. 5 below. Kuepper also found considerable regional variation in news accounts of medical opinion, with the opposition of doctors highlighted in Boston, Baltimore, Philadelphia, and St. Louis newspapers.

52. For more on gender politics and eugenics, see chap. 5 below.

53. Anna Blount, *CN* November 17, 1915, p. 3; Lathrop, *CT* November 18, 1915.

54. National Board of Review of Motion Pictures Records, Controversial Film Correspondence, Box 103, Rare Books and Manuscripts Division, The New York Public Library Astor, Lenox and Tilden Foundations. For a full list of the advisory committee, see 1917 list of "Personnel of the National Board of Review" in the file for the film *Enlighten Thy Daughter*. Not all the replies came from solicited individuals. Those who sent clippings of their published comments are counted among the public statements dis-

cussed above. For a brief introduction to the NBRMP, see Garth Jowett, *Film: The Democratic Art* (Boston: Little, Brown, 1976), pp. 126–30; and Daniel Czitrom, "The Redemption of Leisure: The National Board of Censorship and the Rise of Motion Pictures in New York City, 1900–1920," unpublished paper, American Studies Association, November 4, 1983, Philadelphia. I am grateful to him for sharing this manuscript and bringing the NBRMP papers to my attention, as well as to Robert Giroux for permission to use them.

Chapter 3

1. *Independent* January 3, 1916, p. 23; *CT* December 20, 1915, p. 7; *NYS* November 21, 1915, sect. 7, p. 8; *CA* December 3, 1915, p. 6; *Motography* February 17, 1917, advertising p. 2; see also Fig. 9.

2. Charles Rosenberg, "The Bitter Fruit: Heredity, Disease, and Social Thought," in *No Other Gods: On Science and American Social Thought* (Baltimore: Johns Hopkins University Press, 1976), pp. 25–53. Rosenberg quotes William Buchan's 1797 equation of biological and financial inheritance, pp. 31–32. See also Mary Bogin, "The Meaning of Heredity in American Medicine and Popular Health Advice, 1771–1860," Ph.D. diss., Cornell University, 1990; William Stanton, *The Leopard's Spots: Scientific Attitudes toward Race in America 1815–59* (Chicago: University of Chicago Press, 1960), Chaps. 1–2.

3. Ludmilla Jordanova, *Lamarck* (Oxford: Oxford University Press, 1984).

4. Genesis 30:25–43.

5. Paul–Gabriel Boucé, "Imagination, Pregnant Women, and Monsters in Eighteenth-Century England and France," in *Sexual Underworlds of the Enlightenment*, ed. G. S. Rousseau and Roy Porter (Chapel Hill: University of North Carolina Press, 1988) pp. 86–100; Park and Daston, "Unnatural Conceptions."

6. Yet even very good historians sometimes do so, e.g., Hamilton Cravens, *The Triumph of Evolution*, 2d ed. (Baltimore: Johns Hopkins University Press, 1988), p. 36.

7. Bernard Wishy, *The School and the Republic* (Philadelphia: University of Pennsylvania Press, 1968), esp. Chaps. 7–8, 10–11.

8. *OED*, "breed," verb senses 9–11.

9. Kevles, *Name of Eugenics;* David Joravsky, *The Lysenko Affair* (Cambridge: Harvard University Press, 1970); Loren Graham, *Science in Russia and the Soviet Union* (New York: Cambridge University Press, 1993); Stanton, *Leopard's Spots* on Rush; Adrian Desmond, *The Politics of Evolution* (Chicago: University of Chicago, 1989).

10. Stanton, *Leopard's Spots.*

11. Daniel Pick, *Faces of Degeneration: A European Disorder* (New York: Cambridge University Press, 1989); Rosenberg, "Bitter Fruit" is especially good on this irony. For one example of the resulting gloom in Lamarckian eugenics, see Smith, "Shall Degenerates Be Condemned," p. 51. For stimu-

lating comparison with modern concepts of atavism, see the title essay in Stephen Jay Gould, *Hen's Teeth and Horse's Toes* (New York: Norton, 1983).

12. For an American example, see Charles J. Bayer, *Maternal Impressions*, 2d ed. (Winona, Minn.: Jones & Kroger, 1897). Peter J. Bowler, "E. W. MacBride's Lamarckian Eugenics," *Annals of Science* 41 (1984): 245–60.

13. For nineteenth-century fears, see Dane Kennedy, "The Perils of the Midday Sun: Climatic Anxieties in the Colonial Tropics," in *Imperialism and the Natural World*, ed. John Mackenzie (Manchester: Manchester University Press, 1990), pp. 118–40. For Pasteur on anthrax vaccine, see De Kruif, *Microbe Hunters*. For more on final solutions, see the section on perfectionism later in this chapter, esp. note 115. Opposition both to the inheritance of acquired characteristics and to spontaneous generation was based in part on Virchow's 1858 doctrine that all cells come from other cells.

14. Bayer, *Maternal Impressions* exemplifies the links between this belief and late-nineteenth-century purity and eugenics movements. For continuing popular concern, see Mrs. E. G. to Children's Bureau, June 18, 1918, and reply by Anna Rude, excerpted in Ladd-Taylor, *Raising a Baby the Government Way*, pp. 51–52. For the late nineteenth century, see esp. E. J. Overend in *Pacific Medical Journal* (February 1890), p. 70, cited in Erin McLeary, "Late Victorian Explanations for Deformity," unpublished undergraduate paper, University of Michigan, April 24, 1992.

For an important debate on the relation between embryology and evolutionary biology in this period, see Stephen Jay Gould, *Ontogeny and Phylogeny* (Cambridge: Harvard University Press, 1977); Robert Richards, *The Meaning of Evolution* (Chicago: University of Chicago Press, 1992).

15. Race Betterment Conference *Proceedings* 1 (1914): 497, and 3 (1928): 88; Aldred Scott Warthin, *Creed of a Biologist* (New York: P. B. Hoeber, 1930), p. 18. For other examples, see *New York Medical Journal* 99 (January 31, 1914): 216, and 100 (December 26, 1914): 1252. See Kevles, *Name of Eugenics;* Peter Bowler, *Eclipse of Darwinism* (Baltimore: Johns Hopkins University Press, 1983); Bowler, *The Non-Darwinian Revolution* (Baltimore: Johns Hopkins University Press, 1988); Bowler, *The Mendelian Revolution* (London: Athlone, 1989); Edward J. Pfeiffer in *The Comparative Reception of Darwinism*, ed. Thomas Glick (Austin: University of Texas Press, 1974), pp. 168–206.

16. This section is based largely on Garland Allen, *Life Science in the Twentieth Century* (New York: Cambridge University Press, 1978); Ernst Mayr, *The Growth of Biological Thought* (Cambridge: Harvard University Press, 1982); Arnold Ravin, "Genetics in America: A Historical Overview," *Perspectives in Biology and Medicine* 21 (Winter 1978): 214–31; *Genetics, Eugenics and Evolution*, ed. Jonathan Harwood, *British Journal for the History of Science* 22 (1989): 257–375; and *Classic Papers in Genetics*, ed. James A. Peters (Englewood Cliffs, N.J.: Prentice-Hall, 1959). On Johannsen, see Allen; Sapp, "Struggle for Authority," pp. 320–36.

17. David Barker, "The Biology of Stupidity: Genetics, Eugenics, and Mental Deficiency in the Inter-War Years," *British Journal for the History of Science* 22 (1989): 370.

18. Robert Olby, "The Dimensions of Scientific Controversy: The

Biometric-Mendelian Debate," *British Journal for the History of Science* 22 (1989): 314; Jones, *Social Hygiene.*

19. Sapp, "Struggle for Authority," esp. pp. 321 and 328, n. 48; Jones, *Social Hygiene*, p. 98.

20. Fisher in National Conference on Race Betterment, *Proceedings* 2 (1915): 64. Irving Fisher and Eugene Lyman Fisk, *How to Live*, 12th ed. (New York: Funk & Wagnalls, 1917), p. 294; *Fourth Annual Report of the State Charities Commission [Illinois], Institution Quarterly* 5 (June 1914): p. 65, as quoted in Curtis, "Eugenic Reformers," p. 91.

For many similar comments, see Mrs. Melvil Dewey, National Conference on Race Betterment, *Proceedings* 1 (1914): 349; Michael Guyer, *Being Well-Born: An Introduction to Heredity and Eugenics* (Indianapolis: Bobbs-Merrill, 1927), p. 426; S. J. Holmes, "Misconceptions of Eugenics," *Atlantic* 115 (February 1915): 222–27; Kevles, *Name of Eugenics*, esp. p. 58; William J. Robinson, *Eugenics, Marriage and Birth Control*, 2d ed. (New York: Critic & Guide, 1922), pp. 91–93.

For the occasional less hostile view of mass cultural meanings, see National Conference on Race Betterment, *Proceedings* 1 (1914): p. 272; *Good Health Magazine* 50 (1915), pp. 485–88, and 51 (1916), pp. 594–95.

21. *CA* November 13, 1917; *DN* November 17, 1915; *CA* December 27, 1915, magazine page; *CT* November 17, 1915; *NYT* November 17, 1915. See also *Popular Science Monthly* 88 (1916): 83; *Boston Herald* November 21, 1915, p. C-7.

22. *WP* November 17, 1915. Speaking of the Bollinger baby, Haiselden claimed, "Defectives are prolific. It would reproduce its kind." Yet if the physical defects were as severe as Haiselden portrayed, this baby's future ability to reproduce seems questionable. The infant reportedly lacked a testicle, had other genito-urinary defects, and allegedly needed lifelong institutional care. Fear that defectives were prolific marked one of the key points on which eugenicists disagreed with Social Darwinism, some versions of which held that defects eventually led to sterility. Haiselden believed that physical defects were almost always associated with mental and moral defects that destroyed inhibitions against sexual promiscuity; see the section on mental and physical defects in this chapter.

23. *CA* December 6, 1915, magazine page; December 8, 1915, pp. 1–2; *WP* July 25, 1917, p. 5; *NYT* July 25, 1917, p. 11. For Haiselden's views on maternal impressions as a cause of defects, see *NYT* July 25, 1917, p. 11; *WP* July 25, 1917, p. 5; *CA* December 8, 1915, afternoon ed., p. 2; though he had second thoughts about how important such factors might be, *CE* July 25, 1917, p. 6.

Belief in maternal impressions remained particularly strong among midwest purity advocates. The works of Charles J. Bayer, author of *Maternal Impressions*, were featured prominently in the National Purity Alliance's *Purity Journal and the Christian Life.* The *Purity Journal* was published in Morton Park, Illinois, which may have been in or near the North Chicago suburb of Morton Grove, where Haiselden ran the Bethesda Industrial Home for Incurables. Unlike Haiselden, however, the National Purity Alliance was bitterly anti–birth control. *Purity Journal*, January 1901, pp. 2–3, 26; McDonough, *Physicians Blue Book* (1897), pp. 31, 73. On the social purity movement in general, see David J. Pivar, *Purity Crusade* (Westport, Conn.: Greenwood, 1973).

24. Some of Haiselden's critics also believed in maternal impressions, arguing that by publicizing birth defects Haiselden might cause more of them. See chap. 6 below.

25. The lengthy subplot concerning tuberculosis was eliminated from the film by 1927, although this may have been done for aesthetic as well as medical reasons; see chapter 8. LC-MBRS; UM-HHFC. Haiselden repeated the spitting-kissing metaphor in his lectures to film audiences, *MPN* April 28, 1917, p. 2675.

26. *MPN* May 19, 1917, p. 3133. Though Haiselden's film did not use the word "syphilis," the euphemisms employed were widely understood, and the *Moving Picture World* reviewer, for one, explicitly made the identification, *MPW* February 24, 1917, p. 1211.

27. *Call* November 29, 1915, p. 3. Haller, *Eugenics*, pp. 141–43; Kevles, *In the Name of Eugenics*, p. 100.

28. Arthur B. Reeve, "The Eugenic Bride," *Cosmopolitan* 56 (April 1914): 642. Thanks to Peter Laipson for the story. Davenport in *NYT* October 2, 1921, sect. II, p. 4.

29. Ross, *G. Stanley Hall*, pp. 362–63, 413. Thanks to Alice Smuts for this reference. For more on Wedd, see chap. 7 below.

30. In Britain, historian Greta Jones has concluded, eugenics and social hygiene were so intertwined as to be indistinguishable, Jones, *Social Hygiene*, chap. 1. Whether or not this was true in Britain, the relationship was more complex in the United States.

31. American Film Institute *Catalog of Feature Films, 1911–20* (Berkeley: University of California Press, 1989), p. 794; Brandt, *No Magic Bullet*, pp. 19, 27, 39, and *passim*.

32. Kevles, *Name of Eugenics*, pp. 99–100.

33. Fisher and Fisk, *How to Live*, pp. 293–94; *Good Health* 54 (1919): 658; *Social Hygiene Bulletin* January 1916, p. 3, and November 1916, p. 4.

34. *Popular Science Monthly* 88 (1916): 84–85; Brandt, *No Magic Bullet*, pp. 14–15; *Eugenics in Race and State: Scientific Papers of the Second International Congress of Eugenics . . . New York 1921* (Baltimore: Williams & Wilkins, 1923), pp. 309, 346–47.

Anti-Lamarckian prohibitionist John Harvey Kellogg gave extensive publicity to alcohol as a germ poison: *Good Health* 51 (1916): 75–76; 52 (1917): 502–503; 54 (1919): 164, 219–24, 273–78, 717. For a Lamarckian view of this research, see Warthin, *Creed*, pp. 57–58.

Jean-Charles Sournia, *A History of Alcoholism* (Oxford: Basil Blackwell, 1990), chap. 7; L. Crowe, "Alcohol and Heredity: Theories About the Effects of Alcohol Use on Offspring," *Social Biology* 32 (1985): 146–61; R. H. Warner and H. L. Rosett, "Effects of Drinking on Offspring: An Historical Survey of the American and British Literature," *Journal of Studies of Alcohol* 36 (November 1975): 1395–1420.

35. Garrod described the idea in 1902 and popularized it in his 1909 *Inborn Errors of Metabolism* (London: Oxford University Press, 1963); Alexander Bearn, *Archibald Garrod and the Individuality of Man* (New York: Oxford University Press, 1993).

36. Rene and Jean Dubos, *The White Plague: Tuberculosis, Man and Society* (London: Victor Gollancz, 1953), pp. 28–43, 125–28; Proctor, *Racial Hygiene*, pp. 215–17; *Eugenics in Race and State*, pp. 300–301.

37. Attacks on the reproduction of supposedly hereditary defectives often drew on images of quarantine and infection. For one early example, see *Physical Culture* 21 (January 1909): 50. In upholding compulsory sterilization of those with supposedly hereditary diseases, the U.S. Supreme Court relied on the precedent of involuntary vaccination to protect society against smallpox epidemics, *Buck v. Bell* 274 U.S. 200 (1927). See also Susan Sontag, *Illness as Metaphor* (New York: Farrar, Straus and Giroux, 1978); Lucy Dawidowicz, *The War Against the Jews, 1933–1945* (New York: Holt, Rinehart and Winston, 1975), pp. 21, 25, 41, 54; Proctor, *Racial Hygiene*, pp. 194–202; Howard Markel, "The Stigma of Disease: Implications of Genetic Screening," *American Journal of Medicine* 93 (August 1992): 209–15; Alan M. Kraut, *Silent Travelers: Germs, Genes and the 'Immigrant Menace'* (New York: Basic, 1994).

For general background on the late-nineteenth-century "social purity" roots of progressive "social hygiene," see Pivar, *Purity Crusade*. For a perceptive theoretical discussion, see Mary Douglas, *Purity and Danger: An Analysis of Concepts of Pollution and Taboo* (New York: Praeger, 1966).

38. *NYT* June 2, 1914, p. 11. " 'The Black Stork' is not a sex picture," *MPN* February 14, 1917, p. 1244; for more alluring disclaimers, see *Baltimore American* January 5, 1919, sect. 11, pp. 22, 23.

On eugenics and "sex problem" films, see chap. 7 below. Also see Kevin Brownlow, *Behind the Mask of Innocence* (New York: Knopf, 1990); Annette Kuhn, *Cinema, Censorship, and Sexuality 1909–1925* (London: Routledge, 1988); Kuhn, *The Power of the Image* (London: Routledge & Kegan Paul, 1985); Kay Sloan, *The Loud Silents* (Urbana: University of Illinois Press, 1988). For much more on eugenics and sexuality, see "Defects and Desires" section in this chapter.

39. This meaning is the subject of the old joke that "insanity is hereditary—you get it from your children." See also OED.

40. On the link between causality and morality, see Thomas Haskell, *The Emergence of Professional Social Science* (Urbana: University of Illinois Press, 1977), esp. chap. 11; and Sylvia Tesh, *Hidden Arguments: Political Ideology and Disease Prevention Policy* (New Brunswick: Rutgers University Press, 1988).

41. *Good Health* 52 (1917): 106; see also 51 (1916): 594.

42. *ExTrR* February 24, 1917, p. 817 for "Fit to Marry" ad. For fitness without ancestry, see *The Eugenic Girl*, in *MPW* September 12, 1914, p. 1547; *Eugenics at the Bar "U" Ranch, MPW* June 6, 1914, p. 1438; *Eugenics Versus Love, MPW* May 2, 1914, p. 724, and LC-MBRS paperprint #L2732.

43. A scene script of *Birth* is in LC-MBRS copyright records #MU-835; quotes are from *Wid's Film Daily* April 19, 1917, pp. 244–45. See also *MPW* April 28, 1917, p. 609; *MPN*, April 28, 1917, p. 2687; *NYAm* April 8, 1917, p. 7M, and April 15, 1917, p. 4M; *Motography* April 28, 1917, p. 915; *DN* April 29, 1917, p. 6, and May 6, 1917, p. 5. See also *New York Evening Journal* April 9, 1917, p. 8, and ads April 11–14, 1917, movie page; AFI, *Catalog 1911–20*, pp. 69–70.

A synopsis of *Well Born* is in *Child Health Magazine*, December 1923, pp. 571–72. See also *ibid.*, September 1924, p. 407; *Educational Screen*, February 1924, p. 80; *American Journal of Public Health* 14 (1924): 276; *Bulletin of the National Tuberculosis Association*, January 1924, p. 4. Other Children's Bureau films of the 1920s are available at the National Archives, but no surviving copies of this one are known.

44. *Eugenics in Race and State* pp. 318, 464–65; *A Decade of Progress in Eugenics: Scientific Papers of the Third International Congress of Eugenics* (Baltimore: Williams & Wilkins, 1934), p. 202; for similar views of the American Eugenics Society in 1935, see Ellsworth Huntington, *Tomorrow's Children* (New York: Wiley, 1935), pp. 41–42, quoted in Barry Mehler, "Eliminating the Inferior," *Science for the People*, November–December 1987, p. 16.

Such views may have become more common in the scientific and economic world of the mid-1930s, but they were clearly present throughout the history of eugenics. See also Kathy Cooke, "Heredity and Environment: Partners in Eugenic Reform," unpublished paper, History of Science Society, New Orleans, October 14, 1994.

45. *The Eugenic Boy*, in *MPW* March 21, 1914, p. 1584. The Race Betterment Foundation made a number of films that they considered "eugenic," but none are known to have dealt with genetics or ancestry. They ranged instead from physical exercise to smoking and alcohol, though the latter two may well have been depicted as "germ poisons." See chap. 7 below.

This quick summary is both too cynical about Chicago voters, and not cynical enough about the candidate. Frederick Wallace Patterson, a machinist and self-made pioneer auto manufacturer not known to have previously held public office, was running against an incumbent who had been part of Mayor Big Bill Thompson's political machine. But despite his "eugenic" protestations, Patterson was the machine candidate. His rival had recently turned against the Thompson organization, and in a close primary, Patterson unseated him. But Patterson lost the general election in a citywide Democratic landslide fueled by charges the Thompson machine had driven the respected head of the tuberculosis sanitarium to commit suicide. Even by Chicago standards, the campaign was considered unusually violent, including two shootings just during the primary. *CA* December 6, 1915, p. 4; *CT* March 1, 1916, and April 5, 1916; *The Book of Chicagoans* (Chicago: Marquis, 1917), p. 527; *NYT* February 29, 1916, p. 5.

For a socialist cartoon suggesting sterilization of munitions manufacturers as defectives, see *Call*, November 27, 1915, p. 6.

46. *CA* December 1, 1915, 2d ed.; *CH* December 15, 1915, p. 2; For Haiselden's citation of this and other similar murder cases, see *CA* December 8, 1915, magazine page; *DFP* November 18, 1915.

Police efforts to "round up" all Chicago defectives continued for some time. See *CH* July 29, 1916, reprinted in *Medical Freedom* (September 1916): 3; *Survey* 36 (August 12, 1916): 494–95.

The head of the Jersey City, New Jersey, Health Department praised Haiselden for helping fight the "menace" of "feeblemindedness," *DN* November 23, 1915. On the "menace of the feebleminded" in general, see Haller, *Eugenics*, Chap. 7; Steven A. Gelb, "Not Simply Bad and Incorrigible: Science, Morality, and Intellectual Deficiency," *History of Education Quarterly* 29 (Fall 1989): 359–79.

47. *DFP* December 20, 1915, p. 11; *NYT* November 19, 1915, p. 22; *NYAm* November 23, 1915, p. 7; *CA* December 7, 1915, magazine page; *CT* November 17, 1915, p. 7.

48. *CT* and *Washington Star* November 17, 1915; *TNR* November 18, 1915, p. 173.

49. Charles S. Bacon, "The Race Problem," *Medicine* [Detroit] 9 (1903): 341. See John Haller, *Outcasts from Evolution: Scientific Attitudes of Racial Inferiority 1859–1900* (Urbana: University of Illinois Press, 1971); George Fredrickson, *The Black Image in the White Mind* (New York: Harper & Row, 1972); Allan Chase, *The Legacy of Malthus* (New York: Knopf, 1977).

50. Hollander, "Euthanasia," p. 57.

51. Karen C. Lund, *American Indians in Silent Film: Motion Pictures in the Library of Congress* (Washington: Library of Congress, 1992).

52. J. G. Wilson, "A Study in Jewish Psychopathology," *Popular Science Monthly* 82 (1913): 265, 271. For more examples, see Stephen Jay Gould, "Science and Jewish Immigration," in *Hen's Teeth*, pp. 291–309. On eugenic immigration restrictions, see Ludmerer, *Genetics;* Kevles, *Name of Eugenics;* Kraut, *Silent Travelers.*

53. *DFP* November 29, 1915, p. 4; Wiley, "The Rights of the Unborn," *Good Housekeeping,* October 1922, p. 32; Grant, *The Passing of the Great Race* (New York: Scribner's, 1916), pp. 45, 47. Thanks to Juan Leon for the Wiley article.

54. Quote is from paper print of December 1916 version, which I recently located at the LC-MBRS, #LU-9978, Box 109. *MPW* February 24, 1917, p. 1211; *MPN* February 24, 1917, p. 1256; Commissioner to H. J. Brooks, April 4, 1923, NYSA-MPD, Box 2565, Folder 383. In response to *Birth of a Nation* in 1917, Illinois banned any film or publication that incited race hatred, Allan Spear, *Black Chicago* (Chicago: University of Chicago Press, 1967), p. 191.

55. *CA* November 24, 1915. See also *CA* November 30, 1915, p. 2; December 1, 1915, p. 3; December 2, 1915, p. 2. For other similarities between race and physical handicap, see Leonard Kriegel, "Uncle Tom and Tiny Tim: Reflections on the Cripple as Negro," *American Scholar* 38 (Summer 1969): 412–30.

56. Larry Wayne Ward, *The Motion Picture Goes to War: The U.S. Government Film Effort during World War I* (Ann Arbor: UMI Research Press, 1985), pp. 116–17.

57. For more on class and race in *The Black Stork*, see the section on "Defects and Desires" in this chapter; see also chap. 8 below.

58. Cynthia Eagle Russett, *Sexual Science* (Cambridge: Harvard University Press, 1989); Allison Carey, "The Changing Role of Gender in Compulsory Sterilization Programs, 1907–1950," unpublished graduate seminar paper, University of Michigan, 1992.

59. Amartya Sen, "More Than 100 Million Women Are Missing," *New York Review of Books,* December 20, 1990, pp. 61–66.

60. One reviewer of *The Black Stork* consistently mistakenly referred to the Bollinger baby as "her" and "she". Perhaps this reflected some tendency

to associate nontreatment with girl babies, although any number of other explanations are also plausible. *MPN* March 3, 1917, p. 1349. For current concerns, see Mary Anne Warren, *Gendercide: The Implications of Sex Selection* (Totowa, N.J.: Rowman & Allanheld, 1985).

61. Kraut, *Silent Travelers;* JoAnne Brown, *The Definition of a Profession: The Authority of Metaphor in the History of Intelligence Testing* (Princeton, N.J.: Princeton University Press, 1992), esp. pp. 78–81. For similar use of bacteriology in Nazi race theory, see Proctor, *Racial Hygiene.*

62. Of fifteen Haiselden supporters with German-American Hospital affiliations, four were immigrants (German, Russian, French, and Canadian), one was the son of immigrants (Bohemian), and five others had Jewish-Germanic surnames. Haiselden was the only one to claim old-stock American ancestry.

Quote is from *CT* November 17, 1915, p. 7. The Japanese did practice infanticide since at least the early 1700s, largely for reasons of economics, convenience, and sex selection. William LaFleur, *Liquid Life: Abortion and Buddhism in Japan* (Princeton, N.J.: Princeton University Press, 1992); Kuhse and Singer, *Should the Baby Live?*, pp. 105–107, 209. I have been unable to verify that not tying the umbilical cord was a common method, or that disabled infants were particular targets.

Of course being pro-Japanese was not incompatible with racial prejudice. At the First National Conference on Race Betterment, both an advocate and an opponent of eugenics agreed it was an injustice to the Japanese to equate them with the inferior colored races. See the Conference *Proceedings* 1 (1914): 502, 549.

On Fenger, see Bonner, *Medicine in Chicago,* p. 155. On Roberts, see *Dictionary of American Medical Biography,* ed. Martin Kaufman, Stuart Galishoff, and Todd L. Savitt (Westport, Conn.: Greenwood, 1984), vol. 2, p. 641; *CH* July 24, 1917, p. 14. For the abolition comparison, see *CA* December 16, 1915, magazine page.

63. *Christian Science Monitor* reprinted in *Medical Freedom* 5 (December 1915): 56; *Independent* January 3, 1916: p. 27; *Chicago Medical Recorder* 38 (1916), 592; *NYT* July 26, 1917, p. 10; W. P. Manton in *MRR* 22 (February 1916): 100; *New World* December 24, 1915, p. 4.

64. Haller, *Outcasts;* Fredrickson, *Black Image;* Winthrop Jordan, *White Over Black: American Attitudes toward the Negro 1550–1812,* 2d ed. (Baltimore: Penguin, 1969); Stanton, *Leopard's Spots.*

65. *ExTrR* February 24, 1917, p. 836; *Are You Fit to Marry?*, Historical Health Film Collection, University of Michigan. Mrs. Bollinger, an Irish woman married to a German man, was named Anna, *New York Medical Journal* 102 (December 4, 1915): 1132.

66. *Science of Life* reel 12, *General Hygiene,* NA reel number 90.26. The following discussion is also based on two versions of reel 11, *Personal Hygiene for Young Men* and *Personal Hygiene for Young Women,* NA reels 90.24 and 90.25.

NYT November 15, 1923, p. 10; *American Journal of Public Health,* December 1922, p. 1033, and September 1923, p. 737; *Journal of Social Hygiene,* January 1928, p. 14; NYSA-MPD Box 2565, Folders 12,471 and 12,493, including a clipping from the *New York Herald* April 15, 1923; Records of the United States Public Health Service, National Archives, Record Group 90, File 1350. Thanks to Peter Laipson and Aloha South for locating the NA material.

On the eugenic goals of this film series, see chap. 7 below, esp. note 28.

67. Eagle, *Sexual Science*, pp. 78–92; Kevles, *Name of Eugenics*, p. 12; Albert E. Wiggam, *The Fruit of the Family Tree* (Garden City: Garden City Publishing, 1924); "Jackie Swims to Increase Beauty," *Call* November 24, 1915, p. 5.

See also Lawrence Birken, *Consuming Desire: Sexual Science and the Emergence of a Culture of Abundance 1871–1914* (Ithaca: Cornell University Press, 1989); Trombley, *Right to Reproduce*, p. 79; and H. G. Wells, *Modern Utopia* (London: Chapman & Hall, 1905).

68. *Portrait of the Artist as a Young Man*, first published in 1916, quoted in Kevles, *Name of Eugenics*, p. 119.

Historians of Germany pioneered the recognition of this aesthetic dimension of eugenics, especially George Mosse, *Toward the Final Solution: A History of European Racism* (London: J. M. Dent, 1978), p. 2; Mosse, *Nationalism and Sexuality* (New York: H. Fertig, 1985); Weindling, *Health Race and German Politics;* Willibrald Saürländer, "The Nazis' Theater of Seduction," *New York Review of Books* April 21, 1994, pp. 16–19; Hillel Tryster, "The Art and Science of Pure Racism," *Jerusalem Post International* August 17, 1991, p. 13; Sander Gilman, *Picturing Health and Illness: Images of Identity and Difference* (Baltimore, Md.: Johns Hopkins University Press, 1995).

69. Wiggam, *Fruit of the Family Tree*, pp. 272, 279.

70. *CA* December 2, 1915, p. 2. This view still surfaces in modern evolutionary studies. Natalie Angier, "Why Birds and Bees, Too, Like Good Looks," and "Not Just a Beauty Contest," *NYT* February 8, 1994, pp. B5, B8; Jane Brody, "Ideals of Beauty Seen as Innate," *NYT* March 21, 1994, p. A6.

For more sophisticated current theories on the evolution of beauty, see David M. Buss, *The Evolution of Desire* (New York: Basic, 1994); R. W. Smuts, "Fat, Sex, Class, Adaptive Flexibility, and Cultural Change," *Ethology and Sociobiology* 13 (1992): 523–42; and forthcoming work by Richard Alexander and Robert Trivers. I thank Bob Smuts for discussing these works with me and for saving me from my initial misrepresentation of Darwin's views.

71. Helena Cronin, *The Ant and the Peacock: Altruism and Sexual Selection from Darwin to Today* (New York: Cambridge University Press, 1992); Stephen Jay Gould, "The Great Seal Principle," in *Eight Little Piggies* (New York: Norton, 1993), pp. 371–81.

72. Fisher and Fisk, *How to Live*, 12th ed. (New York: Funk & Wagnalls, 1917), p. 322; Wiggam, *Fruit of the Family Tree*, p. 275. See also Guyer, *Being Well-Born*, p. 438, passage retained from 1916 edition. For similar esthetic efforts in German eugenics, see Weindling, *Health, Race and German Politics*, pp. 410–13.

The presumably unintended implication of communal living or polygamy in Wiggam's quote results from his diction, not my ellipsis.

73. For more on *The Science of Life*, see Martin S. Pernick, "Sex Education Films, U.S. Government," *Isis* 84 (1993): 766–68; and chap. 7 below.

74. Charles Musser, *The Emergence of Cinema* (New York: Scribner's,

1990); Francois Dragognet, *Etienne-Jules Maret* (New York: Zone, 1992); Marta Braun, *Picturing Time: The Work of Etienne-Jules Maret* (Chicago: University of Chicago Press, 1992). Thanks to Rebecca Zurier for prompting these ideas.

75. The film was produced by the UFA and is available from the Bundesarchiv in Cologne and the LC-MBRS. For MacFadden on film, see *Fit: Episodes in the History of the Body* (Straight Ahead Films, 1993). See also Lois Banner, *American Beauty* (New York: Knopf, 1983); Martha Banta, *Imaging American Women* (New York: Columbia University Press, 1987).

76. *CA* December 2, 1915, p. 2.

77. Mann used the phrase to describe "the really characteristic and dangerous aspect of National Socialism," quoted in *New York Review of Books,* January 30, 1986, p. 21.

78. *CA* December 2, 1915, p. 2. *CA* November 29, 1915, and November 30, 1915, p. 2. In many ways, Haiselden's approach to art mimicked that of Thomas Eakins. On art and disfiguration of the canvas, see Michael Fried, *Realism, Writing, Disfiguration* (Chicago: University of Chicago Press, 1987). For other comparisons, see the section on nudes and sexuality in this chapter.

Aesthetic considerations still evoke significant controversy in defining disease and disability. See e.g., T.R.B., "The Tyranny of Beauty," *TNR* October 12, 1987, p. 4.

79. On photographic iconography, see Martin Elks, "Visual Rhetoric: Photographs of the Feeble-Minded during the Eugenics Era, 1900–1930," Ph.D. diss., Syracuse University, 1992. On the disabled in entertainment film, see the forthcoming book by Martin F. Norden (New Brunswick, N.J.: Rutgers University Press). On disability in recent horror films, see Paul K. Longmore, "Screening Stereotypes: Images of Disabled People," *Social Policy* 16 (Summer 1985): 31–37.

80. Wiggam, *Fruit of the Family Tree,* pp. 262, 273–74.

81. *CA* November 24, 1915; November 30, 1915, p. 2; see section on race in this chapter.

82. *CA* December 6, 1915, magazine page.

83. *Eugenics in Race and State,* p. 51.

84. James Whitcomb Riley, *"The Old Swimmin'-hole" and 'Leven More Poems* (Indianapolis: Bowen-Merrill, 1891); Lloyd Goodrich, *Thomas Eakins: His Life and Work* (New York: Whitney Museum, 1933), pp. 86, 88, 109, 176; *CA* November 23, 1915, p. 3. Such images had roots in the social purity movement and the muscular Christianity of the late nineteenth century. These scenes were considerably changed in later editions of the film; see chap. 8 below.

Eakins, like Haiselden, seems to have seen himself as scientifically, dispassionately dissecting the elements of physical beauty.

85. NBRMP, Box 163 "Reviews and Reports" folder, May 24, 1918.

86. Executive Secretary to H. E. Smith, December 2, 1916, NBRMP Box 103. The scene was not completely eliminated in 1916 and continued to provoke censors through the 1920s. NYSA-MPD Box 2565, Folder 383, undated list of cuts [March 1923]; Chicago Film Censorship Board, Review Cards, adult permit for *Are You Fit to Marry?,* November 17, 1927, Illinois

Regional Archives Depository, Northeastern Illinois University Library, Chicago.

87. *ExTrR* February 14, 1917, p. 836.

88. *MPN* February 14, 1917, p. 1244.

89. *Baltimore American* January 5, 1919, sect. 11, p. 23. See similar tone of review, p. 22.

90. NYSA-MPD Box 2565, Folders 383 and 12,421.

91. B. A. Towers, "Health Education Policy 1916–1926: Venereal Disease and the Prophylaxis Dilemma," *Medical History* 24 (1980): 70–87; Kuhn, *Cinema, Censorship and Sexuality* and *Power of the Image.*

92. Such concerns often surfaced in debates over whether sterilization would increase illegitimate sexual behavior, and, if so, whether that had any eugenic implications. John P. Radford, "Sterilization versus Segregation: Control of the 'Feebleminded' 1900–1938," *Social Science and Medicine* 33 (1991): 449–59; Tyor, "Segregation or Surgery"; Kevles, *Name of Eugenics;* Bert Hansen, "American Physicians' 'Discovery' of Homosexuals 1880–1920," in *Framing Disease,* ed. Charles Rosenberg and Janet Golden (New Brunswick, N.J.: Rutgers University Press, 1992), pp. 104–133.

93. Haller, *Eugenics,* p. 86. Similarly, Ludmerer, *Genetics in American Society.*

94. Gordon, *Woman's Body, Woman's Right;* Ruth Hubbard, *The Politics of Women's Biology* (New Brunswick, N.J.: Rutgers University Press, 1990).

95. Kevles, *Name of Eugenics,* pp. 53, 107.

96. Michel Foucault, *History of Sexuality* (New York: Vintage, 1985); Lasch, *Culture of Narcissism.*

97. The questions of power and autonomy are the subject of chap. 5 below. Lewis Perry, "Progress Not Pleasure is Our Aim: The Sexual Advice of an Antebellum Radical," *Journal of Social History* 12 (1979): 354–67; Philip R. Wyatt, "John Humphrey Noyes and the Stirpicultural Experiment," *Journal of the History of Medicine and Allied Sciences* 31 (January 1976): 55–66. For similar sexual aspects of Nazi eugenics, see chap. 9, esp. note 23 below.

98. Nathan G. Hale, Jr., *Freud and the Americans: The Beginnings of Psychoanalysis in the United States, 1876–1917* (New York: Oxford University Press, 1971), p. 271, on William J. Robinson; *MRR* 22 (January 1916): 4–5, for history of the periodical under Frederic H. Robinson.

99. *CT* November 19, 1915, p. 5; *CA* November 23, 1915, p. 3. His mother died several months before the Bollinger case, *CT* November 18, 1915, p. 2. She was only seventy-six according to several decades of census reports; see chap. 1 above.

Before the 1940s, elderly parents often lived with their adult children. In 1910 more than half of whites over age 65 were members of such households. In many cases the responsibility fell to an unmarried adult child, such as Haiselden. However, it was more common for a married daughter, such as Haiselden's sister, to take in a widowed mother, than for an unmarried man to do so. Steven Ruggles, "The Transformation of American Family Structure," *American Historical Review* 99 (February 1994): 103–128, esp. 116, 121, 124.

100. For perceptive comments, see John D'Emilio and Estelle B. Freed-

man, *Intimate Matters: A History of Sexuality in America* (New York: Harper & Row, 1988), chaps. 9 and 10, esp. pp. 204–207.

101. Mary Ware Dennett, "The Sex Side of Life," *MRR* 24 (February 1918): 69; *Notable American Women* I:465; Kevles, *Name of Eugenics*, pp. 52–53.

102. *Three Plays By Brieux* (New York: Brentano's, 1911), pp. xi–xii.

103. Victor Robinson in *MRR* 24 (February 1918): 65–68.

104. *Call* November 23, 1915.

105. Victor Robinson in *MRR* 24 (February 1918): 65–68.

106. For Haiselden's "advanced" views, see *CT* November 17, 1915; *BA* December 9, 1915, p. 12; *Motography* February 24, 1917, p. 424; *ExTrR* February 24, 1917, p. 836. Stanley Coben, *Rebellion Against Victorianism: The Impetus for Cultural Change in 1920s America* (New York: Oxford University Press, 1991); Steven Watson, *Strange Bedfellows: The First American Avant-Garde* (New York: Abbeville, 1991).

107. Brown, *Definition of a Profession;* Kevles, *Name of Eugenics*, pp. 76–77; Linda Gordon, *Woman's Body*, p. 277.

108. *Independent* January 3, 1916, p. 23; *TNR* December 18, 1915, p. 174; *NYT* November 26, 1915, p. 8. For others with similar views, see *NYT* November 18, 1915, p. 4, and November 25, 1915; *CH* November 17, 1915; *CT* November 18, 1915; *NYAm* November 19, 1915, p. 6; *New York Medical Journal*, 100 (December 26, 1914): 1247, 1249.

109. *CA* November 25, 1915.

110. *CA* November 27, 1915, p. 2; see Fig. 1. Since the 1960s, many different distinctive crying sounds have been linked to specific neurologic conditions, including Down syndrome and "cri-du-chat" syndrome. Alan J. Weston and Nancy T. Mader, "Infants' Vocalizations as a Diagnostic Tool," *Perceptual and Motor Skills* 58 (1984): 787–796.

111. *DN* November 18, 1915; *Washington Star* November 18, 1915; *NYT* November 19, 1915, p. 22.

112. *NYAm* November 20, 1915; *DFP* November 20, 1915. For Haiselden's view that the inquest had been stacked against him, and his account of why the jury rejected Reinhardt's findings, see *CA* December 22, 23, and 24, 1915, magazine pages. The full text of the coroner's jury "verdict" was widely reprinted; see e.g., *CH* November 20, 1915.

On history of neonatal assessment, see Selma H. Calmes, "Virginia Apgar: A Woman Physician's Career in a Developing Specialty," *Journal of the American Medical Women's Association* 39 (November–December 1984): 184–88. For discussion of why such predictions are still seen as difficult, see Anthony Gallo, "Spina Bifida: The State of the Art of Medical Management," *Hastings Center Report* 14 (February 1984): 10–13.

113. *NYT* November 25, 1915, p. 4; *Washington Star* November 18, 1915, p. 6. For Wiggam see note 69 above.

114. *CT* January 28, 1918, p. 12; *NYT* January 28, 1918, p. 6; *CE* January 28, 1918; *CT* December 3, 1915, p. 9; *CA* December 28, 1915, magazine; *Call* December 13, 1915; Lary May, *Screening Out the Past*, 2d ed. (Chicago: University of Chicago Press, 1983), p. 87.

115. Wyatt, "John Humphrey Noyes"; Kevles, *Name of Eugenics*, p. 21; Richard A. Soloway, *Demography and Degeneration: Eugenics and the Declin-*

ing Birthrate in Twentieth-Century Britain (Chapel Hill: University of North Carolina Press, 1990). For typical comments on the race between progress and degeneration, see National Conference on Race Betterment, *Proceedings* 1 (1914): 432 (Kellogg); *Proceedings* 3 (1928), 86 (Warthin).

For the allure of permanent solutions, see remarks of Irving Fisher in the same series, *Proceedings* 2 (1915): 64. For Haiselden on "the final solution of the problem," see *CA* December 30, 1915, magazine page. True to its millennial roots, this eugenics would not just speed up evolution, it would bring it to a conclusion, a biological end of time.

For another religious dimension to the determinism of eugenic thought, see David Hollinger, "What is Darwinism? It is Calvinism!" *Reviews in American History* 8 (March 1980): 80–85. One source of Haiselden's perfectionism was his mother, an ardent Methodist prohibitionist. *CA* November 23, 1915, p. 3.

116. Reeve, "The Eugenic Bride," p. 643.

117. *MRR* 22 (February 1916): 124, emphasis added; M. E. Mazur of Sheriott Pictures, quoted in *MPN* April 28, 1917, p. 2676, "both" *sic*.

118. *CA* November 24, 1915, p. 2.

119. *Call*, November 20, 1915; *DFP* December 20, 1915, p. 11. For similar comments, see *CE*, July 25, 1917, p. 6; *NYAm* November 24, 1915, p. 8; *CA* December 6, 1915, magazine page. On sterilization and other preventives versus euthanasia, see chapter 4. Reilly, "The Surgical Solution," pp. 637–56, includes much on Chicago sterilizers.

120. *MPN* February 17, 1917, p. 997. The fluidity and expansiveness of "eugenics" has many similarities with the protean progressive term "efficiency." On the latter term in medicine, see George Rosen, "The Efficiency Criterion in Medical Care 1900–1920," *Bulletin of the History of Medicine* 50 (Spring 1976): 28–44; in engineering, see John M. Jordan, *Machine-Age Ideology* (Chapel Hill: University of North Carolina Press, 1994).

121. McKim, *Heredity*, p. 194; Grant, *Great Race*, pp. 44–49; see also Wiley, "Rights," p. 32.

122. *NYAm* November 19, 1915, p. 6; *New World* December 24, 1915.

123. *New World* November 26, 1915, and November 19, 1915.

124. *Christian Science Monitor* quoted in *Medical Freedom* 5 (December 1915): 56. On natural theology and scientific vitalism, see Herbert Hovenkamp, *Science and Religion in America 1800–1860* (Philadelphia: University of Pennsylvania Press, 1978); James C. Turner, *Reckoning with the Beast* (Baltimore: Johns Hopkins University Press, 1980), chap. 6; Turner, *Without God, Without Creed* (Baltimore: Johns Hopkins University Press, 1985); Pernick, *Calculus of Suffering* and "Back from the Grave: Recurring Controversies Over Defining and Diagnosing Death in History," in *Death: Beyond Whole-Brain Criteria*, ed. Richard M. Zaner, Philosophy and Medicine Series (Dordrecht and Boston: Kluwer Academic Publishers, 1988), pp. 17–74.

125. P. Smith in *Independent* January 3, 1916, p. 27; *Medical Record* November 27, 1915, p. 925. See also Walter Croll in *MRR* 22 (February 1916): 97; and *NYT* November 29, 1915, p. 10. Ralph Waldo Emerson, "Compensation," *Essays, First Series* (Boston: Houghton Mifflin, 1888), pp. 89–122.

126. See for example *WP* November 18, 1915, p. 6.

127. P. Smith in *Independent* January 3, 1916, p. 27. See also *Journal of the American Medical Association* 65 (1915): 2025.

128. *Bentham's Theory of Legislation*, vol. I, trans. Charles Milner Atkinson (Humphrey Milford: Oxford University Press, 1914), pp. 38–39. For good examples from the Bollinger debate, see *New York World* reprinted in *Boston Advertiser* November 19, 1915, p. 6; Judge Henry Neil in *Call* December 12, 1915; New Orleans *Morning Star* November 20, 1915, p. 4.

For modern comment on the implicit rule-utilitarianism of slippery-slope arguments, see Tom L. Beauchamp, "A Reply to Rachels on Active and Passive Euthanasia," in *Ethical Issues in Death and Dying*, ed. Beauchamp and Seymour Perlin (Englewood Cliffs, N.J.: Prentice-Hall, 1978), pp. 246–58.

129. For early use of "slippery slope," see Harry Roberts, *Euthanasia* (London: Constable, 1936), p. 13.

130. A. W. Taylor to Executive Secretary McGuire, November 24, 1916, NBRMP Box 103. For similar wedge metaphors, see *NYT* November 18, 1915, p. 8; *MRR* 22 (February 1916): 97; *Survey* December 4, 1915, p. 266; *New World* December 24, 1915, p. 4.

131. New Orleans *Morning Star* November 20, 1915; *Current Opinion* 60 (January 1916): 43. See also NBRMP Box 103, letter of Felix Adler, November 16, 1916; *NYAm* December 3, 1915, p. 5.

132. *NYAm* November 25, 1915, p. 14; *Good Health* 51 (1916): 8.

133. L. A. Halbert to W. D. McGuire, December 1, 1916; and Edwin H. Jenks quoted in T. F. Sturgess to W. D. McGuire, December 4, 1916, both in NBRMP Box 103. See also comments of Judge Henry Neil in *Call* December 12, 1915; *New World* December 24, 1915, p. 4. Actually, such suggestions had already been made, in both medicine and the movies. See chap. 7 below.

134. *New World* November 19, 1915; *Call* November 21, 1915, magazine p. 16.

135. *NYS* November 19, 1915, p. 6; *Boston Herald* November 21, 1915, p. C7; *WP* November 18, 1915, p. 4.

136. Kevles, *Name of Eugenics*, p. 12. For Karl Pearson's insistence that his diagnosis of Jewish inferiority was based on "the cold light of statistical inquiry" not "prejudice," see his paper in the 1925 inaugural *Annals of Eugenics*, quoted by Gould in *Hen's Teeth*, pp. 296–98. Wiggam, *Fruit of the Family Tree*, pp. 272–79.

137. *NYAm* November 23, 1915, p. 10; *CA* November 29, 1915, p. 2. For others who held monsters were nonhuman, see *Baltimore American* in *Current Opinion* 60 (January 1916): 43.

138. Robinson, *Eugenics, Marriage and Birth Control* (1922), pp. 100, 101, 109–10.

139. T. H. Huxley quoted in Diane Paul, "The Selection of the 'Survival of the Fittest,'" *Journal of the History of Biology* 21 (Fall 1988): 411–24 at 419. This paragraph inevitably oversimplifies complex controversies in theoretical biology. See Richards, *Meaning of Evolution;* Gould, *Ontogeny and Phylogeny*, for debate over the history of teleology in evolution.

140. *Good Health* 52 (1917): 504, 567.

141. Quoted by A. E. Hamilton in *Good Health* 51 (1916): 76; see also Kevles, *Name of Eugenics*, p. 91.

142. For Joseph Kett's incisive criticism of the progressive-era tendency to objectify value judgments about childrearing, see *Which Babies Shall Live?*, ed. Murray and Caplan, pp. 30–31.

On progressivism and objectivity, see Peter Novick, *That Noble Dream: The "Objectivity Question" and the American Historical Profession* (New York: Cambridge University Press, 1988), Haskell, *The Emergence of Professional Social Science;* and David Hollinger, "Justification by Verification: The Scientific Challenge to the Moral Authority of Christianity in Modern America," in *Religion and Twentieth-Century American Intellectual Life,* ed. Michael Lacey (Cambridge: Cambridge University Press, 1989), pp. 116–35. See also chap. 4 below on objectivity as a source of ethical obligations.

143. Peter Steinfels, "Introduction" to issue on "The Concept of Health," *Hastings Center Studies* 1 (1973): 3–88; Charles Rosenberg, "Framing Disease," in *Framing Disease,* ed. Rosenberg and Golden, pp. xiii–xxvi; H. Tristram Engelhardt, "The Concepts of Health and Disease," *Evaluation and Explanation in the Biomedical Sciences* (Dordrecht: D. Reidel, 1975), pp. 125–41; Sander Gilman, *Difference and Pathology* (Ithaca: Cornell University Press, 1985).

Chapter 4

1. Kuepper, "Euthanasia in America," p. 62; National Conference on Race Betterment, *Proceedings* 1 (1914): 500–501; 2 (1915): 89–90, addenda slip for p. 61. For the others, see C. W. Saleeby, 1 (1914): 477; Irving Fisher, 1 (1914): 472, 475. For early supporters of eugenic euthanasia, see chap. 2 above.

2. Leon J. Cole, quoting G. Chatterton-Hill, National Conference on Race Betterment, *Proceedings* 1 (1914): 503. Part of the ugliness of the expression is its equation of impaired babies with excreta.

3. *Call* November 20, 1915; *DFP* December 20, 1915, p. 11; *CE*, July 25, 1917, p. 6; *NYAm* November 24, 1915, p. 8; *CA* December 6, 1915, magazine page.

4. *CA* December 17, 1915, magazine; *CH* November 14, 1917, p. 7; *New York Medical Journal* 102 (December 4, 1915): 1134. For the announcement, *Bulletin of Chicago Medical Society* 15 (February 26, 1916): 19.

5. *MRR* 22 (February 1916): 95, 96, 101.

6. *Chicago Herald and Examiner* June 19, 1919.

7. *MPW* May 2, 1914, p. 661.

8. Elliot S. Valenstein, *Great and Desperate Cures: The Rise and Decline of Psychosurgery and Other Related Treatments for Mental Illness* (New York: Basic, 1986), p. 43; Susan Leigh Star, *Regions of the Mind: Brain Research and the Quest for Scientific Certainty* (Stanford: Stanford University Press, 1989).

"Reform by Surgery," *DFP* May 23, 1903, p. 4, reprinted from *NYT* (London trephining); Thomas Travis, *The Young Malefactor* (New York: Crowell, 1908), p. 210 (New York adenoids); *Medical Freedom* 4 (September 1914): 7 (first Philadelphia trephining); *NYAm* November 18, 1915 (Brooklyn tonsillectomy); *Good Health* 51 (1916): 110 (second Philadelphia trephining); *Good Health* 52 (1917): 5 (Michigan trephining). Thanks to Maris Vinovskis for the Travis reference.

9. AFI, *Catalog 1911–20*, p. 244; *Variety* June 5, 1914, p. 19.

10. *MPW* February 22, 1913, p. 804; the subject's "consent" is obtained by giving him a choice between surgery and jail. *MPW* April 4, 1914, p. 116. In *The Germ* (Research 1923) the cause of crime turns out to be germs not genes, but here too discovery of a biological cause for crime is the basis of therapeutic optimism, not grounds for biological fatalism. See AFI, *Catalog of Motion Pictures Produced in the United States: Feature Films, 1921–1930* (New York: Bowker, 1971), p. 286. Thanks to JoAnne Brown for the reference to *The Germ*.

11. *Ithaca [NY] Daily Journal* September 25, 1916, n.p.

12. Thomas Travis, *The Young Malefactor*, pp. 210–12.

13. *CA* November 24, 1915, p. 2.

14. *Independent* January 3, 1916, p. 23.

15. *Chicago Medical Recorder* 38 (1916): 592; *Illinois Medical Journal* 28 (December 1915): 431. See also Dr. J. H. Hanson Knox in *NYS* November 18, 1915, p. 3.

16. This small group included Lewellys Barker, John Harvey Kellogg, Boston psychiatrists Frankwood Williams and E. E. Southard, and child health leader James Hall Mason Knox.

17. For example, Dr. William Pritchard in *NYS* November 18, 1915, p. 3.

18. *BA* December 10, 1915, p. 16; George Woodcock, *Anarchism* (Cleveland: World, 1962), pp. 328, 336, 462. Parallels with the approach of Dr. Jack Kevorkian today will be developed in chap. 9 below.

19. *NYAm* November 21, 1915; *Independent* January 3, 1916, p. 23; *CA* November 24, 1915, p. 2, and November 30, 1915, p. 2.

20. *CH* November 21, 1915, p. 3; *CT* November 17, 1915.

21. *DN* November 18, 1915, p. 4. *CT* November 20, 1915, p. 8, quoting *Baltimore Catholic Review*, November 19, 1915. For similar views of an obstetrician at Catholic Georgetown University, see *MRR* 22 (February 1916): 99. Non-Catholics found the distinction persuasive as well, *NYAm* November 18, 1915, p. 6; *Independent* January 3, 1916, p. 25. However, Bishop Carroll of Montana replied that surgery had advanced to the point where most lifesaving operations were no longer attended with the degree of pain and danger that had made them extraordinary measures in the past, *New World* December 24, 1915, p. 4.

22. *Call* November 28, 1915, p. 6. On the nineteenth-century uses, see Pernick, *Calculus of Suffering*. Haiselden denied that he was simply passing the buck, *CA* December 1, 1915, p. 3.

On the theoretical issues, see James Rachels, "Active and Passive Euthanasia," *New England Journal of Medicine* 292 (January 9, 1975): 78–80; Beauchamp, "Reply to Rachels"; and K. Danner Clouser, "Allowing or Causing: Another Look," *Annals of Internal Medicine* 87 (1977): 622–24. I am grateful to Yale Kamisar for additional sources and comments.

23. Andrew Somers in *MRR* 22 (February 1916): 102. For identical remarks, see comments by Greer Baughman, Stricker Coles, and Rudolph Holmes, *ibid;* and views of a Philadelphia judge in *NYT* November 18, 1915, p. 6.

24. *NYS* November 19, 1915, p. 6; *NYT* November 19, 1915, p. 10; though the *Times* editors changed their minds on this point, July 26, 1917, p. 10.

25. *New World* November 19, November 26, and December 24, 1915; *NYT* November 17, 1915; *Times* (London) November 18, 1915, p. 7; *MRR* 22 (February 1916): 101; *Boston Herald* November 21, 1915, pp. C7–C8; *NYAm* November 19, 1915, p. 6.

26. For the only exception, and not a very successful one, see *New World* November 26, 1915. In general, see Owsei Temkin, W. K. Frankena, and S. H. Kadish, *Respect for Life in Medicine, Philosophy and Law* (Baltimore: Johns Hopkins University Press, 1977).

27. *NYT* November 19, 1915, p. 10.

28. A. W. Taylor to W. D. McGuire, November 24, 1916, NBRMP, Box 103; *NYAm* November 25, 1915, p. 14. See also *Journal of the American Medical Association* 65 (1915): 2025; *New World* December 24, 1915, p. 4.

29. *CA* December 1, 1915, p. 3.

30. *Call* November 17, 1915, pp. 1–2. On Grimshaw girl, *CA* December 28, 1915, magazine; *Call* December 13, 1915; for a similar "cured or dead" request, see *DFP* November 23, 1915, p. 9.

31. *CT* November 17, 1915, p. 7; *CH* July 24, 1917, p. 14. He described the baby as "microcephalic, undeveloped skull cap," and implied the baby would die from encephalitis unless he operated to cover the exposed brain, *MRR* 22 (February 1916): 95; *NYS* July 25, 1917.

32. *NYT* November 13, 1917, p. 12, and November 16, 1917, p. 4.

33. *Call* November 17, 1915, pp. 1–2. A Catholic bishop denied that this doctrine applied to such cases, without explaining why, *New World* December 24, 1915.

34. *CH* November 19, 1917, p. 5.

35. For Haiselden's use in sterilizations, see *CT* December 20, 1915, p. 7; quote is from *New York Medical Journal,* 100 (September 5, 1914): 476. See Judith Walzer Leavitt, "Birthing and Anesthesia: The Debate Over Twilight Sleep," *Signs* 6 (Autumn 1980): 147–64; Lawrence G. Miller, "Pain, Parturition, and the Profession: Twilight Sleep in America," in *Health Care in America: Essays in Social History,* ed. Susan Reverby and David Rosner (Philadelphia: Temple University Press, 1979), pp. 19–44; and Margarete Sandelowski, *Pain, Pleasure and American Childbirth from the Twilight Sleep to the Read Method 1914–1960* (Westport, Conn.: Greenwood, 1984).

A 1915 German movie, *Twilight Sleep,* helped publicize the method only a few months before the Bollinger case. Although the "twilight treatment" scene lasts less than a minute in Haiselden's film, his movie was advertised as being about twilight sleep as late as 1919. For the 1915 film, see LC-MBRS, copyright files, #LM-561; *NYT* August 26, 1915, p. 9; *MPW* April 17,

1915, p. 396, July 31, 1915, p. 859, and December 4, 1915, p. 1806. For the 1919 ad, see *Baltimore Sun* January 12, 1919, p. B10.

36. *ExTrR* February 14, 1917, p. 850; Chicago Film Censorship Board, adult permit, November 17, 1927. The Board cut the poison reference and it was eliminated in the surviving print.

37. *CT* November 18, 1915, p. 6; *NYS* November 14, 1917, p. 3.

38. *Good Health* 51 (1916): 7; *NYAm* November 23, 1915, p. 10; *New York Medical Journal* 100 (December 26, 1914) 1251.

39. Letter of November 20, 1916, NBRMP Box 103.

40. *CT* November 17, 1915, p. 7; *CN* November 12, 1917, p. 1; *NYT* November 13, 1917, p. 12; *CA* November 12, 1917, afternoon ed.; *CT* November 12, 1917. For passive euthanasia of *adults*, see *CA* December 22, 1915, p. 3.

41. *NYT* November 18, 1915, p. 4.

42. *NYS* November 21, 1915, sect. 7, p. 8.

43. Pernick, *Calculus of Suffering*, pp. 172–73.

44. *CA* November 27, 1915, p. 2.

45. *WP* July 25, 1917, p. 5; see also *CA* December 16, 1915, magazine page.

46. *CA* November 29, 1915; *CA* November 26, 1915, p. 2; see also *CA* November 24, 1915, p. 2; *New York Medical Journal* 102 (December 4, 1915): 1134; *Lancet* editor in *Current Opinion* 60 (January 1916): 43.

47. Pernick, "Back from the Grave."

48. *MRR* 18 (June 1912): 362–63. My colleague Joel Howell graciously supplied this example.

49. *WP* November 18, 1915, p. 4; *WP* November 18, 1915, p. 4. For a recent critique of the claim that defective newborns have interests that we can meaningfully distinguish from our own legitimate concerns, see Howard Brody, "In the Best Interests of. . . ," *Hastings Center Report* 18 (December 1988): 37–39.

50. *Call* November 27, 1915, p. 5; *WP* November 19, 1915, p. 2 ("child who suffers" and "life is hard"). The girl's letter was reprinted repeatedly, including *Call* November 23, 1915; *Independent* January 3, 1916, p. 25; and, with various editorial modifications, *WP* November 23, 1915, p. 4, and *DN* November 22, 1915.

51. *MRR* 23 (October 1917): 698; *DN* July 24, 1917; *DFP* November 12, 1917; *WP* November 14, 1917, p. 2. For a medical defense of therapeutic abortion, see Barton Cooke Hirst, "The Rights of the Unborn Child," *New York Medical Journal* 105 (February 10, 1917): 241–43.

52. *Independent* January 3, 1916, p. 23, including similar comment by Irving Fisher; *MRR* 22 (February 1916): 124. Haiselden agreed: "A surgery that cures the race of mortal sickness is surely a higher art than that which . . . attempt[s] to check the fleeting misery of one individual." *CA* November 24, 1915, p. 2; see also *CT* December 20, 1915, p. 7.

53. *Call* November 26, 1915, p. 5.

54. *MRR* 22 (February 1916): 124.

55. Ronald Numbers, *Almost Persuaded: American Physicians and Compulsory Health Insurance 1912–1920* (Baltimore: Johns Hopkins University Press, 1978); Daniel Fox, "Social Policy and City Politics: Tuberculosis Reporting in New York 1889–1900," *Bulletin of the History of Medicine* 49

(1975): 169–95; Barbara Rosenkrantz, *Public Health and the State: Changing Views in Massachusetts 1842–1936* (Cambridge: Harvard University Press, 1972); Starr, *Social Transformation.* For the role of individualism in nineteenth-century conservative professionalism, see Pernick, *Calculus of Suffering,* esp. Chap. 6.

56. *Survey* December 4, 1915: p. 266; *Good Health* 51 (1916): 8. This section deals only with whose interests eugenic euthanasia should serve. Chapter 5, which focuses on who should have the power to make such decisions, will consider the conflicts over authority among doctors, lay reformers, and the state.

57. *WP* November 18, 1915, p. 4.; *New World* December 24, 1915, p. 4.

58. Graham, "Science and Values."

59. Beauchamp, "Reply to Rachels."

60. *Morning Star* November 20, 1919, p. 4. For another striking example, see P. Smith, *Independent* January 3, 1916, p. 27.

61. Kevles, *Name of Eugenics,* p. 94 for undated denial of rights; *Call* November 28, 1915, magazine sect., p. 13; *NYAm* November 21, 1915, see also November 26, 1915, p. 3; and *DFP* November 18, 1915, pp. 1, 25; *DN* November 18, 1915, p. 25.

62. *Independent* January 3, 1916, p. 25; *WP* November 19, 1915; *Washington Star* November 18, 1915, p. 13. See also Eden Paul, "Eugenics, Birth-Control, and Socialism," p. 142; Engel, *Elements of Child-Protection,* p. 257.

63. Proctor, *Racial Hygiene,* p. 178. The nineteenth-century roots of this connection between utilitarianism and humanitarianism are explored in Pernick, *Calculus of Suffering.* Modern advocates of mercy killing insist on distinguishing the two motives. Russell, *Freedom to Die,* pp. 19–20; Humphry, *Right to Die.*

64. Aldous Huxley, *Brave New World* (New York: Bantam, 1960, 1932); Pernick, *Calculus of Suffering.*

65. For progressivism as the "via media" of "rational benevolence," see Kloppenberg, *Uncertain Victory,* Part One. I am also grateful to George Stocking of the University of Chicago for helping me to clarify this point.

66. *Call* November 20, 1915. For one mother's agreement, see *Call* November 27, 1915, p. 5.

67. *CA* November 12, 1917, afternoon ed., p. 1.

68. *CA* December 8, 1915, magazine page; *CA* December 7, 1915, magazine page; *WP* November 14, 1917, p. 2; *CA* November 26, 1915, p. 2; *CA* December 30, 1915, magazine page.

69. *CA* December 6, 1915, magazine page.

70. *Independent* January 3, 1916, p. 24. For other links between contagion and hereditary disease, see chap. 3 above.

71. *IDJ* September 25, 1916; *MRR* 23 (October 1917): 697. See also *CA* December 7, 1915, magazine page, and December 21, 1915, editorial page.

Similar stark visual contrasts between loathsome expensive defectives and beautiful healthy people fill such Nazi Party films as the 1934 *Erbkrank* [Hereditary Disease], National Archives, Motion Picture Branch #243.3, and University of Michigan Historical Health Film Collection; and the 1940 *Alles Leben ist Kampf* [All Life is Struggle]. See chap. 9 below.

72. *CA* November 27, 1915, p. 2. Kuepper too was struck by the mix of love and hate in Haiselden's writings, "Euthanasia," p. 70.

73. *WP* November 18, 1915; *Call* November 26, 1915. "It is our duty to defend ourselves and the future generations against the mentally defective we allow to . . . suffer among us," Haiselden declared. *WP* November 19, 1915; *Washington Star* November 18, 1915, p. 13.

74. *DN* November 18, 1915, pp. 1, 25; *NYAm* November 16, 1915, p. 6, and November 23, 1915, p. 22; *New York Medical Journal* 102 (December 4, 1915): 1134; *CA* December 3, 1915, p. 6. See also *DFP* November 19, 1915, p. 5.

75. *CA* December 2, 1915, p. 2.

76. Leslie Fiedler, *Freaks: Myths and Images of the Secret Self* (New York: Simon & Schuster, 1978), and "The Tyranny of the Normal," *Hastings Center Report* 14 (April 1984): 40–42.

77. *NYT* July 26, 1917, p. 10; *WP* November 18, 1915, p. 10. See also *NYT* November 18, 1915; *New World* November 19 and 26, 1915. Of course, Frankenstein's science aimed at creating rather than taking life.

78. *CE* November 13, 1917, p. 5; see also *CT* November 17, 1915, p. 7.

79. *CA* December 18, 1915, magazine page; for centrality of ethics, see *New York Medical Journal* 102 (December 4, 1915): 1134.

80. *CA* December 1, 1915, p. 3.; *Current Opinion* 60 (January 1916): 43. See also chap. 7, note 4 below.

81. *CA* November 30, 1915, p. 2; *CT* November 18, 1915, p. 2. For similar views, see *Washington Herald* in *Current Opinion* 60 (January 1916): 43. *The Black Stork* appealed extensively to religious imagery, see note 22 above and chap. 8 below.

82. *CA* November 24, 1915, p. 2, November 29, 1915, and December 29, 1915. "Playing God" is discussed in chap. 5 below.

83. *DN* November 18, 1915, pp. 1, 25.

84. *God and Nature*, ed. David Lindberg and Ronald Numbers (Berkeley: University of California Press, 1986), chaps. 12–15; Frank M. Turner, *Between Science and Religion: The Reaction to Scientific Naturalism in Later Victorian England* (New Haven: Yale University Press, 1974); James Turner, *Without God, Without Creed.*

Renaming the bad as the good was a strategy denounced by the prophet Isaiah.

85. On Galton, see National Conference on Race Betterment, *Proceedings* 2 (1915): 64; McKim, *Heredity*, p. 213. Warthin in *Proceedings* 3 (1928): 86–90.

86. The phrase is David Hollinger's, "Justification by Verification." See also his "Inquiry and Uplift: Late Nineteenth Century American Academics and the Moral Efficacy of Scientific Practice," in *The Authority of Experts*, ed. Thomas Haskell (Bloomington: Indiana University Press, 1984), pp. 142–56. We have each benefitted from the opportunity to share ideas on these issues. While Hollinger's work focuses on science as a source of virtue for scientific practitioners, Haiselden's example illustrates how these concepts also functioned as a source of moral obligation for the masses.

See also Kenneth Ludmerer, "Eugenics: History," *Encyclopedia of Bioethics*, vol. I (New York: Free Press, 1978), pp. 457–62.

Chapter 5

1. Lasch, *Culture of Narcissism;* Foucault, *History of Sexuality;* Barbara Ehrenreich and Deirdre English, *For Her Own Good: 150 Years of the Experts' Advice to Women* (New York: Anchor/Doubleday, 1978); Rothman, *Woman's Proper Place;* Gordon, *Woman's Body;* Leavitt, *Brought to Bed.*

2. *Survey* December 4, 1915: p. 266.

3. *NYT* November 13, 1917, p.12.

4. Keller in *TNR* December 18, 1915, pp. 173–74. *CH* November 20, 1915, p. 2, and November 21, 1915, p. 3. *Call* November 29, 1915, p. 3. A Los Angeles proposal was reported as early as November 20, *CA* November 24, 1915, p. 3. For Haiselden's use of consultants to confirm his nontreatment decisions, see *CA* December 22, 1915, magazine page; *CE,* July 24, 1917; *NYT* November 16, 1917, p. 4; *MRR* 23 (October 1917): 697; *CA* November 16, 1917, p. 3.

For modern parallels, see Mary B. Mahowald, "Baby Doe Committees: A Critical Evaluation," *Clinics in Perinatology* 15 (December 1988): 789–800.

5. *NYT* November 18, 1915, p. 8; Mrs. George W. Crile to Executive Secretary McGuire, November 25, 1916, NBRMP Box 103; *MRR* 22 (February 1916): 96, 99, 100, 102.

6. *WP* November 18, 1917, p. 10; *DN* November 18, 1915, p. 2.

7. *Medical Freedom* 5 (December 1915): 56. He also attacked the female-run Children's Bureau without directly attributing its faults to gender, *BA* December 10, 1915, p. 16.

8. Wald: *Independent* January 3, 1916, p. 25; Keller: *TNR* December 18, 1915, pp. 173–74; Austin: *NYAm* November 23, 1915, p. 10; Davis: *NYT, WP,* and *Call* November 18, 1915; Block, *MRR* 22 (February 1916): 123. It may be significant that only Austin among these five had a child, and that daughter was in a home for the retarded.

One person whose gender could not be identified did not support parental involvement.

9. *TNR* December 18, 1915, pp. 173–74.

10. *CA* December 30, 1915, and December 27, 1915, magazine pages; *BA* December 19, 1915, p. 12. For his defense of publicity see chap. 6 below.

11. *NYAm* November 23, 1915, pp. 7, 10; *MRR* 22 (February 1916): 122–24; *WP* November 23, 1915, p. 4.

12. *Medical Freedom* 5 (December 1915): 55–56.

13. *Catholic World* December 1915, p. 423; *CH* November 18, 1915, p. 4. For similar attacks on playing God, see *Survey* December 4, 1915, p. 266; *NYS* November 19, 1915, p. 6; *New York Tribune* quoted in *Current Opinion* 60 (January 1916): 43.

14. *CH* December 23, 1915. The city's lawyer agreed, *CT* November 18, 1915, p. 2. See also *NYS* November 21, 1915, VII, p. 8.

15. *MRR* 22 (February 1916): 122–24.

16. *MRR* 22 (February 1916): p. 97; NBRMP Box 103, letter of Harris Rall, November 22, 1916. Such concerns played an important role in the decision to ban *The Black Stork;* see chap. 6 below.

17. *NYAm* November 19, 1915, p. 6.

18. This logic applies not only to eugenic selection, birth control, and abortion, but to the marketing of previously unavailable obstetric technologies in normal births as well; see Leavitt, *Brought to Bed.*

19. *NYS* November 18, 1915, p. 3

20. *Catholic World* 102 (December 1915): 421, 424.

21. *MRR* 22 (February 1916): 98.

22. Judy Barrett Litoff, *American Midwives 1860 to the Present* (Westport, Conn.: Greenwood, 1978); James C. Mohr, "Patterns of Abortion and the Response of American Physicians, 1790–1930," in *Women and Health in America,* ed. Judith Walzer Leavitt (Madison: University of Wisconsin Press, 1984), pp. 117–123; Cone, *History of American Pediatrics,* p. 184.

23. All quoted in *MRR* 22 (February 1916): 95–103.

24. *MRR* 22 (February 1916): 95–103; comments by Dorland, DeWitt, Litzenberg, Welz, Belknap, Paddock, and Macon.

25. To varying degrees this criticism applies to Kevles, *Name of Eugenics;* Ludmerer, *Genetics;* and Elazar Barkan, *Retreat of Scientific Racism* (Cambridge: Cambridge University Press, 1992).

Exceptions include Barker, "Biology of Stupidity," p. 368, and Jonathan Harwood, "Genetics, Eugenics, and Evolution, *British Journal of the History of Science* 22 (1989): 264–65; Proctor, *Racial Hygiene* and *Value-Free Science* (Cambridge: Harvard University Press, 1991).

26. For films, see chap. 7 below, and Pernick, "U.S. Government Sex Education Films." *Forum,* April 1915, pp. 533–34.

27. Cott, *Grounding of Modern Feminism,* esp. p. 30; Regina Morantz-Sanchez, *Sympathy and Science* (New York: Oxford University Press, 1985). For divisions among feminists over Haiselden see chap. 2 above.

28. *CT* November 18, 1915, p. 2.

29. LaReine Baker, "Eugenics and the Modern Feminist Movement," *Race Improvement or Eugenics* (New York: Dodd, Mead, 1912), pp. 86–87, 102–104.

30. *Call* November 27, 1915, p. 5.

31. *NYS* November 21, 1915.

32. *WP* November 23, 1915, p. 4; *NYT* November 20, 1915, p. 4.

33. Cone, *History of American Pediatrics,* pp. 184–90; William A. Silverman, "Incubator Baby Side Shows," *Pediatrics* 64 (1979): 127–41; *White City Magazine* 1 (March 1905): 20–23, cited in David Nasaw, *Going Out* (New York: Basic, 1993), p. 71; information on De Lee from work-in-progress by Jeffrey Baker; Meckel, *Save the Babies;* Gretchen A. Condran, Henry Williams, and Rose A. Cheney, "The Decline in Mortality in Philadelphia from 1870 to 1930: The Role of Municipal Services" in *Sickness and Health in America,* ed. Judith Walzer Leavitt and Ronald L. Numbers 2d ed. (Madison: University of Wisconsin Press, 1985), pp. 422–38; and Antler and Fox, "The Movement toward a Safe Maternity."

34. Gritzer and Arluke, *Making of Rehabilitation;* Vogel, *Invention of the Modern Hospital.*

35. *NYS* November 18, 1915, p. 3; W. H. Ballou in *NYAm* November 19, 1915. For similar expressions of faith in therapeutic progress, see *CT* November 17, 1915; *CN* November 17, 1915, p. 3.

36. *CT* November 17, 1915, p. 7; see also *CT* December 11, 1915, sect. 2, p. 1.

37. *CA* July 24, 1917, second ed., and November 24, 1915, pp. 1, 2; see also *CA* December 20, 1915, magazine page; *Independent* January 3, 1916, pp. 24, 27; *Cincinnati Enquirer* April 8, 1917, p. 31.

38. *CA* December 6, 1915, magazine page.

39. *Social Hygiene Bulletin*, November 1915, p. 3. The scene might have been meant as a comic sight-gag, but if so its effectiveness still depended on portraying Haiselden as unfamiliar with well-baby care skills.

40. James Harvey Young, "This Greasy Counterfeit: Butter versus Oleomargarine in the United States Congress, 1886," *Bulletin of the History of Medicine* 53 (1979): 392–414; Manfred Wasserman, "Henry L. Coit and the Certified Milk Movement in the Development of Modern Pediatrics," *Bulletin of the History of Medicine* 46 (1972): 359–90; Oscar Anderson, *The Health of a Nation: Harvey W. Wiley and the Fight for Pure Food* (Chicago: University of Chicago Press, 1958).

41. See chap. 2, note 24 above.

42. Similar fragmentation of both medicine and progressivism resulted from the effort to use motion pictures against venereal diseases during World War I. This story will be told in Pernick, *Bringing Medicine to the Masses*. See also Pernick, "Progressives, Propaganda, and Public Health."

On medical specialization in general, see Rosemary Stevens, *American Medicine and the Public Interest* (New Haven: Yale University Press, 1971). For particular specialties involved with defective infants, see Halpern, *American Pediatrics;* Benison, "Treatment of Crippled Children."

Critics noted the failure of science to speak with one voice on this issue, *New World* December 10, 1915, p. 2.

Chapter 6

1. *NYT* March 15, 1916, p. 5. See also *NYT* December 14, 1915, p. 4. In a November 18, 1915, editorial, the Socialist *Call* claimed the root of most criticism was in Haiselden's "widespread discussion of the case, not in the case itself," p. 6.

2. *CT* December 15, 1915. In response to my telephone inquiries, Bill Verick, Senior Director of the Chicago Medical Society, reported that the Society had no unpublished materials in their collections. When I visited the Society in October 1988, I found that they do have bound typescript minutes of their Council meetings from 1912 on. But the volume(s) covering 1914–22 were not on the shelf, though there appeared to be a small space on the shelf between 1913 and 1923. Mr. Verick suggested the volumes might have been lost, and several subsequent inquiries have turned up nothing. Other scholars who have worked with these documents many years ago do not recall a break in the run, but cannot be sure of their recollections.

3. *Lancet* 1 (1854): 86, cited in Daniel M. Fox and Christopher Law-

rence, *Photographing Medicine: Images and Power in Britain and America since 1840* (Westport, Conn.: Greenwood, 1988), p. 338; Pernick, *Calculus of Suffering,* pp. 63–75.

4. *NYS* November 18, 1915, p. 3.

5. Minutes of the Council for February 11, March 11, November 18, and December 9, 1913, and March 10, 1914, Chicago Medical Society Historical Library. For a slightly later case in which the Chicago Medical Society used the publicity issue to successfully fight both public health reformers and the business elite, see Conrad Siepp, "Organized Medicine and the Public Health Institute of Chicago," *Bulletin of the History of Medicine* 62 (Fall 1988): 429–49. Haiselden criticized the medical society for attacking him more harshly than these other violators of the self-promotion ban, *CA* December 29, 1915, magazine page.

6. *Independent* January 3, 1916, p. 26; Giddings in *NYT* November 18, 1915, p. 4, and letter to W. D. McGuire, November 20, 1916, NBRMP Box 103; *NYT* July 16, 1917, p. 10.

Although the *Times* shifted its position on nontreatment, from arguing that any policy other than an absolute commitment to life would lead to abuses, to declaring that the question was "insoluble," to endorsing nontreatment at the doctor's discretion, from first to last, the editors insisted that in practice the "wise" physician should make such decisions silently. A November 29, 1915, editorial noted with approval a medical article that the *Times* (inaccurately) summarized as saying that Haiselden "should have used his own judgment and said nothing." *NYT* November 18, 1915, p. 8; November 22, 1915, p. 14; November 29, 1915, pt. II, p. 10.

7. *CA* December 30, 1915, editorial page. See also letter *CT* December 26, 1915, p. 6; *Baltimore Star* and *Chicago Post* in *CA* December 24, 1915, editorial page; *CN* in *CA* December 18, 1915, editorial page; *Survey* December 4, 1915, p. 265; *TNR* November 27, 1915, p. 86.

8. *CA* December 23, 1915, p. 5; Lillian Wald, *NYAm* November 18, 1915.

9. Well over 1000 health-related films were made between 1905 and 1927, including many on such morally controversial topics as birth control, abortion, sexual hygiene, childbirth, euthanasia, and eugenics. Pernick, *Bringing Medicine to the Masses.*

Historians are just beginning to realize the significance of mass-media health publicity in this era. For one important interpretation, see John C. Burnham, *How Superstition Won and Science Lost: Popularizing Science and Health in the United States* (New Brunswick, N.J.: Rutgers University Press, 1987). Other significant new studies of aspects of this issue include: Brownlow, *Behind the Mask of Innocence;* Teller, *The Tuberculosis Movement;* Krin Gabbard and Glen O. Gabbard, *Psychiatry and the Cinema* (Chicago: University of Chicago Press, 1987); Terra Ziporyn, *Disease in the Popular American Press* (Westport, Conn.: Greenwood, 1988); Roland Marchand, *Advertising the American Dream: Making Way for Modernity 1920–1940* (Berkeley: University of California Press, 1985); JoAnne Brown, "Policing the Body: Criminological Metaphor in the Popularization of Germ Theories in the United States, 1870–1950," unpublished paper, American Association for the History of Medicine, Philadelphia, May 3, 1987; Patterson, *The Dread Disease;* Fox and Lawrence, *Photographing Medicine;* and Joseph Turow,

Playing Doctor: Television, Storytelling, and Medical Power (New York: Oxford University Press, 1989).

See also Bruce Gebhard, "A Century of Visual Health Education in the United States, 1860–1960: From Sanitary Fairs to Health Museums," *Current Problems in the History of Medicine: XIXth International Congress of the History of Medicine* (Basel: Karger, 1966), pp. 652–59; George Rosen, "Evolving Trends in Health Education," *Canadian Journal of Public Health* 52 (1961): 499–506; Barbara Gutmann Rosenkrantz, "Damaged Goods: Dilemmas of Responsibility for Risk," *Milbank Memorial Fund Quarterly* 57 (1979): 1–37; and Don S. Kirschner, "Publicity Properly Applied: The Selling of Expertise in America," *American Studies* 19 (Spring 1978): 65–78.

Sexual hygiene films have been a particular focus of recent scholarship. Eric Schaefer, "Of Hygiene and Hollywood: Origins of the Exploitation Film," *Velvet Light Trap* 30 (Fall 1992): 37; Stacie Colwell, "*The End of the Road:* Gender, the Dissemination of Knowledge, and the American Campaign Against Venereal Disease during World War I," *Camera Obscura* 29 (May 1992): 91–129; Kuhn, *Cinema, Censorship* and *Power of the Image;* Sloan, *Loud Silents;* Brandt, *No Magic Bullet,* Pernick, "Progressives, Propaganda, and Public Health" and "Sex Education Films"; and Brownlow, *Mask of Innocence.*

10. Karl Spencer Lashley and John B. Watson, *A Psychological Study of Motion Pictures in Relation to Venereal Disease Campaigns* (Washington, D.C.: United States Interdepartmental Social Hygiene Board, 1922); Lashley and Watson, "A Psychological Study of Motion Pictures in Relation to Venereal Disease Campaigns," *Social Hygiene* 7 (1921): 181–219; Watson and Lashley, "A Consensus of Medical Opinion Upon Questions Relating to Sex Education and Venereal Disease Campaigns," *Mental Hygiene* 4 (October 1920): 769–847.

11. Barbara Stafford, *Body Criticism: Imaging the Unseen in Enlightenment Art and Medicine* (Cambridge: M.I.T. Press, 1991); Lorraine Daston, "Baconian Facts, Academic Civility, and the Prehistory of Objectivity," *Annals of Scholarship* 8 (1991): 337–64.

12. "Black Stork Stay Off" from *ExTrR* March 10, 1917, p. 935; "Black Stork Babies Not Treated" from *Motography* April 14, 1917, advertising sect., p. 2. However, *Variety* insisted that the film maintained "careful fidelity so as to leave no loophole for criticism on the charge of resorting to sensationalism at the expense of scientific facts. . . ," March 2, 1917, p. 29.

Following the Bollinger case, the Chicago Medical Society attempted unsuccessfully to distinguish "scientific" from "sensational" uses of medical publicity, *Illinois Medical Journal* 31 (January 1917): 75.

13. Flying stork, *CH* April 1, 1917, p. 7; "World Famous Surgeon," *CT* April 2, 1917, p. 19. For similar shock tactics in modern films on the opposite side of the "right to life" debate, see the 1984 production *Silent Scream* (Anaheim, Calif.: American Portrait Films, 1984), University of Minnesota Medical Library; Jefferson Morley, "Right-to-Life Porn," *TNR* March 25, 1985, pp. 8–10; Rosalind Petchesky, "Fetal Images: The Power of Visual Culture in the Politics of Reproduction," *Feminist Studies* 13 (1987): 263–92.

14. Silverman "Incubator Side Shows." Films of Couney's exhibits at the 1915 Panama-Pacific Exposition and the 1939–40 New York World's

Fair collected by Dr. Silverman are available at the National Library of Medicine, Smithsonian Institution, and University of Michigan Historical Health Film Collection.

15. Martin S. Pernick, "The Ethics of Preventive Medicine: Thomas Edison's Tuberculosis Films: Mass Media and Health Propaganda," *Hastings Center Report* 8 (June 1978): 21–27; Tom Gunning, "An Aesthetic of Astonishment," *Art and Text* 34 (1989): 31–45. My initial ideas on this subject were further developed in conversation with Tom Gunning.

16. *Variety* March 2, 1917, p. 29; *Cleveland Plain Dealer* April 2, 1917, p. 4; *Chicago Post* in *Motography* March 3, 1917, p. 1462. The *Cincinnati Enquirer* in a brief note called the film "wonderful," April 1, 1917, sect. 3, p. 1.

17. *ExTrR* February 24, 1917, p. 836; *Motography* February 24, 1917, p. 424. For similar mixed reviews, see *NYDM* February 17, 1917, p. 32; *MPN* February 24, 1917, p. 1256.

18. *Wid's* April 5, 1917, pp. 220–21.

19. Parsons in *CH* April 2, 1917, p. 11; Kelly in *CE*, April 4, 1917, p. 8; *CT* April 2, 1917, p. 18; *Photoplay* 12 (June 1917): 155. Most reviewers also found Dr. Haiselden a stiff and amateurish actor, e.g., *CN* April 6, 1917, p.21; but there were a few dissenters who praised his performance, *Chicago Post*, in *ExTrR* March 3, 1917, p. 911.

20. *Current Opinion* 60 (January 1916): 43; *NYAm* November 21, 1915, p. 13.

21. *MPW* October 13, 1917, p. 250.

22. *Wid's* June 14, 1917, p. 371.

23. *CN* April 6, 1917, p. 21.

24. For the role of venereal disease and sex education films in the growth of film censorship, see Edward de Grazia and Roger K. Newman, *Banned Films: Movies, Censors and the First Amendment* (New York: Bowker, 1982); and Kuhn, *Cinema, Censorship and Sexuality.* For censorship history of *The Black Stork*, see NBRMP Box 103; NYSA-MPD Box 2565, Folders 383 and 12,421. Quotations are from letter of disapproval, Commissioner to H. J. Brooks, April 4, 1923, NYSA-MPD, Box 2565, Folder 383.

25. The board got 53 responses but one took no position on the film. Of 24 others who took a published stand on the film, 5 advocated banning it.

26. Quotes are from Andrew Edson of New York City's Education Department, in NBRMP Box 103, November 17, 1916. Among the many others using virtually the same language, see especially U. G. Manning, November 18; Jonathan Dean, November 18; Ernest Batchelder, November 22; Maude Levy, November 20; W. L. Percy, November 21; and Robbins Gilman, November 23.

Variety March 2, 1917, p. 29; *Medical Freedom* 4 (September 1914): 11, and 6 (September 1916): 5. Similar views were the subject of several cartoons by Ellison Hoover in *Life Magazine.*

27. NBRMP Box 103. Elkus, November 22, and Peck, November 26, 1916.

28. Gunning, "Aesthetic of Astonishment"; *Little Cripple:* LC-MBRS #FEA 7533; *Variety* February 29, 1908, p. 12; *MPW* February 22, 1908, pp. 145–46. For an unrelated 1911 film also called *the Little Cripple*, see *American Journal of Public Health*, March 1912, p. 213, and September 1916, p.

1019; *MPW* August 11, 1911, p. 475, and September 9, 1911, p. 716. For regulators' growing unease, see comments on *The Paralytic*, John Collier to Executive Secretary, December 20, 1912, NBRMP Box 105.

29. NBRMP Box 103, Jonathan Dean, November 18, 1916. In 1927 the Chicago film censors limited Haiselden's film to adults only, "because it deals with the evils of heredity." Chicago Film Censorship Board, review cards, November 17, 1927.

30. Pennsylvania State Board of Censors, *Rules and Standards* (Harrisburg: J. L. L. Kuhn, 1918), pp. 15–17; Jowett, *Film: The Democratic Art*, chaps. 5, 7, 10. Code of 1930 reprinted pp. 468–72. On pre-code films and the rise of censorship, see also Francis Couvares, "Hollywood, Main Street, and the Church: Trying to Censor the Movies Before the Production Code," *American Quarterly* 44 (December 1992): 584–615; Stephen Vaughn, "Morality and Entertainment: The Origins of the Motion Picture Production Code," *Journal of American History* 77 (June 1990): 39–65; De Grazia and Newman, *Banned Films*.

31. "Memo on Behalf of the Motion Picture Division to the Commissioner of Education," p. 4; and "Court of Appeals Brief for the Respondent," p. 6, both in NYSA-MPD Box 333, Folder 28,361. The censors initially also ruled the film "immoral" for showing audiences "methods that . . . prevent conception" but this argument was soon dropped; see letter of Irving Esmond, August 24, 1934, in Box 296, Folder 27,387.

32. *MPW* February 24, 1917, p. 1211; *CN* April 6, 1917, p. 21. See also *NYDM* February 17, 1917, p. 32; NBRMP Box 103, Robert W. de Forest, November 17, 1916.

33. For a typical use of the "non-theatrical" label, and for educational filmmaker John Bray's unease with these hardening categories, see *NYT* November 13, 1921, sect. VI, p. 5.

34. *Deliverance: Variety* August 22, 1919, p. 76; *NYT* August 24, 1919, sect. IV, p. 4. The film was distributed by George Kleine. A partial print is at LC-MBRS #FLA 1996–1997. The rehabilitation films, mostly one or two reelers, produced by the Red Cross, Army Medical Museum, and Ford Educational Weekly included: *Broken Silence; Broken Lives; Heroes All; Little Comrades; Not Charity But a Chance; Paralytic Girl at a Typewriter; Prevention and Treatment of Disability of Legs and Feet; The Reawakening; Reeducation of the Blind; US Army General Hospital #36 Detroit;* and *Vocational Training for Blind Soldiers*.

35. *NYT* July 9, 1932, p. 7; Bogdan, *Freak Show;* Fiedler, *Freaks*.

36. See for example, "Health Propaganda," *Philadelphia Public Ledger* July 8, 1919, p. 11; H. E. Kleinschmidt, "Educational Prophylaxis of Venereal Diseases:" *Social Hygiene* 5 (1919): 27. As late as 1920 a British observer sarcastically defined "propaganda" as meaning movies about venereal disease; see Sir Sidney James Mark Low, "Propaganda Films and Mixed Morals," *Fortnightly Review* 113 (May 1920): 717–28. For the growing negative connotations of the word, see Agnes Repplier, "A Good Word Gone Wrong," *Independent* October 1, 1921, p. 5; Lee William Huebner, "The Discovery of Propaganda: Changing Attitudes Towards Public Communication in America, 1900–1930," unpublished Ph.D. diss., Harvard University, 1968.

37. Memo to Mr. Barrett, and W. A. B[arrett] to Gilman, November 28, 1916; all in NBRMP Box 103.

38. *CE* April 4, 1917, p. 8, and April 17, 1917, p. 7. The manager of the company distributing the film unconvincingly responded to such criticisms: "It is but incidental to the picture that a great moral lesson is taught, but fundamentally the picture has . . . great appeal from a dramatic standpoint. . . ." "[I]f, in addition, a moral lesson was to be taught, that was secondary to the business of the corporation, which is the releasing of pictures which shall produce entertainment for the multitude." *Motography* April 28, 1917, p. 880.

39. Letter of R. H. Edwards, November 21, 1916. Robbins Gilman to Executive Secretary, November 23, 1916; Memo to Mr. Barrett, and W. A. B[arrett] to Gilman, November 28, 1916; all in NBRMP Box 103. See also letter of Festus Foster, November 20, 1916.

40. Pennsylvania State Board of Censors, *Rules and Standards,* p. 16; McGuire to National Advisory Committee, December 15, 1916; and R. Andrew Hamilton letter of November 16, 1916, both in NBRMP Box 103.

41. *NYAm* November 30, 1915; the courts reversed the license commissioner, and the play was shown. This play appears to be quite different from the later anti-abortion movie of the same name. For the play, see *CT* November 21, 1915, sect. 8, p. 1; *NYAm* November 25, 1915, p. 15, and November 30, 1915; *CH* November 30, 1915, p. 9. For the film, see AFI *Catalog 1911–1920,* p. 963.

42. Letters of Franklin H. Giddings, November 20, 1916; R. A[ndrew] Hamilton, November 16, 1916; Rev. John P. Peters, November 18, 1916; and comments of Edwin H. Jenks, in T. F. Sturgess to W. D. McGuire, December 4, 1916. See also letters of Franklin H. Sargent, November 16, 1916; Robert W. de Forest, November 17, 1916; Harris Franklin Rall, November 22, 1916. All in NBRMP Box 103.

43. *NYAm* December 3, 1915, p. 5. Similar arguments are still made today, Robert Burt, "Authorizing Death for Anomalous Newborns," in *Genetics and the Law,* ed. Aubrey Milunsky and George Annas (New York: Plenum, 1976).

44. NBRMP *Special Bulletin,* March 3, 1917, and memo McGuire to National Advisory Committee, December 15, 1916; both in NBRMP Box 103. NYSA-MPD Box 2565, Folder 12,421.

MPW February 24, 1917, p. 1211. For similar movie industry sensitivity to medical professional concerns raised by this film, see *Variety* March 2, 1917, p. 24; *CT* April 2, 1917, p. 18.

45. *BA* December 14, 1915, p. 12; *CA* December 21, 1915, magazine page.

46. In the 1915 Roberts case, in which Haiselden was only indirectly involved, the father and grandmother made all the parental decisions about nontreatment and publicity. While the mother's name was on the front pages of newspapers nationwide, she was kept completely ignorant of the baby's fate because of concern that such knowledge would worsen her own medical condition. See *WP* November 26, 1915, p. 2. For Haiselden's similar actions in the Meter case, see *CE* July 24, 1917, p. 1. For the claim Mrs. Bollinger was not able to give truly voluntary consent, see *Independent* Jan-

uary 3, 1916, p. 27, although the quoted passage does not criticize the use of her name.

47. For example, *NYT* November 24, 1915.

Chapter 7

1. On the conflict in general, see Kathy Peiss, *Cheap Amusements: Working Women and Leisure in Turn-of-the-Century New York* (Philadelphia: Temple University Press, 1986), pp. 144–62; and Roy Rosenzweig, *Eight Hours for What We Will: Workers and Leisure in an Industrial City 1870–1920* (Cambridge: Cambridge University Press, 1983), Chap. 8. For another example of cinematic lampooning of reformers, see Will Rogers's 1920 Goldwyn feature, *Water, Water Everywhere*, Craig W. Campbell, *Reel America and World War I: A Comprehensive Filmography and History of Motion Pictures in the United States, 1914–1920* (Jefferson, N.C.: McFarland, 1985), p. 127.

2. Only a few of the films mentioned in this chapter are known to still exist; those copies will be cited in the notes. *Strenuous Life:* Museum of Modern Art (MOMA), New York; see also American Federation of Arts, *Before Hollywood: Turn-of-the-Century Film from American Archives* (New York: American Federation of Arts, 1986), p. 118. *Case of Eugenics:* LC-MBRS #FEA 3355. *Eugenic Boy:* MPW March 21, 1914, p. 1584. *Bar "U":* LC-MBRS copyright records #LP-2754; *MPW* June 6, 1914, p. 1438. *Wedd:* Edison *Kinetogram* #7763; MOMA Edison Script Collection #1994, scene script and title script. *Snakeville:* MPW November 20, 1915, pp. 1538, 1543; and November 27, 1915, p, 1663. *Versus Love:* LC-MBRS paperprint and copyright records #LU-2732, and *MPW* May 2, 1914, p. 724. *Very Idea:* AFI *Catalog 1911–1920*, p. 986, AFI *Catalog 1921–1930*, pp. 857–58; *Foe to Race Suicide: Motography* September 28, 1912, ad p. 2. *Mutual Child:* AFI *Catalog 1911–1920*, based on a novel by P. G. Wodehouse. For Fitzgerald song, see Kevles, *Name of Eugenics*, p. 58. A related satire is *The Scientific Mother* (Mutual-Falstaff, 1915), see *MPW* May 8 and May 15, 1915, in Foster scrapbooks, LC-MBRS.

3. *Girl:* LC-MBRS copyright file #LP-3303, and *MPW* September 12, 1914, p. 1547. *Born or Made: MPW* January 2, 1917, in Foster scrapbooks, LC-MBRS. *Daughter's Strange Inheritance:* LC-MBRS copyright files #LP-4467, and *MPN* February 27, 1915, in Foster scrapbooks, LC-MBRS. *Victim: MPW* May 24, 1913, p. 832. *Power of Mind: MPW* August 19, 1916, in Foster scrapbooks, LC-MBRS. *Disciple: Motography* October 9, 1915, pp. 749–50. *MPW* September 25, 1915, pp. 2246–47, and October 2, 1915, pp. 80, 94; *Reel Life* September 18, 1915, quoted in David Bowers, *Thanhouser Films: An Encyclopedia and History* (manuscript of work in progress, 1988). I am grateful to Mr. Bowers for sharing this work with me.

The Battle of Life (Fox, 1916) concerned the efforts of a criminal girl to go straight, and it featured a character called "the defective," but I've not been able to determine what role heredity played in the plot; see *Wid's Film Daily* December 14, 1916, pp. 1170–71.

See also the strongly Lamarckian comments of film critic Louis Reeves Harrison in *MPW* May 29, 1915, p. 1440.

4. Michael Guyer, *Being Well-Born*, p. 426. See also Fisher and Fisk, *How to Live*, p. 294. *Good Health* 50 (1915): 487. See also "Scheme to Establish Courtship on Genetic Foundations," *Current Opinion* 61 (September 1916): 180; "Eugenics as Romance," *NYT* September 25, 1921, sect. II, p. 2; Warthin, *Creed of a Biologist*, pp. 42–43. On eugenics, emotion, sex, and objectivity, see chaps. 3 and 4 above, especially the section "Defects and Desires."

5. *Motography* December 4, 1915, p. 1179, and January 1, 1916, advertising page 23.

6. *MPW* July 1, 1916, pp. 111, 135, and July 22, 1916, p. 654; LC-MBRS copyright file #LP-8551, July 1, 1916. The film was directed by Charles Brabin (who later directed and married "vamp" star Theda Bara) from a screen play by Mary Imlay Taylor; *Variety* November 13, 1957, p. 79.

7. *Buck v. Bell*

8. The copy at the University of Michigan Historical Health Film Collection, obtained from Video Yesteryears/Filmic Archives, Botsford, Connecticut includes a trailer explicitly equating American and Nazi eugenics. However, the original script did not mention Germany, and the date of the trailer is unknown. The script and much additional material is in NYSA-MPD Box 296, Folder 27,387. See also *Motion Picture Herald* May 19, 1934, pp. 68–69.

For the censorship battle, see *Foy Productions v. Frank P. Graves*, 299 N.Y.S. 671 (1937); 3 N.Y.S. 2d 573 (1938); 15 N.E. 2d 435 (1938); *NYT* May 18, 1938, p. 16; De Grazia and Newman, *Banned Films*, pp. 215–17.

9. *Heredity* (1912): *MPW* November 2, 1912, p. 480, and January 1, 1916, p. 128. *Heredity* (1915): *MPW* November 6, 1915, p. 1187, November 13, 1915, p. 1269, and November 27, 1915, p. 1664. *Inherited Sin: MPW* May 1, 1915, pp. 729, 798. *Power of Heredity: MPW* July 26, 1913, p. 460. *Second Generation: MPW* February 28, 1914, p. 1150.

10. May, *Screening Out the Past*, p. 87; *AFI Catalog 1911–1920*, p. 244; *Variety* June 5, 1914, p. 19; *NYT* June 2, 1914, p. 11; William K. Everson, *American Silent Film* (New York: Oxford University Press, 1978), p. 76; Robert Connelly, *The Motion Picture Guide: Silent Film* (Chicago: Cinebooks, 1986), p. 74.

11. *MPW* June 13, 1914, p. 1515; *NYDM* June 10, 1914, p. 42.

12. Quotes from *Wid's* June 14, 1917, pp. 369–71. For promotion, see *MPN* June–August 1917, *passim*.

13. A scene script of *Birth* is in LC-MBRS copyright records #MU-835; *Wid's Film Daily* April 19, 1917, pp. 244–45. See also *MPW* April 28, 1917, p. 609; *MPN* April 28, 1917, p. 2687; *NYAm* April 8, 1917, p. 7M, and April 15, 1917, p. 4M.

14. *MPW* September 6, 1914, p. 1288; Brownlow, *Behind the Mask*, p. 271.

15. *Enlighten:* see chap. 8 below. *Sex Lure:* De Grazia and Newman, *Banned Films*, pp. 191–92.

16. *MPW* October 13, 1917, pp. 182, 250, 293; *Variety* April 26, 1918, p. 44.

17. Robert W. Rydell, "Eugenics Hits the Road: The Popularization of Eugenics at American Fairs and Museums Between the World Wars," unpublished paper, History of Science Society, Chicago, December 1984. For the filmstrip, see John Harvey Kellogg Papers, Box 9, undated memo headed "Dr. Price," Michigan Historical Collections, Bentley Library, University of Michigan. (Note: Kellogg box numbers are as of Fall 1989, but the collection is being reorganized.)

18. National Conference on Race Betterment, *Proceedings* 1 (1914): xv, 598, 603; 2 (1915): 83.

19. Third Race Betterment Conference, *Proceedings* (1928): xxiv, 220, 738.

20. The following journals were searched: *Bulletin of the Eugenics Record Office* 1915–33; *Eugenical News* 1916–33; and *Journal of Heredity* 1915–30. *Journal of Heredity* 8 (February 1917): 95.

None of the Battle Creek films have yet been located. The titles included other Kellogg interests such as *Outdoor Gymnasium, Effect of Alcohol, Tobacco Habit, Tobacco Plague,* a film linking health education with Americanization called *Torchbearer,* and one called *Itinerary of a Breakfast.* National Health Council, *Film List,* 5th ed. (New York: Metropolitan Life Insurance Company, 1928).

21. Originally called simply the *Men's Lecture Film* (1917), it was expanded and rereleased as *Venereal Diseases: Their Origin and Results* (1919). It survives as NA 111.M.163, and with additional footage from the LC can be seen at the UM-HHFC. See Adolf Nichtenhauser Papers, NLM-HMD, esp. Nichtenhauser, "A History of Motion Pictures in Medicine," II:100 ff., unpublished typescript.

22. See chap. 6, note 9 above. A jumbled but fairly complete print of *The End of the Road* is at the NA, #200.200. A much shorter version with full continuity is at the Museum of Modern Art in New York. Copies of each are at UM-HHFC. The surviving portions of 3 reels of *Fit to Win,* the postwar civilian version of *Fit to Fight,* are also at UM-HHFC.

23. Nichtenhauser, "History of Motion Pictures," vol. I, pp. 208–209; *Social Hygiene Bulletin* October 1919, p. 2.

24. Among the sponsored ones: *Damaged Goods* (1917 version); *Know Thy Husband,* or *Some Wild Oats* (Samuel Cummins Public Health Films, 1919); *The Spreading Evil* (J. Keane, 1918); and *Open Your Eyes* (Warner, 1919). Others included: *S.O.S.* (American Standard, 1917); *Enlighten Thy Daughter* (Ivan, 1917); *The Scarlet Trail* (G&L, 1918); and *The Solitary Sin* (Solitary Sin, 1919).

25. *Science of Life* NA reels #90.14–90.26, and UM-HHFC; *Gift of Life* LC #FRA-3072–73 and UM-HHFC; a more complete copy may be at British National Film Institute; *Social Hygiene for Women* LC-MBRS and UM-HHFC; a more complete copy may be at National Film Archive of Canada #N2331–32. Other titles included: *Gonorrhea in the Male* (1920); *Modern Diagnosis and Treatment of Syphilis* (1920); *A Model Clinic Plan* (1920); *American Plan for Combatting VD* (1921); *Locating the Missing Girl* (c. 1922); *Protective Social Measures* (1922).

26. The clinical footage for *T.N.T,* along with much other recycled Cummins footage, is now at the LC-MBRS and UM-HHFC. I am very grate-

ful to Justice Brennan for sharing his reminiscences of the effect of this case on his thinking during several conversations with me in the fall of 1985.

27. *S.O.S: MPN* May 19, 1917, p. 3133; AFI *Catalog 1911–1920*, p. 794. *Damaged Goods:* "Eugenics Play Endorsed," *NYT* February 27, 1913, p. 8; Schaefer, "Of Hygiene and Hollywood," p. 37.

28. The two reels originally planned to be titled "Heredity and Eugenics" were released as three reels on "Personal Hygiene," linking eugenics, sexual diseases, and physical fitness, NA-MPD #s 90.24, 90.25, and 90.26. For title change, see George R. Callender to Surgeon General U.S. Army, June 21, 1921, and J. R. Bray to James F. Coupal, July 11, 1922, Adolf Nichtenhauser Papers, Box 21, NLM-HMD; see also Nichtenhauser, "A History of Motion Pictures in Medicine," II:100 ff., unpublished typescript, also NLM-HMD; Pernick, "U.S. Government Sex Education Films"; and chap. 3, note 66 above.

29. *Eugenics Review* 16 (October 1924): 252; and 17 (January 1926): 334. On *From Generation to Generation*, see Timothy Boon, "Lighting the Understanding and Kindling the Heart: Social Hygiene and Propaganda Film in the 1930s," *Social History of Medicine* 3 (1990): 140–41. Successive editions and documentation are at the Wellcome Institute Contemporary Medical Archives Center, London.

30. Proctor, *Racial Hygiene*, p. 101; Kühl, *Nazi Connection*, pp. 48–50.

31. *Motherhood:* a lengthy but damaged and incomplete script is in LC-MBRS copyright files #LU-10661.

Better Babies: Bulletin of the National Tuberculosis Association February 1921, p. 4; *Educational Film Magazine* 6 (December 1921): 11. For what may have been an earlier film by the same title, perhaps in the Universal Screen Magazine series, see *Good Health* 52 (January 1917): 78; *MPW* December 1, 1917, p. 1320.

32. *Evolution of Man: NYT* December 12, 1922, p. 8; *Evolution:* AFI *Catalog 1921–1930*, p. 220; *NYT* August 2, 1925, sect. VII, p. 4. These may have been the same film, but should not be confused with a 1920 *Evolution of Man*, a mystery about an ape-man; see AFI *Catalog 1911–1920*, p. 252.

33. *Educational Film Magazine*, December 1920, opp. p. 1, and May 1921, p. 13.

34. A scene summary is in LC-MBRS copyright file #LP7516; see also extensive file in Foster scrapbooks. Only one reel of warped, nonstandard gauge film remains of this movie, at George Eastman House in Rochester, N.Y. It is unrelated to the surviving 1937 feature by the same title.

35. Many film historians misunderstand the context in which Weber was using opposition to abortion as an argument for birth control. Their accounts reflect an assumption common both today and among pronatalist film reviewers of the time, that support for birth control necessarily included support for abortion. From that vantage point, Weber's distinction (which mirrored Margaret Sanger's) seemed ambivalent, noncommittal, or confused. See for example Kuhn, *Cinema, Censorship*, pp. 29–47. For a film historian who understands this context, see Brownlow, *Behind the Mask*, pp. 50–56. Most of *Where Are My Children?* is available at the LC-MBRS and UM-HHFC.

36. Not much is known about this film, available at LC-MBRS and UM-

HHFC. Also from 1917 was *The Curse of Eve* (Corona), a pro-abortion film. But whether it dealt with eugenics has not been determined, *Wid's Film Daily*, October 18, 1917, pp. 666–67.

37. Brownlow, *Behind the Mask*, pp. 47–50; *MPN* April 21, 1917, p. 2506.

38. Victor Robinson, *Pioneers of Birth Control* (New York: Voluntary Parenthood League, 1919), p. 78.

39. *MPN* December 23, 1911, p. 9; *Educational Film Magazine* February–March 1922, pp. 18–19.

40. Osler, "The Fixed Period." *Papa:* G. W. Bitzer, *Billy Bitzer: His Story* (New York: Farrar, Straus and Giroux, 1973), p. 249. *Neighbor:* LC-MBRS copyright files #LP8040; AFI *Catalog 1911–1920*, part 1, p. 220, misreads the subtitle.

41. *MPN* April 22, 1916, p. 2385.

42. AFI *Catalog 1911–1920*, pp. 365–66, 1013; *MPW* January 10, 1920, p. 195.

43. Haiselden appeared in *Universal Animated Weekly #194* for 1915, released November 24, 1915, and *#99* for 1917, released November 21, 1917; as well as *Pathé News #94* for 1915, released November 24, 1915. See LC-MBRS "Community Motion Picture Bureau—Foster Scrapbook" microfilm; *Motography* December 11, 1915, p. 1250; *MPW* December 4, 1915, p. 1906, and December 8, 1917; quotes are from the latter.

Chapter 8

1. The 1927 version has been restored and is available for on-site research viewing only, at the UM-HHFC. The 1916 version exists only in unprojectable paperprint format though efforts to reanimate it are underway, LC-MBRS, #LU-9978, Box 109.

2. For a typical photographic contrast between "uncared-for human beings and cared-for cattle" in the public health propaganda of the era, see *Journal of the Outdoor Life* 9 (1912): 194. See also the prologue to D. W. Griffith's *The Escape*. Use of such contrasts was already centuries old; see Burton, *Anatomy of Melancholy*.

3. Haiselden himself claimed to have treated defectives who lived to curse him for saving them. *CA* December 2, 1915, p. 2, and December 3, 1915, p. 6.

4. The idea for the death scene may have originated with a clergyman who wrote that when Jesus said "Suffer the children to come unto Me," he was calling the Bollinger baby to him. *Independent* January 3, 1916, p. 25.

5. *CT* April 2, 1917, p. 18; *NYDM* February 17, 1917, p. 32; *Wid's Film Daily* April 5, 1917, p. 220; *MPN* February 24, 1917, p. 1256.

6. *CA* December 7, 1915, magazine page.

7. Thanks to Peter Laipson for recognizing the multiple readings for this scene.

8. Schaefer, "Hygiene and Hollywood."

9. Shaw, "Preface," *Three Plays by Brieux*, pp. xlvii, xxxii.

10. Marjorie Rosen, *Popcorn Venus* (New York: Coward, McCann & Geoghegan, 1973); Molly Haskell, *From Reverence to Rape* (New York: Holt, Rinehart and Winston, 1974).

11. *CE* April 4, 1917, p. 8.

12. Edward Rothstein, "Don't Shoot the Piano," *TNR* May 1, 1989, pp. 32–35, citing Arthur Loesser, *Men, Women and Pianos: A Social History* (New York: Simon & Schuster, 1954), and Craig H. Roell, *The Piano in America 1890–1940* (Chapel Hill: University of North Carolina Press, 1989).

13. The fireplace as a place for visions conjured by dancing flames and intoxicating smoke was a stock theatrical device since Shakespeare, and had been the justification for early cinematic "special effects" since Edwin Porter's *Fireside Reminiscences* (Edison 1907). Thanks to Tom Gunning for showing me the Edison film.

On hearths and domesticity, see Margaret Hindle Hazen and Robert M. Hazen, *Keepers of the Flame: The Role of Fire in American Culture 1775–1925* (Princeton, N.J.: Princeton University Press, 1993).

14. This absence and several possible interpretations were first pointed out in Hanley Kanar, "Juxtaposed Images and Stereotypes of Disability and Difference in Selected Twentieth-Century Literature," unpublished senior honors thesis in American Culture, University of Michigan, 1989.

15. For film locations, see chap. 7, note 22 above.

16. I am grateful to Roger White of the Smithsonian Institution for identifying the car. See *The New Encyclopedia of Motorcars*, ed. G. N. Georgano (New York: Dutton, 1982).

17. Unlike the 1927 version, the 1916 copy retains the credit titles. They identify Bergman's character as "The Monster," though published reviews call him "The Defective" or "The Cripple," e.g., *ExTrR* February 24, 1917, p. 836.

18. There were several actors of the era with the names Henry or Henri Bergman. This one was a veteran Broadway actor, who died at age 58 in January 1917, shortly after completing *The Black Stork*. See *Ithaca Daily Journal* January 11, 1917; *Wid's Film Daily* April 5, 1917, p. 220; *Variety* January 19, 1917, p. 13. For Davenport, see *Variety* August 2, 1918, p. 15; for Revelle, *Who Was Who in the Theater, 1912–1976*, vol. 4 (Detroit: Gale Research, 1978), pp. 2016–17. For the others, Connelly, *Motion Picture Guide*; AFI *Catalog, 1911–1920* and AFI *Catalog, 1921–1930*.

19. On John T. Miltern, see *MPN* March 3, 1917, p. 1349. On John Miltern, see *NYT* December 28, 1918, sect. IV, p. 2; *Variety* January 20, 1937, p. 62; and AFI *Catalog, 1911–1920*, p. 76, plus *Index* volume for other credits. John Miltern remained active in films until his death in 1937.

Elsie Esmond's husband, Thurlow Bergen, may also have been in the film; his name appears on a group photograph of cast members in the Cody Collection, DeWitt Historical Society of Tompkins County, Ithaca, N.Y.

20. *Illinois Medical Journal* 29 (April 1916): 316. Charles Chaplin and one or two other film stars could earn $10,000 a week at this time. *The American Film Industry*, rev. ed., ed. Tino Balio (Madison: University of Wisconsin Press, 1985), p. 116.

21. *Motography* February 17, 1917, advertising p. 2; *MPN* February 10, 1917, pp. 854–55, and February 17, 1917, p. 997. *CH* April 1, 1917, p. 7; *CT*

April 2, 1917, p. 19: See also Figs. 5–8. The cast did get name billing in the movie trade magazines.

22. *CH* November 17, 1915, p. 4, and November 19, 1915, p. 5. Late editions of the November 19 *CH* carried a different version titled "Hundreds of Cases Like 'Hopeless' Baby in State Hospital," on p. 3. The *Herald* and the *American* were separate Hearst papers at this time. On Lait, see *Dictionary of American Biography* (New York: Scribner's, 1959–), supp. 5, p. 406. Lait's papers are in the Special Collections, University of Oregon at Eugene. They include the undated, unfinished draft of "The Birthright," a stage play about congenital syphilis written with J. C. Nugent, but contain nothing related to *The Black Stork*. I am grateful to Hilary Cummings for searching this collection.

23. *CH* December 14, 1915, p. 18.

24. NBRMP, Box 163, "Rejections and Cut Outs, December 6, 1916. Many of the title frames in the early reels of the 1916 paperprint still have the Rothacker logo.

25. *Ithaca Journal* June 10, 1916, p. 7; September 25, 1916; and June 19, 1919, p. 3. *MPW* July 15, 1916, p. 481; *CE* April 6, 1917, p. 11.

26. *IDJ* July 8, 1916, n.p.; September 13, 1916, p. 5; April 4, 1916, p. 7. The purchase rumors were false, *Motography* April 22, 1916, p. 930. On Whartons, see *MPW* April 18, 1914, p. 349; Einar Lauritzen and Gunnar Lundquist, *American Film-Index 1916–1920* (Stockholm: Film-Index, 1984), pp. xviii, xxx, 359; Ward, *The Motion Picture Goes to War*, pp. 116–17; Walter Stainton, "Pearl White in Ithaca," *Films in Review* 2 (May 1951): 19–25; Anthony Slide, *The American Film Industry: A Historical Dictionary* (Westport, Conn.: Greenwood, 1986), p. 388; Lindsay Chaney and Michael Cieply, *The Hearsts: Family and Empire—The Later Years* (New York: Simon & Schuster, 1981), p. 74. Another well-known Wharton serial made for Hearst was *Beatrice Fairfax*.

For erroneous credit, see *MPW* July 15, 1916, p. 481. For Wharton complaints about a pattern of such credit-stealing, see President [Theodore Wharton] to E. A. MacManus, July 31, 1916; Edward A. MacManus to L. D. Wharton, August 8, 1916; Wharton, Inc. to International Film Service, Inc., August 17, 1916; all in Wharton Corporation Records, Cornell University Archives.

The *IDJ* did not indicate whether Hearst's visit overlapped with Haiselden's, and it is not known if they might have met. Hearst was to have arrived September 14, apparently mainly to discuss *Patria*. Haiselden had arrived by September 24 on a stay of several days.

27. On Patton, see *BA* December 13, 1915, p. 12, and December 14, 1915, p. 12. *New York Medical Journal* 102 (December 4, 1915): 1134; *NYAm* November 23, 1915, p. 22, and November 19, 1915, p. 20; and many other examples. *Pathé News #94* for 1915, released November 24, 1915; *MPW* December 4, 1915, p. 1906.

28. William Randolph Hearst to George Hearst, ca. 1884, quoted in Mrs. Fremont Older, *William Randolph Hearst: American* (New York: D. Appleton-Century, 1936), p. 62. The William Randolph Hearst papers at the Bancroft Library in Berkeley contain only six folders of correspondence for 1915–19, none to or from Haiselden, Lait, the Whartons, or Hadfield.

29. Chaney and Cieply, *The Hearsts*, esp. chap. 3; W. A. Swanberg, *Citizen Hearst* (New York: Scribner's, 1961), esp. chaps. 8–10.

30. *IDJ* February 3, 1917; Peter F. McAllister to Howard Cobb, August 9, 1919, Wharton Corporation Records, Cornell University Archives. Hearst apparently tried to resolve the dispute. The August 9, 1919, *MPW* announced that Pathé was planning a new serial to be produced by Theodore Wharton, p. 820. I can find no record of whether Wharton actually continued to work for Pathé, nor what was the outcome of the threatened suit. The Whartons became increasingly marginal filmmakers and may have left the business in the 1920s.

31. *CH* April 1, 1917, p. 7; April 2, 1917, p. 11. Unfortunately, no copies of the early April 1917 *CA* could be located.

32. Slide, *American Film Industry*, pp. 169, 293; AFI *Catalog 1911–1920* and *Catalog 1921–1930, Index* volumes. For a typical later Rothacker production, see *Educational Screen*, January 1925, p. 48.

33. For locations of studios, see Lauritzen, *American Film-Index*, pp. xi–xxx. For trade press, see *International Film, Radio, and Television Journals*, ed. Anthony Slide (Westport, Conn.: Greenwood, 1985).

On Ithaca and the Whartons, see the exhibit "Hollywood on Cayuga," DeWitt Historical Society of Tompkins County, Ithaca N.Y., Summer 1989; Stainton, "Pearl White in Ithaca"; Slide, *American Film Industry*, p. 388; and the following small collections at the Division of Rare and Manuscripts Collections, Cornell University Library: Mame Hennessy Photograph Collection, Walter Stainton Papers, and Wharton Releasing Corporation Records.

34. *Custer's Last Fight*, copyright 1925, #LP-21,952; AFI *Catalog 1921–1930*, p. 159. Office was at 29 South LaSalle, as recorded in copyright office application log files, LC-MBRS; my thanks to Pat Sheehan for finding it. Ince died in 1924, and his studio was disbanded. Richard Koszarski, *Hollywood Directors 1914–1940* (London: Oxford University Press, 1976), p. 61.

35. Information gleaned from the movie theater listings in the Chicago papers, especially the *CT*. That paper contained a directory listing theaters by neighborhood and ownership. For information on Balaban & Katz, see the forthcoming work of Douglas Gomery, portions of which were presented at the University of Michigan Institute for the Humanities, 1989–90; and his contribution to *Seeing Through Movies*, ed. Mark Crispin Miller (New York: Pantheon, 1990). See also David Naylor, *Great American Movie Theaters* (Washington, D.C.: Preservation Press, 1987); Charlotte Herzog, "The Archaeology of Cinema Architecture: Origins of the Movie Theater," *Quarterly Review of Film Studies* 9 (Winter 1984): 11–32. For working class identity of West Madison Street theaters by the 1920s, see Lizabeth Cohen, "Encountering Mass Culture at the Grassroots: The Experience of Chicago Workers in the 1920s," *American Quarterly* 41 (March 1989): 6–33, at pp. 13, 15.

36. *Cincinnati Enquirer* April 1, 1917, sect. 3, p. 3; *Cleveland Plain Dealer* April 1, 1917, photoplay sect., p. 4; *Baltimore American* January 5, 1919, sect. 11, p. 23; *Baltimore Sun* January 12, 1919, p. B10. Although it was advertised as coming to both theaters, I have only been able to confirm that the film actually played at the Little Pickwick.

37. Interview with John Allen Sr., April 6, 1973, Park Ridge, N.J. On

road shows in silent-era New York State, see Kathryn Fuller, "Shadowland: American Audiences and the Movie-Going Experience in the Silent Film Era," chap. 3, Ph.D. diss., Johns Hopkins University, 1992. For the later era, see Mark E. Swartz, "Motion Pictures on the Move," *Journal of American Culture* (Winter 1986): 1–7. On traveling health films, see *Journal of the Outdoor Life* 15 (1917): 305.

38. Telegram H. E. Smith to W. D. McGuire, December 9, 1916; R. H. Hadfield to W. D. McGuire, December 19, 1916; Executive Secretary to M. E. Mazur, February 15, 1917; Nat S. Strange to National Board of Review, February 17, 1917; and R. H. Hadfield letter of January 23, 1918; all in NBRMP Box 103. *Motography* February 17, 1917, advertising p. 2. Applications and letters of H. J. Brooks, March 26, 1923; I. Brody, November 7 and 20, 1928; A. Kremicier, November 14, 1928; all in NYSA-MPD Box 2565, file number 383 and 12,421; Bland Brothers in Chicago Film Censorship Board application, November 17, 1927.

For background on state-rights sales, see Everson, *American Silent Film*, pp. 103–106. Western Import Co. to Leading Features Co., November 10, 1914, D. W. Griffith Papers, Museum of Modern Art, microfilm, reel 2. A second Griffith feature, *Avenging Conscience*, was sold by state at the same time.

39. On Bulliet, who later became an important art critic, see *WWW*, vol. 3 (Chicago: Marquis, 1981–)p. 121. R. H. Hadfield may have been Harry Hadfield, a film actor in 1915.

40. Telephone interview with Leander Bulliet, December 29, 1991. The substantial C. J. Bulliet collections at Columbia University and the Archives of American Art contain nothing related to *The Black Stork*. The family retained only a poster and several clippings related to the film, Prof. Richard W. Bulliet, personal correspondence, August 25, 1991. For Selznick, see *MPN* March 17, 1917, pp. 1650–51.

41. *Wid's Film Daily* April 5, 1917, p. 220; *ExTrR* March 24, 1917, p. 1072; *Motography* March 24, 1917, p. 636, and March 17, 1917, p. 583; *Cincinnati Enquirer* April 3, 1917, p. 5. For other claims of strong exhibitor interest in the film, see *ExTrR* February 14, 1917, p. 850; *MPN* May 3, 1917, p. 1348. Western Import Co. to Leading Features Co., November 10, 1914, D. W. Griffith Papers, Museum of Modern Art, microfilm reel 2.

In 1916 urban film theaters charged between ten and fifty cents for feature films, Everson, *American Silent Film*, p. 106. For typical production costs, see Balio, *American Film Industry*, pp. 116–17.

42. *Motography* March 24, 1917, p. 636; Balio, *American Film Industry*, pp. 95–96.

43. *IDJ* September 25, 1916; *Ithaca Weekly Journal* September 28, 1916; original records of the Chicago Film Censorship Board's 1916–1925 decisions have not yet been located, but are mentioned in the board's November 17, 1927, denial of a general audience permit to *Are You Fit to Marry?*; NBRMP Boxes 103, 163; LC-MBRS #LU-9978; *Variety* March 2, 1917, p. 29; *Motography* March 3 and 24, 1917; *MPN* March 3, 1917, p. 1405.

The Ohio legislative showing was not reported in the *Journals* of the House of Representatives or the Senate, though these were largely confined to daily listings of bills considered and the actions taken on them. But on

March 9, the legislature was in a frantic rush to adjourn; scores of bills were disposed of in a session that lasted until early the next morning. The film may well have been shown, but it seems unlikely any legislators would have had time to notice it.

44. NBRMP Box 103, 163; *CT* March 31, 1917, p. 13, and April 9–14, 1917, p. 15; *Cincinnati Enquirer* April 1, 1917, sect. 3, p. 3, and April 8, 1917, sect. 3, p. 3; *Cleveland Plain Dealer* April 1, 1917, photoplay sect., p. 4, April 2, 1917, p. 4, and April 8, 1917, photoplay sect., p. 4; *MPN* April 28, 1917, p. 2675; *ExTrR* January 25, 1919, p. 640.

45. *Baltimore Sun* January 12, 1919, p. B10; Chicago Film Censorship Board denial of general audience permit, November 17, 1927, and adult permits #56450, December 3, 1927, and #56452, February 7, 1928; *ExTrR* January 25, 1919, p. 640; NYSA-MPD Box 2565, Folders 383 and 12,421. John D. Stoeckle and George Abbott White, in *Plain Pictures of Plain Doctoring: Vernacular Expression in New Deal Medicine and Photography* (Cambridge: M.I.T. Press, 1985), p. 170, report the film title as *Are You Fit to Marry?*, but they do not give a source for that information. The actual photo (Fig. 25) does not appear to include the title of the film being advertised, but is headlined IF YOU ARE FIT TO MARRY SEE THIS VITAL PRODUCTION. Library of Congress Prints and Photographs Division #USF 33 13256–M3. The surviving version of the 1927 film runs about 65 minutes.

Chapter 9

1. For eugenic successes, see Ludmerer, *Genetics;* Kevles, *Name of Eugenics.* For alleged decline in euthanasia debate, see Russell, *Freedom to Die,* pp. 60 ff.; Kuepper, "Euthanasia," p. 95; Van der Sluis, "Euthanasia," p. 148; and most other historians of the subject.

However, the latter claim may be overstated. The *Reader's Guide to Periodical Literature* lists two articles on mercy killing (under "homicide") during 1925–28, although there were none a decade earlier. The AFI *Catalog* lists three feature films under "mercy killing" during 1921–30, compared to only two for 1911–20, though the 1910s catalog is much more fully indexed overall. If these indexes are any guide, the level of media attention to euthanasia was fairly low in the 1920s, but it's not clear that there was a decline compared to the 1910s. Mary Jane Ballou claims that discussions of mercy killing were fairly common in the newspapers and magazines of the 1920s, and that the links between euthanasia and eugenics were still visible in these articles: "Bestowing Painless Death: Eugenics and Euthanasia in the 1920s," unpublished paper, History of Science Society, October 15, 1994, New Orleans.

2. Fisher and Fisk, *How to Live,* 12th ed., p. 294.

3. William J. Robinson, *Eugenics and Marriage* (New York: Critic & Guide, 1917), p. 138, see also pp. 73–76. For similar disavowals, see Wiggam, *Fruit,* p. 283; Eden Paul, "Eugenics, Birth-Control, and Socialism," p. 142.

4. These figures are not directly comparable, however, since the latter volume is about one-third less comprehensively indexed overall. On "aesthetic censorship," see chap. 6 above.

5. *Heredity* is available at the Archives of Factual Film, Ames, Iowa. For others, see AFI *Catalog of Feature Films 1931–1940* (Berkeley: University of California Press, 1994). Extensive details on the censorship of *The Mercy Killer* are on pp. 420–21.

6. Kuepper, "Euthanasia," chap. 4; *NYT* September 30, 1924, p. 25; *Fortune* 16 (July 1937): 106; *American Review* 237 (1934): 239–42; *Reader's Digest* 34 (May 1939): 19–22; Triche and Triche, *The Euthanasia Controversy; NYT* February 14, 1939, p. 2; Kennedy, "Euthanasia," *Collier's* May 20, 1939, pp. 15–16, 57–58; Kennedy, "Sterilization and Eugenics," *American Journal of Obstetrics and Gynecology* 34 (September 1937): 519–20.

7. *Fortune* 16 (July 1937): 106. See also Humphry, *Right to Die*, p. 18; J. M. Ostheimer, "The Polls: Changing American Attitudes toward Euthanasia," *Public Opinion Quarterly* 44 (1980): 123–28.

In a related case, a man who killed his thirteen-year-old retarded son received only a suspended sentence from a sympathetic judge and jury in 1941, *Repouille v. US* 165 F.2d 152 (1947). For a similar postwar example, see *Commonwealth v. Noxon* 66 N.E. 2d 814 (Massachusetts 1946). Thanks to Yale Kamisar for discussing these cases with me.

8. *NYT* May 9, 1931, p. 4; Hollander, "Euthanasia and Mental Retardation," p. 58.

9. William W. Gregg, "The Right to Kill," *North American Review* 237 (1934): 242–43.

10. Henry Roberts, "May Doctors Kill?" *Living Age* 347 (October 1934): 160.

11. *NYT* November 8, 1935. There is a discrepancy in the number of infants involved, see *Time*, November 25, 1935, pp. 39–40.

12. Paul Popenoe, *Practical Applications of Heredity* (Baltimore: Williams & Wilkins, 1930), p. 84; Warthin, *Creed*, pp. 37, 51.

13. Jay G. Wanner, "The Privilege of Death," *Colorado Medicine* 30 (1933): 71–72.

14. *NYT* September 30, 1924, p. 25; *CT* May 7, 1938, p. 2; see also *NYT* January 8, 1950, sect. IV, p. 2.

15. Anthony M. Turano, "Murder by Request," *American Mercury* 36 (December 1935): 423–29. Many references in the above paragraph were first located by Kuepper, "Euthanasia," pp. 100, 120.

16. See chap. 6 above for the censorship. See chap. 4 above for reluctance to discuss Haiselden's increasingly active methods of killing. On the role of forgetting and erasure in history, see David William Cohen, *The Combing of History* (Chicago: University of Chicago Press, 1994).

17. While he opposed active killing, Glaser supported withholding treatment and endorsed *The Black Stork. Good Health* 52 (1917): 568, 571. See also Mitman, "Evolution as Gospel"; Paolo Coletta, *William Jennings Bryan* (Lincoln: University of Nebraska Press, 1969); Edward J. Larson, *Trial and Error: The American Controversy Over Creation and Evolution* (New York: Oxford University Press, 1985), p. 47; Stephen Jay Gould, *Bully for Brontosaurus* (New York: Norton, 1991), pp. 416–30.

18. *New York World* reprinted in *Boston Daily Advertiser* November 19, 1915, p. 6.

19. Binding and Hoche, *On Permitting the Destruction of Unworthy Human Lives,* trans. Walter Wright (forthcoming), of *Die Freigabe der Vernichtung lebensunwerten Lebens, ihr Mass und ihre Form;* Weindling, *Health Race and German Politics,* pp. 393–98; and "The 'Sonderweg' of German Eugenics," *British Journal of the History of Science* 22 (1989): 321–33. Mann was the pen name of Gerhard Hoffmann.

Rolf Winau, "Die Freigabe der Vernichtung 'lebensunwerten Lebens'," *Deutsches Ärzteblatt,* 16 February 1989, pp. 1–6; Van der Sluis, "Euthanasia," p. 142; Jonathan Harwood, "National Styles in Science: Genetics in Germany and the United States between World Wars," *Isis* 78 (1987): 390–414; Cornelie Usborne, *The Politics of the Body in Weimar Germany: Women's Reproductive Rights and Duties* (Ann Arbor: University of Michigan Press, 1993).

20. Nichtenhauser, "Motion Pictures," vol. III, pp. 1–21; Weindling, *Health Race and German Politics,* pp. 380, 411–13; see also the compilation-documentary *Desire* (Stuart Marshall, distributed by MayaVision, London, 1990), *NYT* June 21, 1990, p. B4, national ed. Ulf Schmidt of the Wellcome Medical History Unit at Oxford is also researching Weimar and Nazi health films. A copy of *Survival of the Fittest* is at the LC, but it has not yet been copied for viewing.

Weimar entertainment films also supposedly emphasized negative portrayals of the mentally retarded. James M. Gardner, "Contribution of the German Cinema to the Nazi Euthanasia Program," *Mental Retardation* 20 (August 1982): 174–75; Siegfried Kracauer, *From Caligari to Hitler: A Psychological History of the German Film* (Princeton, N.J.: Princeton University Press, 1947); David Weinberg, "Approaches to the Study of Film in the Third Reich: A Critical Appraisal," *Journal of Contemporary History* 19 (1984): 105–26.

21. NYSA-MPD Box 2565, Folders 383 and 12,421. See also chap. 3 above.

22. Kühl, *Nazi Connection;* Weindling, " 'Sonderweg' "; Proctor, *Racial Hygiene.* For example, virtually every issue of the Weimar eugenics journal *Volksaufartung—Erbkunde—Eheberatung* contained news on American practice. Thanks to Lora Wildenthal for the reference.

While many American scientists expressed misgivings about eugenics by the 1930s, many who denounced its methods as unscientific had no quarrel with its goals. On this point, see chap. 5 above.

23. The precise contribution of medicine and biology is too complex and controversial to cover here. Compare: Proctor, *Racial Hygiene;* Weindling, *Health, Race and German Politics;* Peter Weingart, "German Eugenics between Science and Politics," *Osiris* 5 (1989): 260–82; Benno Müller-Hill, *Murderous Science: Elimination by Scientific Selection of Jews, Gypsies, and Others, Germany 1933–1945* (Oxford: Oxford University Press, 1988); Graham, "Science and Values"; Adams, *Wellborn Science;* Sheila Weiss, "The Race Hygiene Movement in Germany," *Osiris* 3 (1987): 193–236; Harwood, "National Styles"; Götz Aly and Karl-Heinz Roth, *Die restlose Erfassung:*

volkszählen, identifizieren, aussondern im Nationalsozialismus (Berlin: Rotbuch, 1984); Christian Pross and Götz Aly, *The Value of the Human Being: Medicine in Germany 1918–45*, exhibition catalog (Berlin: Ärtzkammer, 1991). Also see the work in progress of Bernd Walter and the criticisms of Hans-Walter Schmuhl.

When Biology Became Destiny: Women in Weimar and Nazi Germany, ed. Renate Bridenthal, Atina Grossmann, and Marion Kaplan (New York: Monthly Review, 1984); Claudia Koontz, *Nazi Bodies: Race, Eugenics and Gender in the Third Reich* (in progress 1994); Gisela Bock, "Racism and Sexism in Nazi Germany," *Signs* 8 (1983): 400–421.

This literature is largely separate from important works on the Nazi medical profession by Michael H. Kater, Robert Jay Lifton, and others. For a brief and generally fair introduction, see Weindling, "Essay Review: Medicine in Nazi Germany and Its Aftermath," *Bulletin of the History of Medicine* 65 (Fall 1991): 416–19.

24. *Erbkrank:* NA #243.3, and UM-HHFC.

25. A copy of *Alles Leben ist Kampf* is in the possession of Professor Sharon Herbert of the University of Maryland Baltimore County History Department. I am grateful to her for providing a translation of the narration script.

Portions of the other films mentioned above are shown in *Selling Murder: The Killing Films of the Third Reich* (Domino Films, for British Channel Four, 1991), written by Michael Burleigh. They are discussed in his "Euthanasia and the Third Reich," *History Today* 40 (February 1990): 11–16. Thanks to Laurie Block for helping me locate *Selling Murder*. Much additional information on the Nazi films is in Weindling, *Health, Race*.

For Himmler, see Burleigh, "Euthanasia," p. 14; and Proctor, *Racial Hygiene*, pp. 191–92. For a provocative interpretation of *Ich Klage An*, see Karl-Heinz Roth, "Filmpropaganda für Vernichtung der Geisteskranken und Behinderten im 'Dritten Reich'," *Beiträge zur Nationalsozialistischen Gesundheits- und Sozialpolitik* 2 (1985): 125–193.

26. Kennedy, "The Problem of Social Control of the Congenital Defective: Education, Sterilization, Euthanasia," *American Journal of Psychiatry* 99 (July 1942): 13; Gregg, "Right to Kill," pp. 237, 242. In general, Kuepper, "Euthanasia," chap. 5.

27. Kühl, *Nazi Connection*, p. 59. Perhaps this was *Opfer der Vergangenheit*.

28. Proctor, *Racial Hygiene*, pp. 100–101; Barry Mehler, "Foundations for Fascism: The New Eugenics Movement in the United States," *Patterns of Prejudice* 23 (Winter 1989–90): 21; Kühl, *Nazi Connection*, pp. 49–50.

29. *Eugenical News* 22 (July–August 1937): 65–66. Thanks to Barry Mehler and Stefan Kühl for the reference.

30. *CA* November 12, 1917, afternoon ed., p. 1.

31. Wo den Nachkommen von Säufern, Verbrechern und Schwachsinnigen Paläste gebaut werden, indes der Arbeiter und Bauer mit einer kümmerlichen Hütte vorlieb nehmen muss, da geht ein solches Volk mit Riesenschritten seinem Ende entgegen.

In halb verfallenen Hütten und dumpfen Hinterhäusern brachte man gesunde Familien unter. Aber für Irre, die völlig Stumpf sind für ihre Umgebung baute man Paläste.

Thanks to Hugh Lane for help with the translation.

32. I am grateful to Professor Sharon Herbert for the translation. For a similar scene from *Opfer der Vergangenheit*, plus an early 1990s interview with an orderly from Hademar who found the point especially persuasive in the 1930s, see *Selling Murder*. On similar rhetoric in *Ich Klage An*, see Burleigh, "Euthanasia," p. 14.

33. *Archiv für Rassen- und Gesellschafts-Biologie* did not refer to Haiselden between 1915 and 1920, although their international news section did include other American events. Felix Dietrich, *Bibliographie der deutschen Zeitschriften literatur* (New York: Kraus, 1961) vols. 39–47 and Beilage vols. 37b, 39a, 40a, 42b, 44c, and 46c contained no entries under Haiselden, and nothing about him turned up in articles listed under "Eugenik," "Euthanisie," or "Chicago." I am grateful to Hugh Lane for conducting this search.

Binding and Hoche, *On Permitting the Destruction of Unworthy Human Lives;* Winau, "Die Freigabe der Vernichtung 'lebensunwerten Lebens.' "

Inquiries to several scholars familiar with German eugenics also produced no recollection of references to Haiselden in German sources. Replies were received from Rolf Winau, Robert Proctor, Paul Weindling, Stefan Kühl, Daniel Kevles, Loren Graham, Mark Haller, Walter Wright, and Garland Allen.

34. Proctor, *Racial Hygiene*, pp. 99, 173; Kühl, *Nazi Connection*, p. 85. See also chap. 3 above.

35. However, while the Nazis tried Grant's method, in an important sense it did not work. The killing of impaired Germans provoked far more public opposition than did the killing of other races. See Proctor, *Racial Hygiene*, chap. 7.

36. For an earlier example arguing the cross-class appeal of better babies and maternalism, see *Child Welfare Magazine*, January 1912, p. 158. Thanks to Jo Goodwin for the example. To indicate the sweeping scope of his work on domestic architecture the sixteenth-century architect Sebastiano Serlio used the subtitle, "from palace to hovel." *Erbkrank* attributed the expression to "Dr. Gross," probably race hygienist Walter Gross, but he was only thirteen years old when Haiselden's film was released.

37. National Conference on Race Betterment, *Proceedings* 2 (1915): 76, 79.

38. For an account of the issue from the Johns Hopkins case to the Andrew Stinson case, see David J. Rothman, *Strangers at the Bedside: A History of How Law and Bioethics Transformed Medical Decision Making* (New York: Basic Books, 1991), pp. 190–221.

Russell, *Right to Die*, pp. 246, 257; Rene Anspach, *Deciding Who Lives* (Berkeley: University of California Press, 1993), p. 8 on *Maine Medical Center v. Houle*, no. 74–145 (S.Ct. Maine, February 14, 1974). See also In re Phillip B., 156 Cal. Reporter 48 (Ct. Appeals 1979). Raymond Duff and A.G.M. Campbell, "Moral and Ethical Dilemmas in the Special-Care Nursery," *New England Journal of Medicine* 289 (1973): 890; John Lorber, "Early Results of Selective Treatment of Spina Bifida Cystica," *British Medical Journal* 4 (1973): 201–204.

Notes to pp. 168–169

Pediatrics 60 (1977): 588–90, cited in *Bowen* v. *American Hospital Association*, 476 U.S. 610, White, J., dissenting, 659–60; C. Everett Koop, "Pediatric Surgery: The Newest Specialty for the Youngest Patient," *Transactions and Studies of the College of Physicians of Philadelphia*, ser. 5, v. 3 (September 1981), 198, 208. Of course, before 1920 only one or two Americans considered themselves specialists in pediatric surgery.

39. C. Everett Koop, *Koop* (Grand Rapids, Mich.: Zonderran, 1992), pp. 339ff.; Constance Paige and Elisa Karnofsky, "The Antiabortion Movement and Baby Jane Doe," *Journal of Health Politics, Policy and Law* 11 (Summer 1986): 255–70.

40. The Oklahoma study was published in R. H. Gross, A. Cox, R. Tatyrek, M. Pollay, and W. A. Barnes, "Early Management and Decision Making for the Treatment of Myelomeningocele," *Pediatrics* 72 (October 1983): 450–58. For response to the Oklahoma case, see "Sullivan Reconsidering Choice for Welfare Chief," *NYT* May 18, 1989, national ed., p. 10; Nat Hentoff, "Why Stoney Jackson Smith Died Young," *Ann Arbor News* July 2, 1993, p. A9. Robert and Peggy Stinson, *The Long Dying of Baby Andrew* (Boston: Little, Brown, 1983).

41. *Bowen* v. *American Hospital Association* 476 U.S. 610.

42. Child Abuse Amendments of 1984, Public Law 98–457. With minor subsequent modifications, these amendments appear in the 1994 code as 42 U.S.C.A, section 5106, esp. 5106a(b)(10) and 5106g(10). Thanks to Marie Deveney for helping me track the subsequent codification from the original citation.

43. "Special Issue: Imperiled Newborns," *Hastings Center Report* 17 (December 1987): 9; Anspach, *Deciding*, p. 8.

44. PL 98–457 section 127(b); 42 U.S.C.A. section 5101 historical notes.

45. Daniel Callahan, "Medical Futility, Medical Necessity: The Problem Without a Name," *Hastings Center Report* 21 (July–August 1991): 30–35; E. Haavi Morreim, "Profoundly Diminished Life," *Hastings Center Report* 24 (January–February 1994): 33–42.

46. Baby Terry: *Ann Arbor News* August 12, 1993, p. D6; Baby K: *NYT* September 24, 1993, p. A8, February 12, 1994, p. 6, and February 20, 1994, p. A12.

For similar cases of "Baby Rena," see *WP* July 14–15, 1991; Luis Alvarado, *NYT* October 17, 1989, p. 11; Teresa Hamilton, *NYT* February 12, 1994, p. 6; Ryan Nguyen, *NYT* December 27, 1994.

Variations on the original Baby Doe situations continue as well. See manslaughter charges against Dr. Gregory Messenger of East Lansing, Michigan, *NYT* August 3, 1994, p. A8.

The Indiana "Baby Doe" was allowed to die. The New York "Baby Jane Doe" was treated and ten years later was described as a loving, self-aware child, able to attend special education classes. B. D. Colen, "What Ever Happened to Baby Jane Doe?" *Hastings Center Report* 24 (May–June 1994): 2.

47. E. W. Young and D. K. Stevenson, "Limiting Treatment for Extremely Premature, Low-Birth-Weight Infants," *American Journal of Diseases of Children* 144 (May 1990): 549–52; *CT* May 16, 1990, p. 3. *NYT* March 29, 1992, p. A10, national ed.; and *NYT* May 24, 1995, p. B6, national ed.,

on organ donation. Special series of articles, *NYT* September 29–October 1 and October 6, 1993.

On these issues too the supposed "novelty" is largely the result of the amnesia of the mass media. See *Hastings Center Report* 17 (December 1987): 38.

48. *Who Should Survive?:* LC-MBRS. For comments on the film, see Anthony D'Amato, "Book Review: Ethics at the Edges of Life," *Cardozo Law Review* 2 (Spring 1981): 655–58. For comments on the case itself, see James M. Gustafson, "Mongolism, Parental Desires, and the Right to Life," *Perspectives in Biology and Medicine* 16 (Summer 1973): 529–31.

Born Dying: Carle Medical Communications distributors.

Quincy: Longmore, "Screening Stereotypes," pp. 36–37. On the show in general, see Turow, *Playing Doctor*, pp. 172–74.

Koop, *Koop*, p. 339 ff. On anti–abortion films, see chap. 6, note 13 above.

49. Stephen Klaidman and Tom L. Beauchamp, "Baby Jane Doe in the Media," *Journal of Health Politics, Policy and Law* 11 (Summer 1986): 271–84, at p. 274; mentioned in *Bowen v. American Hospital Association* 476 U.S. 610 at 633–634.

50. Klaidman and Beauchamp, "Baby Jane Doe," p. 274; Kathleen Kerr, "Reporting the Case of Baby Jane Doe," *Hastings Center Report* 14 (August 1984): 7–9; Suzanne Wymelenberg, *Science and Babies: Private Decisions, Public Dilemmas* (Washington D.C.: National Academy of Sciences, 1990).

51. President's Commission for the Study of Ethical Problems in Medicine. . . , *Deciding to Forego Life-Sustaining Treatment* (Washington: Government Printing Office, 1983), pp. 197–98. See also Lawrence Altman, *NYT* quoted in chap. 1 above.

Many major academic studies omit any discussion of pre-1970s precedents, leaving the impression that the issue is a novel outgrowth of modern technology. Some examples include: Norman L. Cantor, *Legal Frontiers of Death and Dying* (Bloomington: Indiana University Press, 1987); Jeanne Harley Guillemin and Lynda Lytle Holmstrom, *Mixed Blessings: Intensive Care for Newborns* (New York: Oxford University Press, 1986); Fred M. Frohock, *Special Care: Medical Decisions at the Beginning of Life* (Chicago: University of Chicago Press, 1986); Stanley J. Reiser, "Survival at What Cost?: Origins and Effects of the Modern Controversy on Treating Severely Handicapped Newborns," *Journal of Health Politics, Policy and Law* 11 (Summer 1986): 199–214.

Many other works do include valuable sections on the history of social and parental infanticide, but overlook past examples of medical nontreatment. Some examples include: *Euthanasia and the Newborn*, ed. McMillan, et al.; *Which Babies Shall Live?*, ed. Murray and Caplan; Lyon, *Playing God;* Weir, *Selective Nontreatment;* Shelp, *Born to Die?;* Kuhse and Singer, *Should the Baby Live?;* "Special Issue: Imperiled Newborns," *Hastings Center Report* 17 (December 1987); and Post, "History, Infanticide, and Imperiled Newborns."

The only ethicist to study both medical and lay precedents is Cynthia

B. Cohen, "The Treatment of Impaired Newborns in American History." I thank Professor Cohen for sharing this manuscript.

52. Russell, *Freedom to Die;* Humphry, *Right to Die.*

53. Derek Humphry, *Final Exit* ([Eugene, Ore.]: Hemlock Society, 1991).

54. For early coverage, see *NYT* June 6, 1990.

55. The only serious study of Haiselden is in Kuepper, "Euthanasia." Scattered and sometimes misleading references to Haiselden also appear in Triche and Triche, *The Euthanasia Controversy,* and Russell, *Freedom to Die,* pp. 63, 241, 255, 260, 330.

However, Ruth Schwartz Cowan is working on a study of eugenics and children that will include material from an earlier draft of this book. And a short article on the ethical implications, perhaps stimulated by a paper I gave at the American Association for the History of Medicine in 1985, recently appeared in a medical journal. Walter J. Friedlander, "The Bollinger Case," *The Pharos* 57 (Spring 1994): 34–37.

56. In response to my inquiry, Kevorkian did not recall ever having heard of Haiselden. Personal communication from Jerry Abrams, February 15, 1994. In mid–1995, Kevorkian awaited trial on several criminal charges. Meanwhile the state of Oregon and Australia's Northern Territory enacted the first laws to permit doctor–assisted suicide for the terminally–ill. *NYT,* November 11, 1994, p. 12 and May 26, 1995, p. 4.

57. All three of the differences cited below are advanced by Kevles, *Name of Eugenics* and "Is the Past Prologue?: Eugenics and the Human Genome Project," *Contention* 2 (Spring 1993): 21–37 for genetics; Humphry, *Right to Die;* and Russell, *Freedom to Die* for euthanasia. On autonomy, see also John Robertson, *Children of Choice* (Princeton, N.J.: Princeton University Press, 1994).

58. This view was presented forcefully by LeRoy Walters, the ethicist in charge of one important watchdog body for genetic research, during a 1991 visit to the University of Michigan; see Walters, "Human Gene Therapy: Ethics and Public Policy," *Human Gene Therapy* 2 (Summer 1991): 115–22. It appears to be shared by Kevles and Ludmerer. For an important critique, see Peter Weingart, "Science Abused: Challenging a Legend," *Science in Context* 6 (Autumn 1993): 555–67.

59. Pernick, "Informed Consent."

60. Brandt, *No Magic Bullet.* On the weakness of modern commitment to autonomy in practice, see Carl Schneider, "Bioethics with a Human Face," *Indiana Law Journal* 69 (Fall 1994): 1075–1104; Alan Meisel and Loren H. Roth, "Toward an Informed Discussion of Informed Consent," *Arizona Law Review* 25 (1983): 265–346.

61. Of the many critics who have raised similar points, I have benefitted most from Hubbard, *The Politics of Women's Biology,* and Troy Duster, *Backdoor to Eugenics* (New York: Routledge, 1990); and Diane Paul and Hamish G. Spencer, "The Hidden Science of Eugenics," *Nature* 374 (March 23, 1995): 302–304.

62. Many critics have contributed to my views on these points, but the essays of Stephen Jay Gould and Richard Lewontin have been particularly

influential. See also Richard Lerner, *Final Solutions* (University Park: Pennsylvania State University Press, 1992).

63. On this point I differ from Robert Proctor, whose comparisons between the present and the past faith in objectivity I otherwise share.

64. The role of values in the current Baby Doe debates has been stressed by Robert Veatch and others; see Warren T. Reich and David E. Ost, "Ethical Perspectives on the Care of Infants," *Encyclopedia of Bioethics,* p. 726; Charles Krauthammer, "What to Do About 'Baby Doe,'" *TNR* September 2, 1985, p. 18. On the possibilities for value consensus see Roger Rosenblatt, *Life Itself: Abortion in the American Mind* (New York: Random House, 1992); Kurt Bayertz, *The Concept of Moral Consensus: the Case of Technological Interventions into Human Reproduction* (Dordrecht and Boston: Kluwer, 1994).

65. In addition to chaps. 3 and 4 above, see Proctor, *Racial Hygiene,* opp. p. 163.

Bibliography

Personal Interviews and Archival Collections

John Allen Sr., Interview, April 6, 1973, Park Ridge, New Jersey
Leander Bulliet, Telephone Interview, December 29, 1991, from Marshfield,
    Massachusetts
Richard W. Bulliet, Personal Correspondence, August 25, 1991
Cabot Family Correspondence, c/o Patricia Spain Ward, Chicago, Illinois
Chicago Medical Society:
    Council Minutes 1912–1914 [1915–1922 reported missing]
Cook County Illinois Death Records, County Clerk's Office, Chicago: 1880–
    1915
Cornell University Library, Division of Rare and Manuscript Collections,
    Ithaca, New York:
    Mame Hennessy Photograph Collection
    Wharton Releasing Corporation Records
    Walter Stainton Papers

DeWitt Historical Society of Tompkins County, Ithaca, New York:
    Cody Collection
    Walter Stainton Collection (custody of Gretchen Sachse)
    Wharton Studios Collection
George Eastman House, Rochester, New York:
    Film Collections
Emma Goldman Correspondence, microfilm edition, reel 9, 1915. Alexandria, Virginia, Chadwick-Healey, 1990.
Illinois Regional Archives Depository, Northeastern Illinois University Library, Chicago:
    Chicago Film Censorship Board review cards
Kendall County Illinois Death Records, County Clerk's Office, Yorkville, Illinois: 1877–1915
Library of Congress, Motion Picture, Broadcast and Recorded Sound Division, Washington, D.C.:
    Motion Picture Copyright Depositions
    Motion Picture Collections
    Motion Picture Paper Prints
    Foster Card Index
    Community Motion Picture Bureau—Foster Clipping Scrapbooks
Library of Congress Prints and Photographs Division
Museum of Modern Art, Film Study Center, New York:
    Edison Kinetograms
    Edison Script Collection
    D. W. Griffith Papers, microfilm edition, reel 2
    Motion Picture Collections
National Archives, Washington D.C.: U.S. Public Health Service Records, RG 90.
National Archives, Motion Picture Branch, College Park, Maryland
National Library of Medicine, History of Medicine Division, Bethesda Maryland:
    Adolf Nichtenhauser Papers
    Adolf Nichtenhauser, "A History of Motion Pictures in Medicine," typescript
    Motion Picture Collections
New York Academy of Medicine, New York:
    Abraham Jacobi papers
New York Public Library Rare Books and Manuscripts Division; Astor, Lenox and Tilden Foundations:
    National Board of Review of Motion Pictures Records, Correspondence and Files
New York State Archives, Albany:
    Motion Picture Division: Scripts, Records
University of Michigan, Ann Arbor:
    Alumni Records Office
    Historical Health Film Collection
    Labadie Collection of Radical Literature, University Library
    Michigan Historical Collections, Bentley Library:
        Royal Copeland Papers

John Harvey Kellogg Papers
Medical School Dean's Correspondence—Victor Vaughan
John Sundwall Papers
University of Minnesota Social Welfare History Archives:
American Social Hygiene Association Records
United States Census, Manuscript Returns, Kendall County, Illinois:
9th Census 1870, Little Rock Township
10th census 1880, Plano
The following collections reported having no material to, from, or about Haiselden, but an item-by-item search for unindexed references has not yet been undertaken:
American Philosophical Society:
American Eugenics Society Collections
Charles B. Davenport Papers
Bancroft Library: William Randolph Hearst Collections
UCLA Film Archive: Hearst Metrotone Collection
University of Oregon: Jack Lait Papers

Newspapers

All available issues of the following newspapers were examined for November 12–December 30, 1915; February 5–7 and March 14–16, 1916; July 22–27 and November 12–20, 1917 (Meter and Hodzima cases); January 25–30, 1918 (Stanke case); and June 18–20, 1919 (obituaries):
Alarm [Chicago, Anarchist]
American Socialist [Chicago]
Appeal to Reason [Girard, Kans., Socialist]
Ann Arbor Daily Times News
Detroit Free Press
Detroit News
Chicago American
Chicago Defender [African-American]
Chicago Herald
Chicago Tribune
Chicago New World [Catholic]
Ithaca Daily Journal
Ithaca Weekly Journal
Michigan Socialist
New York Times
New York American
New York Sun
New York Call [Socialist]
Washington Post

In addition, many specific issues of the following papers were also examined:
Baltimore American
Baltimore Sun

Boston Advertiser
Boston American
Boston Globe
Boston Herald
Chicago Daily News
Chicago Examiner
Cleveland Plain Dealer
Cincinnati Enquirer
New Orleans Morning Star [Catholic]
New York Evening Journal
New York Herald
Philadelphia Ledger
Washington Star
Times (London)

Periodicals

Comparisons between *The Black Stork* and other films on eugenics, birth control, sexuality, and health education, drew heavily on page-by-page searches of numerous medical and film periodicals. This research was conducted as part of my forthcoming overall study of health films, *Bringing Medicine to the Masses*. In most cases, all available issues from 1910–1928 were examined for the following publications:

Motion Picture Trade Publications

Educational Screen 1922–1927
Educational Film Magazine 1920–1922
Exhibitor's Trade Review 1917–1925
Motion Picture News 1913–1928
Motography [Nickelodeon] 1909–1918
Moving Picture World 1910–1928
New York Dramatic Mirror 1910–1922
Photoplay scattered issues 1917 only
Reel and Slide 1918–1922
Variety 1908–1928
Visual Education 1920–1924
Wid's Film Daily [various titles] 1915–1928

Medical Journals

American Journal of Care of Cripples 1914–1919
American Journal of Public Health 1911–1928
Archiv für Rassen- und Gesellschafts-Biologie 1915–1920
Bulletin of the American Social Hygiene Association [Social Hygiene Bulletin]
    1914–1922

Bulletin of the Eugenics Record Office 1915–1933
Bulletin of the National Tuberculosis Association 1913–1928
Child Health Magazine [Child Health Bulletin] 1920–1935
Eugenical News 1916–1933
Eugenics Review [London] 1915–1930
Good Health 1915–1919
Journal of Heredity 1915–1930
Journal of the Outdoor Life 1910–1925, 1930
Proceedings of the National Conference on Race Betterment 1914, 1915, 1928
Social Hygiene [Journal of Social Hygiene] 1914–1928

In addition, all available issues of the following local medical journals were searched for 1915–1919:
Bulletin of Chicago Medical Society
Chicago Medical Recorder
Illinois Medical Journal

Biographical Sources

Appleton's Cyclopedia of American Biography. New York: D. Appleton, 1888.
Biography and Genealogy Master Index. Detroit, Mich.: Gale Research, 1980.
The Book of Chicagoans. Chicago: Marquis, 1917.
Chicago Medical Society. *History of Medicine and Surgery and Physicians and Surgeons of Chicago.* Chicago: Biographical Publishing, 1922.
Chicago telephone directories Summer 1930, Summer 1932, and 1960–61.
Dictionary of American Biography. New York: Scribner's, 1959.
Kaufman, Martin, Stuart Galishoff, and Todd L. Savitt, eds. *Dictionary of American Medical Biography.* Westport, Conn.: Greenwood, 1984.
Kelly, Howard, and Walter Burrage. *Dictionary of American Medical Biography.* New York: D. Appleton, 1928.
Koszarski, Richard. *Hollywood Directors 1914–1940.* London: Oxford University Press, 1976.
Lakeside Annual Directory of the City of Chicago. Chicago: Chicago Directory Company, 1887–1912.
McDonough, Walter R., comp. *Chicago Medical Directory.* Chicago: Chicago Medical Society, 1905, 1917, 1919.
McDonough, Walter R., comp. *Physicians Blue Book.* Chicago: William J. Lowitz, 1897.
Michigan State Gazeteer. Detroit, Mich.: R. L. Polk, 1903.
National Cyclopedia of American Biography. New York: J. T. White, 1898–1984.
New York Times Obituaries Index. New York: New York Times, 1970.
Notable American Women. Cambridge, Mass.: Harvard University Press, 1971.
Polk's Chicago City Directory 1928–1929. Chicago: R. L. Polk, 1928.
Polk's Medical Register. Detroit, Mich.: R. L. Polk, 1915–1917.
Variety Obituaries: An Index. Metuchen, N.J.: Scarecrow, 1980.

Who Was Who in the Theater, 1912–1976. Detroit, Mich.: Gale Research, 1978.

Who Was Who in America. Chicago: Marquis, 1981.

Who's Who in New York. New York: Who's Who, 1918, 1924.

Primary Books and Articles

"A Symposium on Obstetrical Abnormalities." *Medical Review of Reviews* 22 (February 1916): 95–103.

Aristotle. *Politics.* Cambridge, Mass.: Harvard University Press, 1990.

"Ask Medical Board to Pass Life or Death Sentence." *Medical Freedom* 5 (December 1915): 55–56.

Bacon, Charles S. "The Race Problem." *Medicine* [Detroit] 9 (1903): 341.

Baker, LaReine. "Eugenics and the Modern Feminist Movement." In *Race Improvement or Eugenics.* New York: Dodd, Mead, 1912.

Baldwin, Simeon. "The Natural Right to a Natural Death." *Journal of Social Science* 37 (1899): 1–17.

Bayer, Charles J. *Maternal Impressions.* 2d ed. Winona, Minn.: Jones & Kroger, 1897.

Bentham, Jeremy. *Bentham's Theory of Legislation.* Edited and translated by Charles Milner Atkinson. Oxford: Oxford University Press, 1914.

Binding, Karl, and Alfred Hoche. *On Permitting the Destruction of Unworthy Human Lives.* Translated by Walter Wright (forthcoming), of *Die Freigabe der Vernichtung lebensunwerten Lebens, ihr Mass und ihre Form.*

Bitzer, G. W. *Billy Bitzer: His Story.* New York: Farrar, Straus and Giroux, 1973.

Blaikie, William. *How to Get Strong and How to Stay So.* New York: Harper & Bros., 1879, 1902.

Block, Anita C. "The Social Aspects of the Bollinger Baby Case." *Medical Review of Reviews* 22 (1916): 122–24.

Bowen v. American Hospital Association. 476 U.S. 610 (1986).

Buck v. Bell. 274 U.S. 200 (1927).

Burton, Robert. *The Anatomy of Melancholy.* London: George Routledge, 1931.

Catholic World. 102 (December 1915): 421–24.

Child Abuse Amendments of 1984, Public Law 98–457. With minor subsequent modifications, these amendments appear in the 1994 code as 42 U.S.C.A, section 5106, esp. 5106a(b)(10) and 5106g(10).

Commonwealth v. Noxon. 66 N.E. 2d 814 (Massachusetts 1946).

Crane, Stephen. "The Monster." In *Tales of Whilomville.* Charlottesville: University Press of Virginia, 1969.

Darrow, Clarence. "The Eugenics Cult." *American Mercury* 8 (June 1926): 129–37.

A Decade of Progress in Eugenics: Scientific Papers of the Third International Congress of Eugenics. Baltimore: Williams & Wilkins, 1934.

De Kruif, Paul. *Microbe Hunters.* New York: Harcourt, Brace, 1926.

Dennett, Mary Ware. "The Sex Side of Life." *Medical Review of Reviews* 24 (February 1918): 69.

"Destroying Defectives." *Chicago Medical Recorder* 37 (December 15, 1915): 737–38.

Duff, Raymond, and A.G.M. Campbell. "Moral and Ethical Dilemmas in the Special-Care Nursery." *New England Journal of Medicine* 289 (1973): 890.

Emerson, Ralph Waldo. "Compensation." In *Essays, First Series,* pp. 89–122. Boston: Houghton Mifflin, 1888.

Engel, Sigmund. *The Elements of Child-Protection.* Translated by Dr. Eden Paul. New York: Macmillan, 1912.

"Eugenics Again." *Illinois Medical Journal* 28 (December 1915): 454–55.

"Eugenics as Romance." *NYT* September 25, 1921, Sec. II, p. 2.

Eugenics in Race and State: Scientific Papers of the Second International Congress of Eugenics . . . New York 1921. Baltimore: Williams & Wilkins, 1923.

" 'Euthanasia' Again." *Medical Record* [New York], November 27, 1915, p. 925.

Fisher, Irving, and Eugene Lyman Fisk. *How to Live.* 12th ed. New York: Funk & Wagnalls, 1917.

Flexner, Abraham. *Medical Education in the United States and Canada.* New York: Carnegie Foundation, 1910.

Garrod, Archibald. *Inborn Errors of Metabolism.* London: Oxford University Press, 1963 [1909].

Gregg, William W. "The Right to Kill." *North American Review* 237 (1934): 242–43.

Grant, Madison. *The Passing of the Great Race.* New York: Scribner's, 1916.

Gross, R. H., A. Cox, R. Tatyrek, M. Pollay, and W. A. Barnes. "Early Management and Decision Making for the Treatment of Myelomeningocele." *Pediatrics* 72 (October 1983): 450–58.

Guyer, Michael. *Being Well-Born: An Introduction to Heredity and Eugenics.* Indianapolis: Bobbs-Merrill, 1927.

Haeckel, Ernst. *The History of Creation.* New York: D. Appleton, 1876 [1868].

Haeckel, Ernst. *The Wonders of Life.* New York: Harper & Bros., 1905.

Haiselden, Harry J. "The Bollinger Case." *New York Medical Journal* 102 (1915): 1132–34.

Haiselden, Harry J. "Regarding the Meter Baby of Chicago." *Medical Review of Reviews* 23 (1917): 697–98.

Hall, G. Stanley. "What Is to Become of Your Baby?" *Cosmopolitan* 48 (April 1910): 661–68.

"Health Propaganda." *Philadelphia Public Ledger,* July 8, 1919, p. 11.

Hecht, Ben. *A Child of the Century.* New York: Simon & Schuster, 1954.

Hentoff, Nat. "Why Stoney Jackson Smith Died Young." *Ann Arbor News,* July 2, 1993, p. A9.

Hirst, Barton Cooke. "The Rights of the Unborn Child." *New York Medical Journal* 105 (February 10, 1917): 241–43.

Holmes, S. J. "Misconceptions of Eugenics." *Atlantic* 115 (February 1915): 222–27.

Humphry, Derek. *Final Exit.* [Eugene, Ore.]: Hemlock Society, 1991.

Huntington, Ellsworth. *Tomorrow's Children*. New York: Wiley, 1935.

Huxley, Aldous. *Brave New World*. New York: Bantam, 1960 [1932].

In re Phillip B. 156 Cal. Reporter 48 (Ct. Appeals 1979).

Jacobson v. Massachusetts. 197 U.S. 11.

Keith, Arthur. *Menders of the Maimed*. London: H. Frowde, 1919.

Keller, Helen. "Physicians' Juries for Defective Babies." *TNR*, December 18, 1915, pp. 173–74.

Kennedy, Foster. "Euthanasia." *Collier's*, May 20, 1939, pp. 15–16, 57–58.

Kennedy, Foster. "The Problem of Social Control of the Congenital Defective: Education, Sterilization, Euthanasia." *American Journal of Psychiatry* 99 (July 1942): 13–16.

Kennedy, Foster. "Sterilization and Eugenics." *American Journal of Obstetrics and Gynecology* 34 (September 1937): 519–20.

Kleinschmidt, H. E. "Educational Prophylaxis of Venereal Diseases." *Social Hygiene* 5 (1919): 27.

Koop, C. Everett. *Koop*. Grand Rapids, Mich.: Zonderran, 1992.

Krauthammer, Charles. "What to Do About 'Baby Doe.' " *TNR* September 2, 1985, p. 18.

Lashley, Karl Spencer, and John B. Watson. *A Psychological Study of Motion Pictures in Relation to Venereal Disease Campaigns*. Washington, D.C.: United States Interdepartmental Social Hygiene Board, 1922.

Lashley, Karl Spencer, and John B. Watson. "A Psychological Study of Motion Pictures in Relation to Venereal Disease Campaigns." *Social Hygiene* 7 (1921): 181–219.

Lee, Edward Wallace. "Physical Defects a Factor in the Cause of Crime." *New York Medical Journal* 100 (December 26, 1914): 1246–52.

Lorber, John. "Early Results of Selective Treatment of Spina Bifida Cystica." *British Medical Journal* 4 (1973): 201–204.

Low, Sir Sidney James Mark. "Propaganda Films and Mixed Morals." *Fortnightly Review* 113 (May 1920): 717–28.

Maine Medical Center v. Houle. No. 74–145 (S.Ct. Maine, February 14, 1974).

McKim, W. Duncan. *Heredity and Human Progress*. New York: G. P. Putnam's Sons, 1900.

"Misconception of Eugenics." *Chicago Medical Recorder* 38 (1916): 592.

Morley, Jefferson. "Right-to-Life Porn." *TNR* March 25, 1985, pp. 8–10.

National Health Council. *Film List*. New York: Metropolitan Life Insurance Company, 1918, 1924, 1928.

Norris, Kathleen. "The Undefectives." *Literary Digest*, December 11, 1915, p. 1386.

Osler, William. "The Fixed Period." In *Aequanimitas; With Other Addresses*, pp. 391–411. London: H. K. Lewis, 1906.

Paul, Eden. "Eugenics, Birth Control, and Socialism." In *Population and Birth Control*. New York: Critic & Guide, 1917.

Pennsylvania State Board of Censors. *Rules and Standards*. Harrisburg: J. L. L. Kuhn, 1918.

Peters, James A., ed. *Classic Papers in Genetics*. Englewood Cliffs, N.J.: Prentice-Hall, 1959.

Plato, *Republic*. New York: Norton, 1985.

Popenoe, Paul. *Practical Applications of Heredity.* Baltimore: Williams & Wilkins, 1930.

President's Commission for the Study of Ethical Problems in Medicine. . . . *Deciding to Forego Life-Sustaining Treatment.* Washington, D.C.: Government Printing Office, 1983.

Reeve, Arthur B. "The Eugenic Bride." *Cosmopolitan* 56 (April 1914): 637–48.

"Reform that Gets Nowhere." *Medical Freedom* 6 (September 1916): 3.

"Reforming Criminals by Surgery." *Medical Freedom* 4 (September 1914): 7.

Repouille v. U.S. 165 F.2d 152 (1947).

Repplier, Agnes. "A Good Word Gone Wrong." *Independent,* October 1, 1921, p. 5.

"Right and Wrong in the Case of the Baby Who Was Allowed to Die." *Current Opinion* 60 (January 1916): 43–44.

Riley, James Whitcomb. *"The Old Swimmin'-hole" and 'Leven More Poems.* Indianapolis: Bowen-Merrill, 1891.

Roberts, Harry. *Euthanasia.* London: Constable, 1936.

Roberts, Henry. "May Doctors Kill?" *Living Age* 347 (October 1934): 160.

Robertson, John Dill. "The Case of the Bollinger Baby." *Journal of the American Medical Association* 65 (1915): 2025.

Robinson, William J. *Eugenics and Marriage.* New York: Critic & Guide, 1917.

Robinson, William J. *Eugenics, Marriage and Birth Control.* 2d ed. New York: Critic & Guide, 1922.

Robinson, Victor. *Pioneers of Birth Control.* New York: Voluntary Parenthood League, 1919.

Sargent, Dudley. *Health, Strength and Power.* New York: H. M. Caldwell, 1904.

"Scheme to Establish Courtship on Genetic Foundations." *Current Opinion* 61 (September 1916): 180.

Schloendorff v. Society of New York Hospital. 211 N.Y. 125; 105 N.E. 92.

Shaw, George Bernard. "Preface." In *Three Plays By Brieux.* New York: Brentano's, 1911.

Smith, James LeRoy. "Shall Degenerates Be Condemned to Death?" *Physical Culture* 21 (January 1909): 49–52.

Snow, John. "On Asphyxia, and On the Resuscitation of Still-Born Children." *London Medical Gazette* 29 (1841): 222–27.

Soranus. *Gynecology.* Translated Owsei Temkin. Baltimore, Md.: Johns Hopkins University Press, 1956.

Spencer, Herbert. *Facts and Comments.* New York: D. Appleton, 1902.

Stinson, Robert, and Peggy Stinson. *The Long Dying of Baby Andrew.* Boston: Little, Brown, 1983.

"Sullivan Reconsidering Choice for Welfare Chief." *NYT* May 18, 1989, national ed., p. 10.

Talbot, Eugene S. *Degeneracy.* New York: Scribner's [1898].

"The Bollinger Case." *Survey,* December 4, 1915, pp. 265–66.

"The Challenge of a Defective Baby's Life." *Survey,* 4 December 1915, p. 227.

"The Defective Baby." *TNR* November 27, 1915, pp. 85–86.

Travis, Thomas. *The Young Malefactor.* New York: Thomas Y. Crowell, 1908.

Trollope, Anthony. *The Fixed Period*. Ann Arbor: University of Michigan Press, 1990.

Turano, Anthony M. "Murder by Request." *American Mercury* 36 (December 1935): 423–29.

Turnbull, Laurence. *The Advantages and Accidents of Artificial Anaesthesia*. 2d ed. Philadelphia: P. Blakiston, 1885.

Walters, LeRoy. "Human Gene Therapy: Ethics and Public Policy." *Human Gene Therapy* 2 (Summer 1991): 115–22.

Wanner, Jay G. "The Privilege of Death." *Colorado Medicine* 30 (1933): 71–72.

Warthin, Aldred Scott. *Creed of a Biologist*. New York: P. B. Hoeber, 1930.

"Was the Doctor Right?" *Independent*, January 3, 1916, pp. 23–27.

Watson, John B., and Karl Spencer Lashley. "A Consensus of Medical Opinion Upon Questions Relating to Sex Education and Venereal Disease Campaigns." *Mental Hygiene* 4 (October 1920): 769–847.

Wells, H. G. *Modern Utopia*. London: Chapman & Hall, 1905.

Westermarck, Edward. *The Origin and Development of the Moral Ideas*. Vol. 1, pp. 393–413. London: Macmillan, 1906.

Wiggam, Albert E. *The Fruit of the Family Tree*. Garden City: Garden City Publishing, 1924.

Wiley, Harvey. "The Rights of the Unborn." *Good Housekeeping*, October 1922, p. 32.

Wilson, J. G. "A Study in Jewish Psychopathology." *Popular Science Monthly* 82 (1913): 264–71.

Young, E. W., and D. K. Stevenson, "Limiting Treatment for Extremely Premature, Low-Birth-Weight Infants." *American Journal of Diseases of Children* 144 (May 1990): 549–52.

Unpublished Dissertations, Papers, and Works in Progress

Ballou, Mary Jane. "Bestowing Painless Death: Eugenics and Euthanasia in the 1920s." History of Science Society, New Orleans, October 15, 1994.

Bogin, Mary. "The Meaning of Heredity in American Medicine and Popular Health Advice, 1771–1860." Ph.D. diss., Cornell University, 1990.

Bowers, David. *Thanhouser Films: An Encyclopedia and History*. Work in progress, 1988.

Brown, JoAnne. "Policing the Body: Criminological Metaphor in the Popularization of Germ Theories in the United States, 1870–1950." American Association for the History of Medicine, Philadelphia, May 3, 1987.

Carey, Allison. "The Changing Role of Gender in Compulsory Sterilization Programs, 1907–1950." Graduate seminar paper, University of Michigan, 1992.

Cohen, Cynthia B. "The Treatment of Impaired Newborns in American History: Implications for Public Policy." Manuscript, Department of Philosophy, Villanova University, 1985.

Cooke, Kathy. "Heredity and Environment: Partners in Eugenic Reform," History of Science Society, New Orleans, October 14, 1994.

Curtis, Patrick Almond. "Eugenic Reformers, Cultural Perceptions of Dependent Populations, and the Care of the Feebleminded in Illinois, 1909–1920." Ph.D. diss., University of Illinois at Chicago, 1983.

Czitrom, Daniel. "The Redemption of Leisure: The National Board of Censorship and the Rise of Motion Pictures in New York City, 1900–1920." American Studies Association, Philadelphia, November 4, 1983.

Elks, Martin. "Visual Rhetoric: Photographs of the Feeble-Minded during the Eugenics Era, 1900–1930." Ph.D. diss., Syracuse University, 1992.

Fuller, Kathryn. "Shadowland: American Audiences and the Movie-Going Experience in the Silent Film Era." Ph.D. diss., Johns Hopkins University, 1992.

Gomery, Douglas. Presentations of work in progress. University of Michigan Institute for the Humanities, 1989–90.

Huebner, Lee William. "The Discovery of Propaganda: Changing Attitudes Towards Public Communication in America, 1900–1930." Ph.D. diss., Harvard University, 1968.

Kanar, Hanley. "Juxtaposed Images and Stereotypes of Disability and Difference in Selected Twentieth-Century Literature." Senior honors thesis in American Culture, University of Michigan, 1989.

Koontz, Claudia. *Nazi Bodies: Race, Eugenics and Gender in the Third Reich.* Work in Progress, 1994.

Kuepper, Stephen Louis. "Euthanasia in America, 1890–1960." Ph.D. diss., Rutgers University, 1981.

McLeary, Erin. "Late Victorian Explanations for Deformity." Undergraduate paper, University of Michigan, April 24, 1992.

Mehler, Barry Alan. "A History of the American Eugenics Society, 1921–1940." Ph.D. diss., University of Illinois, 1988.

Nichtenhauser, Adolf. "A History of Motion Pictures in Medicine." Typescript, National Library of Medicine, History of Medicine Division, Bethesda, Maryland.

Pernick, Martin S. "Progressives, Propaganda, and Public Health: The Army Venereal Disease Education Films of World War I." Duquesne History Forum, Pittsburgh, Pennsylvania, November 1, 1974.

Rydell, Robert W. "Eugenics Hits the Road: The Popularization of Eugenics at American Fairs and Museums Between the World Wars." History of Science Society, Chicago, December 1984.

Tyor, Peter L. "Segregation or Surgery: The Mentally Retarded in America 1850–1920." Ph.D. diss., Northwestern University, 1972.

Walters, LeRoy. Presentations of work in progress. University of Michigan, 1991.

Secondary Books and Articles

There is an extensive secondary literature on many of the subjects discussed in this book. This bibliography is not intended to be comprehensive, but is almost entirely limited to works cited as documentation of specific points raised in the text.

Adams, Mark B., ed. *The Wellborn Science: Eugenics in Germany, France, Brazil and Russia.* Oxford: Oxford University Press, 1989.

Allen, Garland. "Eugenics and American Social History 1880–1950." *Genome* 31 (1989): 885–89.

Allen, Garland. "Genetics, Eugenics, and Class Struggle." *Genetics* 79 (June 1975), supplement, pp. 29–45.

Allen, Garland. *Life Science in the Twentieth Century.* New York: Cambridge University Press, 1978.

Aly, Götz, and Karl-Heinz Roth. *Die restlose Erfassung: volkszählen, identifizieren, aussondern im Nationalsozialismus.* Berlin: Rotbuch, 1984.

American Federation of Arts. *Before Hollywood: Turn-of-the-Century Film from American Archives.* New York: American Federation of Arts, 1986.

American Film Institute. *Catalog of Feature Films, 1911–1920.* Berkeley: University of California Press, 1989.

American Film Institute. *Catalog of Feature Films 1931–1940.* Berkeley: University of California Press, 1994.

American Film Institute. *Catalog of Motion Pictures Produced in the United States: Feature Films, 1921–1930.* New York: Bowker, 1971.

Amundsen, Darrel W. "Medicine and the Birth of Defective Children: Approaches of the Ancient World." In *Euthanasia and the Newborn,* ed. Richard C. McMillan, H. Tristram Engelhardt Jr., and Stuart F. Spicker, pp. 3–22. Philosophy and Medicine Series, vol. 24, Dordrecht: D. Reidel, 1987.

Anderson, Oscar. *The Health of a Nation: Harvey W. Wiley and the Fight for Pure Food.* Chicago: University of Chicago Press, 1958.

Angier, Natalie. "Why Birds and Bees, Too, Like Good Looks," and "Not Just a Beauty Contest," *NYT* February 8, 1994, pp. B5, B8.

Anspach, Rene. *Deciding Who Lives.* Berkeley: University of California Press, 1993.

Antler, Joyce, and Daniel M. Fox. "The Movement Toward a Safe Maternity: Physician Accountability in New York City, 1915–1940." In *Sickness and Health in America,* 2d ed., ed. Judith Walzer Leavitt and Ronald L. Numbers, pp. 490–506. Madison: University of Wisconsin Press, 1985.

Balio, Tino, ed. *The American Film Industry.* Rev. ed. Madison: University of Wisconsin Press, 1985.

Banner, Lois. *American Beauty.* New York: Knopf, 1983.

Bannister, Robert C. *Social Darwinism: Science and Myth in Anglo-American Social Thought.* Philadelphia: Temple University Press, 1979.

Banta, Martha. *Imaging American Women.* New York: Columbia University Press, 1987.

Barkan, Elazar. *Retreat of Scientific Racism.* Cambridge: Cambridge University Press, 1992.

Barker, David. "The Biology of Stupidity: Genetics, Eugenics, and Mental Deficiency in the Inter-War Years." *British Journal for the History of Science* 22 (1989): 347–75.

Bayertz, Kurt. *The Concept of Moral Consensus: The Case of Technological Interventions into Human Reproduction.* Dordrecht and Boston: Kluwer, 1994.

Bearn, Alexander. *Archibald Garrod and the Individuality of Man.* New York: Oxford University Press, 1993.

Beauchamp, Tom L. "A Reply to Rachels on Active and Passive Euthanasia." In *Ethical Issues in Death and Dying,* ed. Beauchamp and Seymour Perlin, pp. 246–58. Englewood Cliffs, N.J.: Prentice-Hall, 1978.

Beauchamp, Tom L., and Laurence B. McCullough. *Medical Ethics: The Moral Responsibilities of Physicians.* Englewood Cliffs, N.J.: Prentice-Hall, 1984.

Behlmer, George K. "Deadly Motherhood: Infanticide and Medical Opinion in Mid-Victorian England." *JHMAS* 34 (October 1979): 403–27.

Benison, Saul. "An Interpretation of the Early Evolution of Care and Treatment of Crippled Children in the United States." *Birth Defects: Original Article Series,* vol. 12, no. 4 (1976): 103–115.

Benison, Saul A., Clifford Barger, and Elin L. Wolfe. *Walter B. Cannon: The Life and Times of a Young Scientist.* Cambridge, Mass.: Harvard University Press, 1987.

Berkowitz, Edward D. *Disabled Policy: America's Programs for the Handicapped.* Cambridge: Cambridge University Press, 1987.

"Biomedical Ethics and the Shadow of Nazism: A Conference." *Hastings Center Report,* Supplement (August 1976).

Birken, Lawrence. *Consuming Desire: Sexual Science and the Emergence of a Culture of Abundance 1871–1914.* Ithaca, N.Y.: Cornell University Press, 1989.

Bock, Gisela. "Racism and Sexism in Nazi Germany." *Signs* 8 (1983): 400–421.

Bodnar, John. *The Transplanted.* Bloomington: Indiana University Press, 1985.

Bogdan, Robert. *Freak Show.* Chicago: University of Chicago Press, 1988.

Bonner, Thomas. *Medicine in Chicago 1850–1950.* Madison, Wisc.: American History Research Center, 1957.

Boon, Timothy. "Lighting the Understanding and Kindling the Heart: Social Hygiene and Propaganda Film in the 1930s." *Social History of Medicine* 3 (1990): 140–41.

Boswell, John. *The Kindness of Strangers: The Abandonment of Children in Western Europe from Late Antiquity to the Renaissance.* New York: Pantheon, 1989.

Boucé, Paul–Gabriel. "Imagination, Pregnant Women, and Monsters in Eighteenth-Century England and France." In *Sexual Underworlds of the Enlightenment,* ed. G. S. Rousseau and Roy Porter, pp. 86–100. Chapel Hill: University of North Carolina Press, 1988.

Bowler, Peter J. "E. W. MacBride's Lamarckian Eugenics." *Annals of Science* 41 (1984): 245–60.

Bowler, Peter J. *Eclipse of Darwinism.* Baltimore: Johns Hopkins University Press, 1983.

Bowler, Peter J. *The Mendelian Revolution.* London: Athlone, 1989.

Bowler, Peter J. *The Non-Darwinian Revolution.* Baltimore: Johns Hopkins University Press, 1988.

Bowser, Eileen. *The Transformation of Cinema, 1907–1915.* New York: Scribner's, 1990.

Brandt, Allan. *No Magic Bullet.* New York: Oxford University Press, 1987.

Braun, Marta. *Picturing Time: The Work of Etienne-Jules Maret.* Chicago: University of Chicago Press, 1992.

Bremner, Robert H., ed. *Children and Youth in America: A Documentary History.* Cambridge, Mass.: Harvard University Press, 1971.

Bridenthal, Renate, Atina Grossmann, and Marion Kaplan, eds. *When Biology Became Destiny: Women in Weimar and Nazi Germany.* New York: Monthly Review, 1984.

Brody, Howard. "In the Best Interests of . . ." *Hastings Center Report* 18 (December 1988): 37–39.

Brody, Jane. "Ideals of Beauty Seen as Innate." *NYT* March 21, 1994, p. A6.

Brown, JoAnne. *The Definition of a Profession: The Authority of Metaphor in the History of Intelligence Testing.* Princeton, N.J.: Princeton University Press, 1992.

Brownlow, Kevin. *Behind the Mask of Innocence.* New York: Knopf, 1990.

Buhle, Mari Jo. *Women and American Socialism 1870–1920.* Urbana: University of Illinois Press, 1981.

Burleigh, Michael. "Euthanasia and the Third Reich." *History Today* 40 (February 1990): 11–16.

Burnham, John C. *How Superstition Won and Science Lost: Popularizing Science and Health in the United States.* New Brunswick, N.J.: Rutgers University Press, 1987.

Burns, Chester. "Richard Cabot Clarke and the Reformation of American Medical Ethics." *Bulletin of the History of Medicine* 51 (Fall 1977): 353–68.

Burt, Robert. "Authorizing Death for Anomalous Newborns." In *Genetics and the Law,* ed. Aubrey Milunsky and George Annas. New York: Plenum, 1976.

Buss, David M. *The Evolution of Desire.* New York: Basic Books, 1994.

Callahan, Daniel. "Medical Futility, Medical Necessity: The Problem Without a Name." *Hastings Center Report* 21 (July–August 1991): 30–35.

Calmes, Selma H. "Virginia Apgar: A Woman Physician's Career in a Developing Specialty." *Journal of the American Medical Women's Association* 39 (November–December 1984): 184–88.

Campbell, Craig W. *Reel America and World War I: A Comprehensive Filmography and History of Motion Pictures in the United States, 1914–1920.* Jefferson, N.C.: McFarland, 1985.

Cantor, Norman L. *Legal Frontiers of Death and Dying.* Bloomington: Indiana University Press, 1987.

Carrick, Paul. *Medical Ethics in Antiquity: Philosophical Perspectives on Abortion and Euthanasia.* Dordrecht and Boston: D. Reidel, 1985.

Chalmers, David. *Hooded Americanism.* 3d ed. Durham, N.C.: Duke University Press, 1987.

Chaney, Lindsay, and Michael Cieply. *The Hearsts: Family and Empire—The Later Years.* New York: Simon & Schuster, 1981.

Chase, Allan. *The Legacy of Malthus.* New York: Knopf, 1977.

Chesler, Ellen. *Woman of Valor: Margaret Sanger and the Birth Control Movement in America.* New York: Simon & Schuster, 1992.

Clouser, K. Danner. "Allowing or Causing: Another Look." *Annals of Internal Medicine* 87 (1977): 622–24.

Coben, Stanley. *Rebellion Against Victorianism: The Impetus for Cultural Change in 1920s America.* New York: Oxford University Press, 1991.

Cohen, Edward P., ed. *Medicine in Transition: The Centennial of the University of Illinois College of Medicine.* Urbana: University of Illinois Press, 1981.

Cohen, David William. *The Combing of History.* Chicago: University of Chicago Press, 1994.

Cohen, Lizabeth. "Encountering Mass Culture at the Grassroots: The Experience of Chicago Workers in the 1920s." *American Quarterly* 41 (March 1989): 6–33.

Colen, B. D. "What Ever Happened to Baby Jane Doe?" *Hastings Center Report* 24 (May–June 1994): 2.

Coletta, Paolo. *William Jennings Bryan.* Lincoln: University of Nebraska Press, 1969.

Colwell, Stacie. "*The End of the Road:* Gender, the Dissemination of Knowledge, and the American Campaign Against Venereal Disease During World War I." *Camera Obscura* 29 (May 1992): 91–129.

Condran, Gretchen A., Henry Williams, and Rose A. Cheney. "The Decline in Mortality in Philadelphia from 1870 to 1930: The Role of Municipal Services." In *Sickness and Health in America,* 2d ed., ed. Judith Walzer Leavitt and Ronald L. Numbers, pp. 422–38. Madison: University of Wisconsin Press, 1985.

Cone, Thomas E. Jr. *History of American Pediatrics.* Boston: Little, Brown, 1979.

Connelly, Robert. *The Motion Picture Guide: Silent Film.* Chicago: Cinebooks, Inc., 1986.

Cooter, Roger, ed. *In the Name of the Child: Health and Welfare 1880–1940.* New York: Routledge, 1992.

Cott, Nancy. *Grounding of Modern Feminism.* New Haven, Conn.: Yale University Press, 1987.

Couvares, Francis. "Hollywood, Main Street, and the Church: Trying to Censor the Movies Before the Production Code." *American Quarterly* 44 (December 1992): 584–615.

Cravens, Hamilton. *The Triumph of Evolution.* 2d ed. Baltimore: Johns Hopkins University Press, 1988.

Cremin, Lawrence. *Transformation of the School.* New York: Knopf, 1961.

Cronin, Helena. *The Ant and the Peacock: Altruism and Sexual Selection from Darwin to Today.* New York: Cambridge University Press, 1992.

Crowe, L. "Alcohol and Heredity: Theories About the Effects of Alcohol Use on Offspring." *Social Biology* 32 (1985): 146–61.

D'Amato, Anthony. "Book Review: Ethics at the Edges of Life." *Cardozo Law Review* 2 (Spring 1981): 655–58.

D'Emilio, John, and Estelle B. Freedman. *Intimate Matters: A History of Sexuality in America.* New York: Harper & Row, 1988.

Damme, Catherine. "Infanticide: The Worth of an Infant under Law." *Medical History* 22 (January 1978): 1–24.

Daston, Lorraine. "Baconian Facts, Academic Civility, and the Prehistory of Objectivity." *Annals of Scholarship* 8 (1991): 337–64.

Dawidowicz, Lucy. *The War Against the Jews, 1933–1945.* New York: Holt, Rinehart, and Winston, 1975.

De Grazia, Edward, and Roger K. Newman. *Banned Films: Movies, Censors and the First Amendment.* New York: Bowker, 1982.

Degler, Carl N. *In Search of Human Nature: The Decline and Revival of Darwinism in American Thought.* New York: Oxford University Press, 1991.

Desmond, Adrian. *The Politics of Evolution.* Chicago: University of Chicago Press, 1989.

Dietrich, Felix. *Bibliographie der deutschen Zeitschriften literatur.* New York: Kraus, 1961.

Douglas, Mary. *Purity and Danger: An Analysis of Concepts of Pollution and Taboo.* New York: Praeger, 1966.

Dowling, Harry. *Fighting Infection.* Cambridge, Mass.: Harvard University Press, 1977.

Dragognet, Francois. *Etienne-Jules Maret.* New York: Zone, 1992.

Dubos, Rene, and Jean Dubos. *The White Plague: Tuberculosis, Man and Society.* London: Victor Gollancz, 1953.

Duster, Troy. *Backdoor to Eugenics.* New York: Routledge, 1990.

Ehrenreich, Barbara, and Deirdre English. *For Her Own Good: 150 Years of the Experts' Advice to Women.* New York: Anchor/Doubleday, 1978.

Elks, Martin. "The Lethal Chamber." *Mental Retardation* 31 (August 1993): 201–207.

Elsaesser, Thomas, ed. *Early Cinema: Space, Frame, Narrative.* London: British Film Institute, 1991.

Engelhardt, H. Tristram. "The Concepts of Health and Disease." In *Evaluation and Explanation in the Biomedical Sciences*, pp. 125–41. Dordrecht: D. Reidel, 1975.

Everson, William K. *American Silent Film.* New York: Oxford University Press, 1978.

Faulkner, Harold. *The Quest for Social Justice.* New York: Macmillan, 1931.

Ferngren, Gary B. "The Status of Defective Newborns from Late Antiquity to the Reformation." In *Euthanasia and the Newborn*, ed. Richard C. McMillan, H. Tristram Engelhardt Jr., and Stuart F. Spicker, pp. 47–64. Philosophy and Medicine Series, vol. 24. Dordrecht: D. Reidel, 1987.

Fiedler, Leslie. "The Tyranny of the Normal." *Hastings Center Report* 14 (April 1984): 40–42.

Fiedler, Leslie. *Freaks: Myths and Images of the Secret Self.* New York: Simon & Schuster, 1978.

Foucault, Michel. *History of Sexuality.* New York: Vintage, 1985.

Fox, Daniel M. "Social Policy and City Politics: Tuberculosis Reporting in New York 1889–1900." *Bulletin of the History of Medicine* 49 (1975): 169–95.

Fox, Daniel M., and Christopher Lawrence. *Photographing Medicine: Images and Power in Britain and America since 1840.* Westport, Conn.: Greenwood Press, 1988.

Fox, Sanford J. *Science and Justice: The Massachusetts Witchcraft Trials.* Baltimore: Johns Hopkins University Press, 1968.

Fredrickson, George. *The Black Image in the White Mind.* New York: Harper & Row, 1972.

Freeden, Michael. "Eugenics and Progressive Thought: A Study in Ideological Affinity." *The Historical Journal* 22 (1979): 645–71.

Fried, Michael. *Realism, Writing, Disfiguration.* Chicago: University of Chicago Press, 1987.

Friedlander, Walter J. "The Bollinger Case." *The Pharos* 57 (Spring 1994): 34–37.

Frohock, Fred M. *Special Care: Medical Decisions at the Beginning of Life.* Chicago: University of Chicago Press, 1986.

Fye, W. Bruce. "Active Euthanasia: An Historical Survey of Its Conceptual Origins and Introduction to Medical Thought." *Bulletin of the History of Medicine* 52 (1979): 492–502.

Gabbard, Krin, and Glen O. Gabbard. *Psychiatry and the Cinema.* Chicago: University of Chicago Press, 1987.

Gallo, Anthony. "Spina Bifida: The State of the Art of Medical Management." *Hastings Center Report* 14 (February 1984): 10–13.

Gardner, James M. "Contribution of the German Cinema to the Nazi Euthanasia Program." *Mental Retardation* 20 (August 1982): 174–75.

Gasman, Daniel. *The Scientific Origins of National Socialism.* London: MacDonald, 1971.

Gebhard, Bruce. "A Century of Visual Health Education in the United States, 1860–1960: From Sanitary Fairs to Health Museums." *Current Problems in the History of Medicine: XIXth International Congress of the History of Medicine.* Basel: Karger, 1966, pp. 652–59.

Gelb, Steven A. "Not Simply Bad and Incorrigible: Science, Morality, and Intellectual Deficiency." *History of Education Quarterly* 29 (Fall 1989): 359–79.

Genetics, Eugenics and Evolution. Harwood, Jonathan, ed. *British Journal for the History of Science* 22 (1989): 257–375.

Georgano, G. N., ed. *The New Encyclopedia of Motorcars.* New York: Dutton, 1982.

Gerstle, Gary. *Working Class Americanism.* New York: Cambridge University Press, 1989.

Gilman, Sander. *Difference and Pathology.* Ithaca, N.Y.: Cornell University Press, 1985.

Gilman, Sander. *Picturing Health and Illness: Images of Identity and Difference.* Baltimore, Md.: Johns Hopkins University Press, 1995.

Glick, Thomas, ed. *The Comparative Reception of Darwinism.* Austin: University of Texas Press, 1974.

Golden, Mark. *Children and Childhood in Classical Athens.* Baltimore: Johns Hopkins University Press, 1990.

Gomery, Douglas. *Shared Pleasures: A History of Movie Presentation in the United States.* Madison: University of Wisconsin Press, 1992.

Goodrich, Lloyd. *Thomas Eakins: His Life and Work.* New York: Whitney Museum, 1933.

Gordon, Linda. *Woman's Body, Woman's Right: A Social History of Birth Control in America.* New York: Viking, 1976.

Gould, Stephen Jay. *Bully for Brontosaurus.* New York: Norton, 1991.

Gould, Stephen Jay. *Eight Little Piggies.* New York: Norton, 1993.

Gould, Stephen Jay. *Hen's Teeth and Horse's Toes.* New York: Norton, 1983.

Gould, Stephen Jay. *The Mismeasure of Man.* New York: Norton, 1981.

Gould, Stephen Jay. *Ontogeny and Phylogeny.* Cambridge, Mass.: Harvard University Press, 1977.

Graham, Loren. "Science and Values: The Eugenics Movement in Germany and Russia in the 1920s." *American Historical Review* 82 (1977): 1133–64.

Graham, Loren. *Science in Russia and the Soviet Union.* New York: Cambridge University Press, 1993.

Gritzer, Glenn, and Arnold Arluke. *The Making of Rehabilitation: A Political Economy of Medical Specialization 1890–1980.* Berkeley: University of California Press, 1985.

Grob, Gerald. *Mental Illness in American Society 1875–1940.* Princeton, N.J.: Princeton University Press, 1983.

Grossmann, Atina. "Abortion and Economic Crisis: The 1931 Campaign Against Paragraph 218." In *When Biology Became Destiny: Women in Weimar and Nazi Germany,* ed. Renate Bridenthal, Grossmann, and Marion Kaplan, pp. 66–86. New York: Monthly Review Press, 1984.

Grossman, James. *Land of Hope: Chicago, Black Southerners and the Great Migration.* Chicago: University of Chicago, 1989.

Guillemin, Jeanne Harley, and Lynda Lytle Holmstrom. *Mixed Blessings: Intensive Care for Newborns.* New York: Oxford University Press, 1986.

Gunning, Tom. "An Aesthetic of Astonishment." *Art and Text* 34 (1989): 31–45.

Gustafson, James M. "Mongolism, Parental Desires, and the Right to Life." *Perspectives in Biology and Medicine* 16 (Summer 1973): 529–31.

Hale, Nathan G. Jr. *Freud and the Americans: The Beginnings of Psychoanalysis in the United States, 1876–1917.* New York: Oxford University Press, 1971.

Haller, John. *Outcasts from Evolution: Scientific Attitudes of Racial Inferiority 1859–1900.* Urbana: University of Illinois Press, 1971.

Haller, Mark. *Eugenics.* New Brunswick, NJ: Rutgers University Press, 1963.

Halpern, Sydney A. *American Pediatrics: The Social Dynamics of Professionalism 1880–1980.* Berkeley: University of California Press, 1988.

Hansen, Bert. "American Physicians' 'Discovery' of Homosexuals 1880–1920." In *Framing Disease,* ed. Charles Rosenberg and Janet Golden, pp. 104–133. New Brunswick, N.J.: Rutgers University Press, 1992.

Hansen, Miriam. *Babel and Babylon: Spectatorship in American Silent Film.* Cambridge, Mass.: Harvard University Press, 1991.

Harwood, Jonathan. "National Styles in Science: Genetics in Germany and the United States between World Wars." *Isis* 78 (September 1987): 390–414.

Haskell, Molly. *From Reverence to Rape.* New York: Holt, Rinehart, and Winston, 1974.

Haskell, Thomas. *The Emergence of Professional Social Science: The American Social Science Association and the Nineteenth-Century Crisis of Authority.* Urbana: University of Illinois Press, 1977.

Hays, Samuel P. *Conservation and the Gospel of Efficiency.* Cambridge, Mass.: Harvard University Press, 1959.

Hays, Samuel P. *The Response to Industrialism.* Chicago: University of Chicago, 1957.

Hazen, Margaret Hindle, and Robert M. Hazen. *Keepers of the Flame: The Role of Fire in American Culture 1775–1925.* Princeton, N.J.: Princeton University Press, 1993.

Herf, Jeffrey. *Reactionary Modernism: Technology, Culture, and Politics in Weimar and the Third Reich.* Cambridge: Cambridge University Press, 1984.

Herzog, Charlotte. "The Archaeology of Cinema Architecture: Origins of the Movie Theater." *Quarterly Review of Film Studies* 9 (Winter 1984): 11–32.

History of Childhood Quarterly. 1 (Winter 1974).

Hoffer, P. C., and N.E.H. Hull. *Murdering Mothers: Infanticide in England and New England 1558–1803.* New York: New York University Press, 1981.

Hofstadter, Richard. *Social Darwinism in American Thought.* Philadelphia: University of Pennsylvania Press, 1944.

Hollander, Russell. "Euthanasia and Mental Retardation." *Mental Retardation* 27 (April 1989): 53–61.

Hollander, Russell. "Mental Retardation and American Society: The Era of Hope." *Social Service Review* (September 1986): 395–420.

Hollinger, David. "Inquiry and Uplift: Late Nineteenth Century American Academics and the Moral Efficacy of Scientific Practice." In *The Authority of Experts,* ed. Thomas Haskell, pp. 142–56. Bloomington: Indiana University Press, 1984.

Hollinger, David. "Justification by Verification: The Scientific Challenge to the Moral Authority of Christianity in Modern America." In *Religion and Twentieth-Century American Intellectual Life,* ed. Michael Lacey, pp. 116–35. Cambridge: Cambridge University Press, 1989.

Hollinger, David. "What is Darwinism? It is Calvinism!" *Reviews in American History* 8 (March 1980): 80–85.

Hovenkamp, Herbert. *Science and Religion in America 1800–1860.* Philadelphia: University of Pennsylvania Press, 1978.

Howell, Joel. "Early Use of X-ray Machines and Electrocardiographs at the Pennsylvania Hospital, 1897–1927." *Journal of the American Medical Association* 255 (1986): 2320–23.

Howell, Joel. "Machines and Medicine: Technology Transforms the American Hospital." In *The American General Hospital: Communities and Social Contexts,* ed. Diana Long and Janet Golden, pp. 109–134. Ithaca, N.Y.: Cornell University Press, 1989.

Hubbard, Ruth. *The Politics of Women's Biology.* New Brunswick, N.J.: Rutgers University Press, 1990.

Humphry, Derek. *The Right to Die: Understanding Euthanasia.* New York: Harper & Row, 1986.

Jones, Greta. "Eugenics and Social Policy Between the Wars." *The Historical Journal* 25 (1982): 718–28.

Jones, Greta. *Social Hygiene in 20th Century Britain.* London: Croom Helm, 1986.

Joravsky, David. *The Lysenko Affair.* Cambridge, Mass.: Harvard University Press, 1970.

Jordan, John M. *Machine-Age Ideology.* Chapel Hill: University of North Carolina Press, 1994.

Jordan, Winthrop. *White Over Black: American Attitudes toward the Negro 1550–1812.* 2d ed. Baltimore: Penguin, 1969.

Jordanova, Ludmilla. *Lamarck.* Oxford: Oxford University Press, 1984.

Jowett, Garth. *Film: The Democratic Art.* Boston: Little, Brown, 1976.

Kennedy, Dane. "The Perils of the Midday Sun: Climatic Anxieties in the Colonial Tropics." In *Imperialism and the Natural World,* ed. John Mackenzie, pp. 118–40. Manchester: Manchester University Press, 1990.

Kennedy, David M. *Birth Control in America.* New Haven, Conn.: Yale University Press, 1970.

Kerr, Kathleen. "Reporting the Case of Baby Jane Doe." *Hastings Center Report* 14 (August 1984): 7–9.

Kessler-Harris, Alice. *Out to Work: A History of Wage-Earning Women in the United States.* New York: Oxford University Press, 1982.

Kevles, Daniel. "Is the Past Prologue?: Eugenics and the Human Genome Project." *Contention* 2 (Spring 1993): 21–37.

Kevles, Daniel. *In the Name of Eugenics: Genetics and the Uses of Human Heredity.* Berkeley: University of California Press, 1985.

Kirschner, Don S. "Publicity Properly Applied: The Selling of Expertise in America." *American Studies,* 19 (Spring 1978): 65–78.

Klaidman, Stephen, and Tom L. Beauchamp. "Baby Jane Doe in the Media." *Journal of Health Politics, Policy and Law* 11 (Summer 1986): 271–84.

Klaus, Alisa. *Every Child a Lion: Origins of Maternal and Infant Health Policy in the United States and France 1890–1920.* Ithaca, N.Y.: Cornell University Press, 1993.

Kloppenberg, James T. *Uncertain Victory: Social Democracy and Progressivism in European and American Thought.* New York: Oxford University Press, 1986.

Kolko, Gabriel. *Triumph of Conservatism.* Glencoe, Ill.: Free Press, 1963.

Koop, C. Everett. "Pediatric Surgery: The Newest Specialty for the Youngest Patient." *Transactions and Studies of the College of Physicians of Philadelphia,* 5th ser. vol. 3 (September 1981): 198–208.

Koszarski, Richard. *An Evening's Entertainment: The Age of the Silent Feature Picture, 1915–1928.* New York: Scribner's, 1990.

Kracauer, Siegfried. *From Caligari to Hitler: A Psychological History of the German Film.* Princeton, N.J.: Princeton University Press, 1947.

Kraut, Alan M. *Silent Travelers: Germs, Genes and the 'Immigrant Menace'.* New York: Basic, 1994.

Kriegel, Leonard. "Uncle Tom and Tiny Tim: Reflections on the Cripple as Negro." *American Scholar* 38 (Summer 1969): 412–30.

Kühl, Stefan. *The Nazi Connection: Eugenics, American Racism, and German National Socialism.* New York: Oxford University Press, 1994.

Kuhn, Annette. *Cinema, Censorship and Sexuality 1909–1925.* London: Routledge, 1988.

Kuhn, Annette. *The Power of the Image.* London: Routledge & Kegan Paul, 1985.

Kuhse, Helga, and Peter Singer. *Should the Baby Live?* Oxford: Oxford University Press, 1985.

Ladd-Taylor, Molly. *Raising a Baby the Government Way: Mothers' Letters to the Children's Bureau 1915–1932.* New Brunswick, N.J.: Rutgers University Press, 1986.

LaFleur, William. *Liquid Life: Abortion and Buddhism in Japan.* Princeton, N.J.: Princeton University Press, 1992.

Larson, Edward J. *Trial and Error: The American Controversy Over Creation and Evolution.* New York: Oxford University Press, 1985.

Lasch, Christopher. *The Culture of Narcissism.* New York: Norton, 1979.

Lauritzen, Einar, and Gunnar Lundquist. *American Film-Index 1916–1920.* Stockholm: Film-Index, 1984.

Lears, T. J. Jackson. *No Place of Grace: Antimodernism and the Transformation of American Culture 1880–1920.* New York: Pantheon, 1981.

Leavitt, Judith Walzer. "Birthing and Anesthesia: The Debate Over Twilight Sleep." *Signs* 6 (Autumn 1980): 147–64.

Leavitt, Judith Walzer. *Brought to Bed: Childbearing in America.* New York: Oxford University Press, 1986.

Leavitt, Judith Walzer, and Ronald L. Numbers, eds. *Sickness and Health in America.* 2nd ed. Madison: University of Wisconsin Press, 1985.

Lerner, Richard. *Final Solutions.* University Park: Pennsylvania State University Press, 1992.

Lederer, Susan E. "The Right and Wrong of Making Experiments on Human Beings: Udo J. Wile and Syphilis." *Bulletin of the History of Medicine* (1984): 380–97.

LeVay, David. *The History of Orthopedics.* Park Ridge, N.J.: Parthenon, 1990.

Liachowitz, Claire H. *Disability as a Social Construct: Legislative Roots.* Philadelphia: University of Pennsylvania Press, 1988.

Library of Congress. *Motion Pictures: Catalog of Copyright Entries 1912–1939.* Washington, D.C.: Library of Congress, 1951.

Lindberg, David, and Ronald L. Numbers, eds. *God and Nature.* Berkeley: University of California Press, 1986.

Litoff, Judy Barrett. *American Midwives 1860 to the Present.* Westport, Conn.: Greenwood, 1978.

Lloyd, G.E.R. *Science, Folklore, and Ideology: Studies in the Life Sciences in Ancient Greece.* Cambridge: Cambridge University Press, 1983.

Loesser, Arthur. *Men, Women, and Pianos: A Social History.* New York: Simon & Schuster, 1954.

Lomax, Elizabeth. "Infantile Syphilis as an Example of Nineteenth Century Belief in the Inheritance of Acquired Characteristics." *JHMAS* 34 (January 1979): 23–39.

Longmore, Paul K. "A Note on Language and the Identity of Disabled People." *American Behavioral Scientist* 28 (January–February 1985): 419–23.

Longmore, Paul K. "Screening Stereotypes: Images of Disabled People." *Social Policy* 16 (Summer 1985): 31–37.

Longstreet, Stephen. *Chicago 1860–1919.* New York: David McKay, 1973.

Ludmerer, Kenneth. "Eugenics: History." In *Encyclopedia of Bioethics,* vol. I, pp. 457–62. New York: Free Press, 1978.

Ludmerer, Kenneth L. *Genetics and American Society.* Baltimore: Johns Hopkins University Press, 1972.

Ludmerer, Kenneth. *Learning to Heal.* New York: Basic Books, 1985.

Luker, Kristen. *Abortion and the Politics of Motherhood.* Berkeley: University of California Press, 1984.

Lund, Karen C. *American Indians in Silent Film: Motion Pictures in the Library of Congress.* Washington, D.C.: Library of Congress, 1992.

Lyon, Jeff. *Playing God in the Nursery.* New York: Norton, 1984.

Lyons, Albert S., and R. Joseph Petrucelli. *Medicine: An Illustrated History.* New York: Abrams, 1978.

MacAdams, William. *Ben Hecht.* New York: Scribner's, 1990.

Macnicol, Ian. "Eugenics and the Campaign for Voluntary Sterilization in Britain." *Social History of Medicine* 2 (August 1989): 147–70.

Mahowald, Mary B. "Baby Doe Committees: A Critical Evaluation." *Clinics in Perinatology* 15 (December 1988): 789–800.

Marchand, Roland. *Advertising the American Dream: Making Way for Modernity 1920–1940.* Berkeley: University of California Press, 1985.

Markel, Howard. "The Stigma of Disease: Implications of Genetic Screening." *American Journal of Medicine* 93 (August 1992): 209–15.

May, Lary. *Screening Out the Past.* 2d ed. Chicago: University of Chicago Press, 1983.

Mayr, Ernst. *The Growth of Biological Thought.* Cambridge, Mass.: Harvard University Press, 1982.

Mazumdar, Pauline M. H. *Eugenics, Human Genetics and Human Failings.* London: Routledge, 1992.

McCormick, Richard L. *The Party Period and Public Policy.* New York: Oxford University Press, 1986.

McMillan, Richard C., H. Tristram Engelhardt Jr., and Stuart Spicker, eds. *Euthanasia and the Newborn.* Philosophy and Medicine, vol. 24. Dordrecht: D. Reidel, 1987.

Meckel, Richard. *Save the Babies: American Public Health Reform and the Prevention of Infant Mortality.* Baltimore: Johns Hopkins University Press, 1990.

Mehler, Barry. "Eliminating the Inferior." *Science for the People* (November–December 1987): 14–18, 32.

Mehler, Barry. "Foundations for Fascism: The New Eugenics Movement in the United States." *Patterns of Prejudice* 23 (Winter 1989–90): 17–25.

Meisel, Alan, and Loren H. Roth, "Toward an Informed Discussion of Informed Consent," *Arizona Law Review* 25 (1983): 265–346.

Miller, Lawrence G. "Pain, Parturition, and the Profession: Twilight Sleep in America." In *Health Care in America: Essays in Social History*, ed. Susan Reverby and David Rosner, pp. 19–44. Philadelphia: Temple University Press, 1979.

Miller, Mark Crispin, ed. *Seeing Through Movies*. New York: Pantheon, 1990.

Mitman, Greg. "Evolution as Gospel: William Patten, the Language of Democracy and the Great War." *Isis* 81 (September 1990): 446–63.

Mohr, James C. "Patterns of Abortion and the Response of American Physicians, 1790–1930." In *Women and Health in America*, ed. Judith Walzer Leavitt, pp. 117–123. Madison: University of Wisconsin Press, 1984.

Montgomery, David. *The Fall of the House of Labor*. New York: Cambridge University Press, 1987.

Morantz-Sanchez, Regina. *Sympathy and Science*. New York: Oxford University Press, 1985.

Morreim, E. Haavi. "Profoundly Diminished Life." *Hastings Center Report* 24 (January–February 1994): 33–42.

Mosse, George L. *Nationalism and Sexuality*. New York: H. Fertig, 1985.

Mosse, George L. *Towards the Final Solution: A History of European Racism*. London: J. M. Dent & Sons, 1978.

Müller-Hill, Benno. *Murderous Science: Elimination by Scientific Selection of Jews, Gypsies, and Others, Germany 1933–1945*. Oxford: Oxford University Press, 1988.

Murray, Thomas H., and Arthur L. Caplan, eds. *Which Babies Shall Live?* Clifton, N.J.: Humana Press, 1985.

Musser, Charles. *The Emergence of Cinema*. New York: Scribner's, 1990.

Nasaw, David. *Going Out*. New York: Basic Books, 1993.

Naylor, David. *Great American Movie Theaters*. Washington, D.C.: Preservation Press, 1987.

Nelkin, Dorothy and M. Susan Lindee. *The DNA Mystique: The Gene as a Cultural Icon*. New York: W. H. Freeman, 1995.

Nelson, Daniel. *Frederick W. Taylor and the Rise of Scientific Management*. Madison: University of Wisconsin Press, 1980.

Noble, David. *America by Design: Science, Technology and the Rise of Corporate Capitalism*. New York: Oxford University Press, 1977.

Novick, Peter. *That Noble Dream: The "Objectivity Question" and the American Historical Profession*. New York: Cambridge University Press, 1988.

Numbers, Ronald. *Almost Persuaded: American Physicians and Compulsory Health Insurance 1912–1920*. Baltimore: Johns Hopkins University Press, 1978.

Olby, Robert. "The Dimensions of Scientific Controversy: The Biometric-Mendelian Debate." *British Journal for the History of Science* 22 (1989): 299–320.

Older, Mrs. Fremont. *William Randolph Hearst: American*. New York: D. Appleton-Century, 1936.

Ostheimer, J. M. "The Polls: Changing American Attitudes toward Euthanasia." *Public Opinion Quarterly* 44 (1980): 123–28.

Oxford English Dictionary. Compact ed. Oxford: Oxford University Press, 1971.

Paige, Constance, and Elisa Karnofsky. "The Antiabortion Movement and Baby Jane Doe." *Journal of Health Politics, Policy and Law* 11 (Summer 1986): 255–70.

Palmer, Richard. "The Church, Leprosy and Plague in Medieval and Early Modern Europe." In *The Church and Healing*, ed. W. J. Sheils, pp. 79–99. Oxford: Basil Blackwell, 1982.

Park, Katharine, and Lorraine Daston. "Unnatural Conceptions: The Study of Monsters in 16th- and 17th-Century France and England." *Past and Present* 92 (1981): 20–54.

Patterson, James T. *The Dread Disease: Cancer and Modern American Culture.* Cambridge, Mass.: Harvard University Press, 1987.

Paul, Diane. "Eugenics and the Left." *Journal of the History of Ideas* 45 (1984): 561–90.

Paul, Diane. "The Selection of the 'Survival of the Fittest.' " *Journal of the History of Biology* 21 (Fall 1988): 411–24.

Paul, Diane and Hamish G. Spencer. "The Hidden Science of Eugenics. *Nature* 374 (March 23, 1995): 302–304.

Pauly, Philip J. "Development of High School Biology: New York City, 1900–1925." *Isis* 82 (December 1991): 662–88.

Peiss, Kathy. *Cheap Amusements: Working Women and Leisure in Turn-of-the-Century New York.* Philadelphia: Temple University Press, 1986.

Pernick, Martin S. "Back from the Grave: Recurring Controversies Over Defining and Diagnosing Death in History." In *Death: Beyond Whole-Brain Criteria*, ed. Richard M. Zaner, pp. 17–74. Philosophy and Medicine Series vol. 31. Dordrecht and Boston: Kluwer Academic Publishers, 1988.

Pernick, Martin S. *A Calculus of Suffering: Pain, Professionalism and Anesthesia in Nineteenth Century America.* New York: Columbia University Press, 1985.

Pernick, Martin S. "The Ethics of Preventive Medicine: Thomas Edison's Tuberculosis Films: Mass Media and Health Propaganda." *Hastings Center Report* 8 (June 1978): 21–27.

Pernick, Martin S. "Medical Professionalism." In *Encyclopedia of Bioethics*, vol. III, pp. 1028–1034. New York: Free Press, 1978.

Pernick, Martin S. "The Patient's Role in Medical Decisionmaking: A Social History of Informed Consent in Medical Therapy." In *Making Health Care Decisions: Studies on the Foundations of Informed Consent*, vol. III, pp. 1–35. President's Commission for the Study of Ethical Problems in Medicine. Washington, D.C.: Government Printing Office, 1982.

Pernick, Martin S. "Sex Education Films, U.S. Government." *Isis* 84 (1993): 766–68.

Perry, Lewis. "Progress Not Pleasure is Our Aim: The Sexual Advice of an Antebellum Radical." *Journal of Social History* 12 (1979): 354–67.

Petchesky, Rosalind. "Fetal Images: The Power of Visual Culture in the Politics of Reproduction." *Feminist Studies* 13 (1987): 263–92.

Phillips, William R., and Janet Rosenberg, eds. *The Origins of Modern Treatment and Education of Physically Handicapped Children: An Anthology.* New York: Arno, 1980.

Pick, Daniel. *Faces of Degeneration: A European Disorder.* New York: Cambridge University Press, 1989.

Pickens, Donald K. *Eugenics and the Progressives.* Nashville, Tenn.: Vanderbilt University Press, 1968.

Piers, Maria W. *Infanticide.* New York: Norton, 1978.

Pivar, David J. *Purity Crusade: Sexual Morality and Social Control 1868–1900.* Westport, Conn.: Greenwood, 1973.

Post, Stephen G. "History, Infanticide, and Imperiled Newborns." *Hastings Center Report* 18 (August–September 1988): 14–17.

President's Commission for the Study of Ethical Problems in Medicine. . . . *Deciding to Forego Life-Sustaining Treatment.* Washington, D.C.: Government Printing Office, 1983.

Preston, Samuel H. and Michael R. Haines. *Fatal Years: Child Mortality in Late Nineteenth-Century America.* Princeton, N.J.: Princeton University Press, 1991.

Proctor, Robert N. *Racial Hygiene: Medicine Under the Nazis.* Cambridge, Mass.: Harvard University Press, 1988.

Proctor, Robert N. *Value-Free Science.* Cambridge, Mass.: Harvard University Press, 1991.

Pross, Christian, and Götz Aly. *The Value of the Human Being: Medicine in Germany 1918–45.* Exhibition catalog. Berlin: Ärtzkammer, 1991.

Rachels, James. "Active and Passive Euthanasia." *New England Journal of Medicine* 292 (January 9, 1975): 78–80.

Radford, John P. "Sterilization versus Segregation: Control of the 'Feebleminded' 1900–1938." *Social Science and Medicine* 33 (1991): 449–59.

Ravin, Arnold. "Genetics in America: A Historical Overview." *Perspectives in Biology and Medicine* 21 (Winter 1978): 214–31.

Reed, James. *From Private Vice to Public Virtue: The Birth Control Movement and American Society Since 1830.* New York: Basic, 1978.

Reich, Warren T., and David E. Ost. "Ethical Perspectives on the Care of Infants." In *Encyclopedia of Bioethics,* vol. II, pp. 724–35. New York: The Free Press, 1978.

Reilly, Philip. *Genetics, Law, and Social Policy.* Cambridge, Mass.: Harvard University Press, 1977.

Reilly, Philip. "The Surgical Solution: The Writings of Activist Physicians in the Early Days of Eugenical Sterilization." *Perspectives in Biology and Medicine* 26 (1983): 637–56.

Reilly, Philip. *The Surgical Solution.* Baltimore: Johns Hopkins University Press, 1991.

Reiser, Stanley J. "Survival at What Cost?: Origins and Effects of the Modern Controversy on Treating Severely Handicapped Newborns." *Journal of Health Politics, Policy and Law* 11 (Summer 1986): 199–214.

Richards, Robert. *The Meaning of Evolution.* Chicago: University of Chicago Press, 1992.

Robertson, John. *Children of Choice.* Princeton, N.J.: Princeton University Press, 1994.

Rodgers, Daniel. "In Search of Progressivism." *Reviews in American History* (December 1982): 113–32.

Roell, Craig H. *The Piano in America 1890–1940.* Chapel Hill: University of North Carolina Press, 1989.

Roper, Allen G. *Ancient Eugenics.* Oxford: B. H. Blackwell, 1913.

Rosen, George. "Christian Fenger: Medical Immigrant." *Bulletin of the History of Medicine* 48 (1974): 129–45.

Rosen, George. "The Efficiency Criterion in Medical Care 1900–1920." *Bulletin of the History of Medicine* 50 (Spring 1976): 28–44.

Rosen, George. "Evolving Trends in Health Education." *Canadian Journal of Public Health* 52 (1961): 499–506.

Rosen, Marjorie. *Popcorn Venus.* New York: Coward, McCann & Geoghegan, 1973.

Rosenberg, Charles. "The Bitter Fruit: Heredity, Disease, and Social Thought." In *No Other Gods: On Science and American Social Thought,* pp. 25–53. Baltimore: Johns Hopkins University Press, 1976.

Rosenberg, Charles. *The Care of Strangers.* New York: Basic, 1987.

Rosenberg, Charles. "Charles Benedict Davenport and the Irony of American Eugenics." In *No Other Gods: On Science and American Social Thought,* pp. 89–97. Baltimore: Johns Hopkins University Press, 1976.

Rosenberg, Charles and Janet Golden, eds. *Framing Disease.* New Brunswick, N.J.: Rutgers University Press, 1992.

Rosenblatt, Roger. *Life Itself: Abortion in the American Mind.* New York: Random House, 1992.

Rosenkrantz, Barbara Gutmann. "Damaged Goods: Dilemmas of Responsibility for Risk." *Milbank Memorial Fund Quarterly* 57 (1979): 1–37.

Rosenkrantz, Barbara Gutmann. *Public Health and the State: Changing Views in Massachusetts 1842–1936.* Cambridge, Mass.: Harvard University Press, 1972.

Rosenzweig, Roy. *Eight Hours for What We Will: Workers and Leisure in an Industrial City 1870–1920.* Cambridge: Cambridge University Press, 1983.

Rosner, David, and Gerald Markowitz, eds. *Dying for Work.* Bloomington: Indiana University Press, 1987.

Ross, Dorothy. *G. Stanley Hall.* Chicago: University of Chicago Press, 1972.

Roth, Karl-Heinz. *Die restlose Erfassung: volkszählen, identifizieren, aussondern im Nationalsozialismus.* Berlin: Rotbuch, 1984.

Rothman, David. *Conscience and Convenience: The Asylum and Its Alternatives in Progressive America.* Boston: Little, Brown, 1980.

Rothman, David J. *Strangers at the Bedside: A History of How Law and Bioethics Transformed Medical Decision Making.* New York: Basic Books, 1991.

Rothman, Sheila. *Woman's Proper Place.* New York: Basic Books, 1978.

Rothstein, Edward. "Don't Shoot the Piano." *TNR* May 1, 1989, pp. 32–35.

Ruggles, Steven. "The Transformation of American Family Structure." *American Historical Review* 99 (February 1994): 103–128.

Russell, O. Ruth. *Freedom to Die: Moral and Legal Aspects of Euthanasia.* New York: Human Sciences Press, 1975.

Russett, Cynthia Eagle. *Sexual Science.* Cambridge, Mass.: Harvard University Press, 1989.

Sandelowski, Margarete. *Pain, Pleasure and American Childbirth from the Twilight Sleep to the Read Method 1914–1960.* Westport, Conn.: Greenwood, 1984.

Sapp, Jan. "The Struggle for Authority in the Field of Heredity 1900–1932: New Perspectives on the Rise of Genetics." *Journal of the History of Biology* 16 (1983): 311–42.

Saürländer, Willibrald. "The Nazis' Theater of Seduction." *New York Review of Books,* April 21, 1994, pp. 16–19.

Schaefer, Eric. "Of Hygiene and Hollywood: Origins of the Exploitation Film." *Velvet Light Trap* 30 (Fall 1992): 34–47.

Schneider, Carl. "Bioethics with a Human Face." *Indiana Law Journal* 69 (Fall 1994): 1075–1104.

Searle, G. R. *Eugenics and Politics in Britain.* Leyden: Noordhof, 1976.

Sen, Amartya. "More Than 100 Million Women Are Missing." *New York Review of Books,* December 20, 1990, pp. 61–66.

Shelp, Earl. *Born to Die?* New York: Free Press, 1986.

Shryock, Richard. *The National Tuberculosis Association 1904–1954.* New York: Tuberculosis Association, 1957.

Siepp, Conrad. "Organized Medicine and the Public Health Institute of Chicago." *Bulletin of the History of Medicine* 62 (Fall 1988): 429–49.

Silverman, William A. "Incubator Baby Side Shows." *Pediatrics* 64 (1979): 127–41.

Sklar, Martin. *Corporate Reconstruction of American Capitalism.* New York: Cambridge University Press, 1988.

Skocpol, Theda. *Protecting Soldiers and Mothers: Origins of Social Policy in the United States.* Cambridge, Mass.: Harvard University Press, 1992.

Skowronek, Stephen. *Building a New American State.* New York: Cambridge University Press, 1982.

Slide, Anthony. *The American Film Industry: A Historical Dictionary.* Westport, Conn.: Greenwood, 1986.

Slide, Anthony, ed. *International Film, Radio, and Television Journals.* Westport, Conn.: Greenwood, 1985.

Sloan, Kay. *The Loud Silents.* Urbana: University of Illinois Press, 1988.

Smuts, R. W. "Fat, Sex, Class, Adaptive Flexibility, and Cultural Change." *Ethology and Sociobiology* 13 (1992): 523–42.

Soloway, Richard A. *Demography and Degeneration: Eugenics and the Declining Birthrate in Twentieth-Century Britain.* Chapel Hill: University of North Carolina Press, 1990.

Sontag, Susan. *Illness as Metaphor.* New York: Farrar, Straus and Giroux, 1978.

Sournia, Jean-Charles. *A History of Alcoholism.* Oxford: Basil Blackwell, 1990.

Spear, Allan. *Black Chicago.* Chicago: University of Chicago Press, 1967.

"Special Issue: Imperiled Newborns." *Hastings Center Report* 17 (December 1987).

Stafford, Barbara. *Body Criticism: Imaging the Unseen in Enlightenment Art and Medicine.* Cambridge, Mass.: M.I.T. Press, 1991.

Staiger, Janet. *Interpreting Film: Studies in the Historical Reception of American Cinema.* Princeton, N.J.: Princeton University Press, 1992.

Stainton, Walter. "Pearl White in Ithaca." *Films in Review* 2 (May 1951): 19–25.

Stanton, William. *The Leopard's Spots: Scientific Attitudes toward Race in America 1815–59.* Chicago: University of Chicago Press, 1960.

Star, Susan Leigh. *Regions of the Mind: Brain Research and the Quest for Scientific Certainty.* Stanford: Stanford University Press, 1989.

Starr, Paul. *The Social Transformation of American Medicine.* New York: Basic, 1982.

Steinfels, Peter. "Introduction." Issue on "The Concept of Health." *Hastings Center Studies* 1 (1973): 3–88.

Stepan, Nancy. *The Idea of Race in Science: Great Britain, 1800–1960.* London: Macmillan, 1982.

Stevens, Rosemary. *American Medicine and the Public Interest.* New Haven, Conn.: Yale University Press, 1971.

Stoeckle, John D., and George Abbott White. *Plain Pictures of Plain Doctoring: Vernacular Expression in New Deal Medicine and Photography.* Cambridge, Mass.: M.I.T. Press, 1985.

Stone, James L. "The Development of Neurological Surgery at Cook County Hospital." *Neurosurgery* 34 (January 1994): 97–102.

Swanberg, W. A. *Citizen Hearst.* New York: Scribner's, 1961.

Swartz, Mark E. "Motion Pictures on the Move." *Journal of American Culture* (Winter 1986): 1–7.

Takaki, Ronald. *Strangers from a Different Shore: A History of Asian-Americans.* Boston: Little, Brown, 1989.

Teller, Michael E. *The Tuberculosis Movement: A Public Health Campaign in the Progressive Era.* Westport, Conn.: Greenwood, 1988.

Temkin, Owsei, W. K. Frankena, and S. H. Kadish. *Respect for Life in Medicine, Philosophy and Law.* Baltimore: Johns Hopkins University Press, 1977.

Tesh, Sylvia. *Hidden Arguments: Political Ideology and Disease Prevention Policy.* New Brunswick, N.J.: Rutgers University Press, 1988.

Tifflin, Susan. *In Whose Best Interest? Child Welfare Reform in the Progressive Era.* Westport, Conn.: Greenwood, 1982.

Towers, B. A. "Health Education Policy 1916–1926: Venereal Disease and the Prophylaxis Dilemma." *Medical History* 24 (1980): 70–87.

"T.R.B." "The Tyranny of Beauty." *TNR* October 12, 1987, p. 4.

Trent, James W. *Inventing the Feeble Mind.* Berkeley: University of California Press, 1994.

Triche, C. W., and S. D. Triche. *The Euthanasia Controversy 1812–1974, A Bibliography.* Troy, N.Y.: Whitston, 1975.

Trombley, Stephen. *The Right to Reproduce: A History of Coercive Sterilization.* London: Weidenfeld and Nicolson, 1988.

Tryster, Hillel. "The Art and Science of Pure Racism." *Jerusalem Post International,* August 17, 1991, p. 13.

Turner, Frank M. *Between Science and Religion: The Reaction to Scientific Naturalism in Later Victorian England.* New Haven, Conn.: Yale University Press, 1974.

Turner, James C. *Reckoning with the Beast.* Baltimore: Johns Hopkins University Press, 1980.

Turner, James C. *Without God, Without Creed.* Baltimore: Johns Hopkins University Press, 1985.

Turow, Joseph. *Playing Doctor: Television, Storytelling, and Medical Power.* New York: Oxford University Press, 1989.

Tyor, Peter L., and Leland V. Bell. *Caring for the Retarded in America: A History.* Westport, Conn.: Greenwood, 1984.

Usborne, Cornelie. *The Politics of the Body in Weimar Germany: Women's Reproductive Rights and Duties.* Ann Arbor: University of Michigan Press, 1993.

Valenstein, Elliot S. *Great and Desperate Cures: The Rise and Decline of Psychosurgery and Other Related Treatments for Mental Illness.* New York: Basic, 1986.

van der Sluis, I. "The Movement for Euthanasia, 1875–1975." *Janus* 66 (1979): 131–72.

Vaughn, Stephen. "Morality and Entertainment: The Origins of the Motion Picture Production Code." *Journal of American History* 77 (June 1990): 39–65.

Vecoli, Rudolph. "Sterilization: A Progressive Measure?" *Wisconsin Magazine of History* 43 (Spring 1960): 190–202.

Vogel, Morris. *Invention of the Modern Hospital.* Chicago: University of Chicago Press, 1980.

Wangensteen, Owen, and Sarah Wangensteen. *The Rise of Surgery.* Minneapolis: University of Minnesota Press, 1978.

Ward, Larry Wayne. *The Motion Picture Goes to War: The U.S. Government Film Effort during World War I.* Ann Arbor: UMI Research Press, 1985.

Ward, Patricia Spain. "The Medical Brothers Cabot: Of Truth and Consequence." *Harvard Medical Alumni Bulletin* 56 (Fall 1982): 30–39.

Ward, Patricia Spain. "The Other Abraham: Flexner in Illinois." *Caduceus: Museum Quarterly for the Health Sciences* 2 (Spring 1986): 1–66.

Ward, Patricia Spain. *Simon Baruch.* Tuscaloosa: University of Alabama Press, 1994.

Warner, R. H., and H. L. Rosett. "Effects of Drinking on Offspring: An Historical Survey of the American and British Literature." *Journal of Studies of Alcohol* 36 (November 1975): 1395–1420.

Warren, Mary Anne. *Gendercide: The Implications of Sex Selection.* Totowa, N.J.: Rowman & Allanheld, 1985.

Wasserman, Manfred. "Henry L. Coit and the Certified Milk Movement in the Development of Modern Pediatrics." *Bulletin of the History of Medicine* 46 (1972): 359–90.

Watson, Steven. *Strange Bedfellows: The First American Avant-Garde.* New York: Abbeville Press, 1991.

Weinberg, David. "Approaches to the Study of Film in the Third Reich: A Critical Appraisal." *Journal of Contemporary History* 19 (1984): 105–26.

Weindling, Paul. "Essay Review: Medicine in Nazi Germany and Its After-math." *Bulletin of the History of Medicine* 65 (Fall 1991): 416–19.

Weindling, Paul. *Health, Race and German Politics between National Unification and Nazism 1870–1945.* Cambridge: Cambridge University Press, 1989.

Weindling, Paul. "The 'Sonderweg' of German Eugenics." *British Journal of the History of Science* 22 (1989): 321–33.

Weingart, Peter. "German Eugenics between Science and Politics." *Osiris* 5 (1989): 260–82.

Weingart, Peter. "Science Abused: Challenging a Legend." *Science in Context* 6 (Autumn 1993), 555–67.

Weir, Robert F. *Selective Nontreatment of Handicapped Newborns: Moral Dilemmas in Neonatal Medicine.* New York: Oxford University Press, 1984.

Weiss, Sheila. "The Race Hygiene Movement in Germany." *Osiris* 3 (1987): 193–236.

Wessling, Mary. "Infanticide Trials and Forensic Evidence: Wurttemberg 1757–1793." In *Legal Medicine in History,* ed. Michael Clark and Catherine Crawford. Cambridge: Cambridge University Press, 1994.

Weston, Alan J. and Nancy T. Mader. "Infants' Vocalizations as a Diagnostic Tool." *Perceptual and Motor Skills* 58 (1984): 787–796.

Wiebe, Robert. *The Search for Order 1877–1920.* New York: Hill & Wang, 1976.

Wiedmann, Thomas. *Adults and Children in the Roman Empire.* New Haven, Conn.: Yale University Press, 1990.

Williamson, Joel. *The Crucible of Race.* New York: Oxford University Press, 1984.

Winau, Rolf. "Die Freigabe der Vernichtung 'lebensunwerten Lebens.'" *Deutsches Ärzteblatt,* 16 February 1989, pp. 1–6.

Wishy, Bernard. *The School and the Republic.* Philadelphia: University of Pennsylvania Press, 1968.

Woodcock, George. *Anarchism.* Cleveland: World, 1962.

Wyatt, Philip R. "John Humphrey Noyes and the Stirpicultural Experiment." *JHMAS* 31 (January 1976): 55–66.

Wymelenberg, Suzanne. *Science and Babies: Private Decisions, Public Dilemmas.* Washington D.C.: National Academy of Sciences, 1990.

Young, James Harvey. "This Greasy Counterfeit: Butter versus Oleomargarine in the United States Congress, 1886." *Bulletin of the History of Medicine* 53 (1979): 392–414.

Ziporyn, Terra. *Disease in the Popular American Press.* Westport, Conn.: Greenwood, 1988.

Zunz, Olivier. *Making America Corporate, 1870–1920.* Chicago: University of Chicago Press, 1990.

Subject Index

Index of Film Titles